NATIONAL STRATEGY FOR
PANDEMIC INFLUENZA

IMPLEMENTATION PLAN

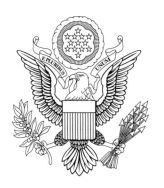

HOMELAND SECURITY COUNCIL

MAY 2006

For sale by the Superintendent of Documents, U.S. Government Printing Office
Internet: bookstore.gpo.gov   Phone: toll free (866) 512-1800;   DC area (202) 512-1800
Fax: (202) 512-2250 Mail: Stop IDCC, Washington, DC 20402-0001

ISBN 0-16-076075-5

My fellow Americans,

On November 1, 2005, I announced the *National Strategy for Pandemic Influenza,* a comprehensive approach to addressing the threat of pandemic influenza. Our *Strategy* outlines how we are preparing for, and how we will detect and respond to, a potential pandemic.

Since then, our Nation has taken a series of historic steps to address the pandemic threat. In December, the Congress appropriated $3.8 billion. The International Partnership for Avian and Pandemic Influenza, which we launched at the United Nations in September 2005, has encouraged openness and coordinated action by the international community. Here at home, we have made major investments in vaccine and antiviral development, research into the influenza virus, surveillance for disease in animals and humans, and the local, State, and Federal infrastructure necessary to respond to a pandemic. By making these critical investments, the Federal Government has begun strengthening our ability to safeguard the American people in the event of a devastating global pandemic and helping to prepare the Nation's public health and medical infrastructure.

Building upon these efforts, the *Implementation Plan for the National Strategy for Pandemic Influenza* ensures that our efforts and resources will be brought to bear in a coordinated manner against this threat. The *Plan* describes more than 300 critical actions, many of which have already been initiated, to address the threat of pandemic influenza.

Our efforts require the participation of, and coordination by, all levels of government and segments of society. State and local governments must be prepared, and my Administration will work with them to provide the necessary guidance in order to best protect their citizens. No less important will be the actions of individual citizens, whose participation is necessary to the success of these efforts.

Our Nation will face this global threat united in purpose and united in action in order to best protect our families, our communities, our Nation, and our world from the threat of pandemic influenza.

GEORGE W. BUSH
THE WHITE HOUSE
May 2006

TABLE OF CONTENTS

PREFACE

In the last century, three influenza pandemics have swept the globe. In 1918, the first pandemic (sometimes referred to as the "Spanish Flu") killed over 500,000 Americans and more than 20 million people worldwide. One-third of the U.S. population was infected, and average life expectancy was reduced by 13 years. Pandemics in 1957 and 1968 killed tens of thousands of Americans and millions across the world. Scientists believe that viruses from birds played a role in each of those outbreaks.

Today, we face a new threat. A new influenza strain — influenza A (H5N1) — is spreading through bird populations across Asia, Africa, and Europe, infecting domesticated birds, including ducks and chickens, and long-range migratory birds. The first recorded appearance of H5N1 in humans occurred in Hong Kong in 1997. Since then, the virus has infected over 200 people in the Eastern Hemisphere, with a mortality rate of over 50 percent.

At this time, avian influenza is primarily an animal disease. Human infections are generally limited to individuals who come into direct contact with infected birds. If the virus develops the capacity for sustained, efficient, human-to-human transmission, however, it could spread quickly around the globe. In response to this threat, the President issued the *National Strategy for Pandemic Influenza* on November 1, 2005. The *Strategy* outlines the coordinated Federal Government effort to prepare for pandemic influenza. Of equal importance, the Strategy underscores the critical roles that State, local, and tribal authorities, the private sector, and communities must play to address the threat of a pandemic, and the concrete steps that individuals can and should take to protect themselves and their families.

This Implementation Plan for the *National Strategy for Pandemic Influenza* further clarifies the roles and responsibilities of governmental and non-governmental entities, including Federal, State, local, and tribal authorities and regional, national, and international stakeholders, and provides preparedness guidance for all segments of society. The Plan addresses the following topics:

- **Chapters 2 and 3 (U.S. Government Planning and Response)** describe the unique threat posed by a pandemic that would spread across the globe over a period of many months; the specific and coordinated actions to be taken by the Federal Government as well as its capabilities and limitations in responding to the sustained and distributed burden of a pandemic; and the central importance of comprehensive preparation at the State, local, and community levels to address medical and non-medical impacts with available resources.

- **Chapters 4 and 5 (International Efforts and Transportation and Borders)** outline steps we will take to work with our international partners to prevent, slow, or limit the spread of infection globally and in the United States, and describe proposed measures for effective management of our borders and the transportation sector during a pandemic.

- **Chapter 6 (Protecting Human Health)** details the critical actions that public health authorities, non-governmental organizations, the private sector, and individuals should take to protect human health and reduce the morbidity and mortality caused by a pandemic.

- **Chapter 7 (Protecting Animal Health)** highlights the actions necessary to prevent and contain outbreaks in animals with the aim of reducing human exposure and the opportunity for viral mutation that could result in efficient human-to-human transmission.

- **Chapter 8 (Law Enforcement, Public Safety, and Security)** outlines the support that State and local law enforcement and public safety agencies must provide, with appropriate Federal assistance, to public health efforts and essential public safety services, and to maintain public order.

- **Chapter 9 (Institutional Considerations)** provides guidance for the preparation of essential pandemic plans by Federal, State, local, and tribal authorities, businesses, schools, and non-governmental organizations to ensure continuity of operations and maintenance of critical infrastructure. It also provides guidance for families and individuals to ensure appropriate personal protection. To address the threat of pandemic influenza, it is essential that such plans be put in place as soon as possible.

The Implementation Plan represents a comprehensive effort by the Federal Government to identify the critical steps that must be taken immediately and over the coming months and years to address the threat of an influenza pandemic. It assigns specific responsibilities to Departments and Agencies across the Federal Government, and includes measures of progress and timelines for implementation to ensure that we meet our preparedness objectives.

This Plan will be revised over time. The pandemic threat is constantly evolving, as is our level of preparedness. The actions, priorities, timelines and measures of progress will be reviewed on a continuous basis and revised as appropriate to reflect changes in our understanding of the threat and the state of relevant response capabilities and technologies. Additional details regarding the implementation of this Plan are included at the conclusion of Chapter 1.

The active engagement and full involvement of all levels of government and all segments of society, including at the community level, are critical for an effective response. Ultimately, however, the actions of individuals will be the key to our response.

CHAPTER 1 — EXECUTIVE SUMMARY

The Pandemic Threat

Influenza viruses have threatened the health of animal and human populations for centuries. Their diversity and propensity for mutation have thwarted our efforts to develop both a universal vaccine and highly effective antiviral drugs. A pandemic occurs when a novel strain of influenza virus emerges that has the ability to infect and be passed between humans. Because humans have little immunity to the new virus, a worldwide epidemic, or pandemic, can ensue. Three human influenza pandemics occurred in the 20th century, each resulting in illness in approximately 30 percent of the world population and death in 0.2 percent to 2 percent of those infected. Using this historical information and current models of disease transmission, it is projected that a modern pandemic could lead to the deaths of 200,000 to 2 million people in the United States alone.

The animal population serves as a reservoir for new influenza viruses. Scientists believe that avian, or bird, viruses played a role in the last three pandemics. The current concern for a pandemic arises from an unprecedented outbreak of H5N1 influenza in birds that began in 1997 and has spread across bird populations in Asia, Europe, and Africa. The virus has shown the ability to infect multiple species, including long-range migratory birds, pigs, cats, and humans. It is impossible to predict whether the H5N1 virus will lead to a pandemic, but history suggests that if it does not, another novel influenza virus will emerge at some point in the future and threaten an unprotected human population.

The economic and societal disruption of an influenza pandemic could be significant. Absenteeism across multiple sectors related to personal illness, illness in family members, fear of contagion, or public health measures to limit contact with others could threaten the functioning of critical infrastructure, the movement of goods and services, and operation of institutions such as schools and universities. A pandemic would thus have significant implications for the economy, national security, and the basic functioning of society.

Chapter 2 — U.S. Government Planning for a Pandemic

The President announced the *National Strategy for Pandemic Influenza (Strategy)* on November 1, 2005. The *Strategy* provides a high-level overview of the approach that the Federal Government will take to prepare for and respond to a pandemic, and articulates expectations of non-Federal entities to prepare themselves and their communities. The *Strategy* contains three pillars: (1) preparedness and communication; (2) surveillance and detection; and (3) response and containment.

Preparedness for a pandemic requires the establishment of infrastructure and capacity, a process that can take years. For this reason, significant steps must be taken now. The Strategy affirms that the Federal Government will use all instruments of national power to address the pandemic threat. The Federal Government will collaborate fully with international partners to attempt containment of a potential pandemic wherever sustained and efficient human-to-human transmission is documented, and will make every reasonable effort to delay the introduction of a pandemic virus to the United States. If these efforts fail, responding effectively to an uncontained pandemic domestically will require the full participation of all levels of government and all segments of society. The Implementation Plan (Plan) for the *Strategy* makes it clear that every segment of society must prepare for a pandemic and will be a part of the response. The Plan further recognizes that the Federal Government must provide clear criteria and decision tools to inform State, local, and private sector planning and response actions, and that Federal agencies must be prepared to supplement and support State and local efforts where necessary and feasible.

The *Strategy* must be translated into tangible action that fully engages the breadth of the Federal Government. This Plan provides a common frame of reference for understanding the pandemic threat and summarizes key planning considerations for all partners. It also proposes that Federal departments and agencies take specific, coordinated steps to achieve the goals of the *Strategy* and outlines expectations of non-Federal stakeholders in the United States and abroad. Joint and integrated planning across all levels of government and the private sector is essential to ensure that available national capabilities and authorities produce detailed plans and response actions that are complementary, compatible, and coordinated.

The Federal Government has already taken a historic series of actions, domestically and internationally, to address the pandemic threat. The actions include the development of a promising human vaccine against the H5N1 avian influenza virus, the submission of a $7.1 billion budget request over several years to support pandemic preparedness, the establishment of the International Partnership on Avian and Pandemic Influenza, and the first Cabinet-level exercise to assess the Federal Government response to a naturally occurring threat.

Chapter 3 — Federal Government Response to a Pandemic

The goals of the Federal Government response to a pandemic are to: (1) stop, slow, or otherwise limit the spread of a pandemic to the United States; (2) limit the domestic spread of a pandemic, and mitigate disease, suffering and death; and (3) sustain infrastructure and mitigate impact to the economy and the functioning of society (see *Stages of Federal Government Response* between Chapters 5 and 6).

Unlike geographically and temporally bounded disasters, a pandemic will spread across the globe over the course of months or over a year, possibly in waves, and will affect communities of all sizes and compositions. In terms of its scope, the impact of a severe pandemic may be more comparable to that of war or a widespread economic crisis than a hurricane, earthquake, or act of terrorism. In addition to coordinating a comprehensive and timely national response, the Federal Government will bear primary responsibility for certain critical functions, including: (1) the support of containment efforts overseas and limitation of the arrival of a pandemic to our shores; (2) guidance related to protective measures that should be taken; (3) modifications to the law and regulations to facilitate the national pandemic response; (4) modifications to monetary policy to mitigate the economic impact of a pandemic on communities and the Nation; (5) procurement and distribution of vaccine and antiviral medications; and (6) the acceleration of research and development of vaccines and therapies during the outbreak.

The center of gravity of the pandemic response, however, will be in communities. The distributed nature of a pandemic, as well as the sheer burden of disease across the Nation over a period of months or longer, means that the Federal Government's support to any particular State, Tribal Nation, or community will be limited in comparison to the aid it mobilizes for disasters such as earthquakes or hurricanes, which strike a more confined geographic area over a shorter period of time. Local communities will have to address the medical and non-medical effects of the pandemic with available resources. This means that it is essential for communities, tribes, States, and regions to have plans in place to support the full spectrum of their needs over the course of weeks or months, and for the Federal Government to provide clear guidance on the manner in which these needs can be met.

Command, Control, and Coordination of the Federal Response during a Pandemic

It is important that the Federal Government have a defined mechanism for coordination of its response. The *National Response Plan* (NRP) is the primary mechanism for coordination of the Federal Government's response to Incidents of National Significance, and will guide the Federal pandemic response. It defines Federal departmental responsibilities for sector-specific responses, and provides the structure and mechanisms for effective coordination among Federal, State, local, and tribal authorities, the private sector, and non-governmental organizations (NGOs). Pursuant to the NRP and Homeland Security Presidential Directive 5 (HSPD-5), the Secretary of Homeland Security is responsible for coordination of Federal operations and resources, establishment of reporting requirements, and conduct of ongoing communications with Federal, State, local, and tribal governments, the private sector, and NGOs.

A pandemic will present unique challenges to the coordination of the Federal response. First and foremost, the types of support that the Federal Government will provide to the Nation are of a different kind and character than those it traditionally provides to communities damaged by natural disasters. Second, although it may occur in discrete waves in any one locale, the national impact of a pandemic could last for many months. Finally, a pandemic is a sustained public health and medical emergency that will have sustained and profound consequences for the operation of critical infrastructure, the mobility of people and freight, and the global economy. Health and medical considerations will affect foreign policy, international trade and travel, domestic disease containment efforts, continuity of operations within the Federal Government, and many other aspects of the Federal response.

Pursuant to the NRP, as the primary agency and coordinator for Emergency Support Function #8 (Public Health and Medical Services), the Secretary of Health and Human Services will lead Federal health and medical response efforts and will be the principal Federal spokesperson for public health issues, coordinating closely with DHS on public messaging pertaining to the pandemic. Pursuant to HSPD-5, as the principal Federal official for domestic incident management, the Secretary of Homeland Security will provide coordination for Federal operations and resources, establish reporting requirements, and conduct ongoing communications with Federal, State, local, and tribal governments, the private sector, and NGOs. In the context of response to a pandemic, the Secretary of Homeland Security will coordinate overall non-medical support and response actions, and ensure necessary support to the Secretary of Health and Human Services' coordination of public health and medical emergency response efforts.

The NRP stipulates mechanisms for coordination of the Federal response, but sustaining these mechanisms for several months to over a year will present unique challenges. Day-to-day situational monitoring will occur through the national operations center, and strategic policy development and coordination on domestic pandemic response issues will be accomplished through an interagency body composed of senior decision-makers from across the government and chaired by the White House. These and other considerations applicable to response to a pandemic will be incorporated in the NRP review process and will inform recommendations on revisions and improvements to the NRP and associated annexes.

Pursuant to the NRP, policy issues that cannot be resolved at the department level will be addressed through the Homeland Security Council/National Security Council (HSC/NSC)-led policy coordination process.

Chapter 4 — International Efforts

Pandemic influenza is a global threat requiring an international response. Given the rapid speed of transmission and the universal susceptibility of human populations, an outbreak of pandemic influenza anywhere poses a risk to populations everywhere. Our international effort to contain and mitigate the effects of an outbreak of pandemic influenza beyond our borders is a central component of our strategy to stop, slow, or limit the spread of infection to the United States.

Substantial obstacles exist to implementing a rapid response to an incipient human pandemic in many nations. The threat of pandemic influenza may not be widely recognized or understood. Many countries do not have sufficient resources or expertise to detect and respond to outbreaks independently, and lack a robust public health and communications infrastructure, pandemic preparedness plans, and proven logistics capability. International mechanisms to support effective global surveillance and response, including coordinated provision of accurate and timely information to the public, are also inadequate.

To address the international dimension of the pandemic threat, the United States will build upon a series of recent actions. The International Partnership on Avian and Pandemic Influenza was launched by the President in September 2005 to heighten awareness of the pandemic threat among governments, to promote the development of national capacity to detect and respond to a pandemic, and to encourage transparency, scientific cooperation, and rapid reporting of outbreaks in birds and humans. We will work through the Partnership, with international health organizations and bilaterally to increase global commitment, cooperation, and capacity to address the threat of avian influenza. At the Beijing Donors Conference in January 2006, the United States committed $334 million to international efforts to prevent and counter the spread of avian and human pandemic influenza, representing approximately one-third of all international grants pledged[1]

Actions to Implement the National Strategy for Pandemic Influenza

The Federal Government will work to increase awareness of the threat by foreign governments and their citizens, and promote the development of national and international capacity to prevent, detect, and limit the spread of animal and human pandemic influenza within and beyond national borders. We will work through bilateral and multilateral channels to assist priority countries, especially those in which highly pathogenic H5N1 avian influenza is endemic or emerging, to develop and exercise plans for an effective response.

Establish Surveillance Capability in Countries at Risk

A country's ability to respond quickly to a human outbreak requires a broad surveillance network to detect cases of influenza-like illnesses in people, coupled with rapid diagnostic and response capabilities. To help address these challenges, the Federal Government and international partners will work together to assist countries at risk to build and improve infrastructure at the central, provincial, and local levels. Building this capability in countries at risk will facilitate monitoring of disease spread and rapid response to contain influenza outbreaks with pandemic potential.

[1] Does not include loans of approximately $1 billion pledged at conference

Expand Capacity for Animal Health Activities and Press for a Strong International Leadership Role

We will press for a strong leadership role for international animal health organizations, particularly the World Organization for Animal Health (OIE) and the United Nations (UN) Food and Agriculture Organization (FAO), to assess the animal health/veterinary services infrastructure of affected, high-risk, and at-risk countries, in order to determine areas of need that must be addressed. We will work to assist the FAO to establish a resident rapid response capability and a network that can be drawn upon to provide technical assistance to address the immediate needs of countries with incipient or advanced outbreaks of avian influenza.

Support a Coordinated Response by the International Community in Support of National Efforts

A series of actions will be necessary to contain an outbreak of a virus with pandemic potential, including rapid characterization of a potential outbreak, immediate and coordinated deployment of rapid reaction teams, deployment of international stocks of antiviral medications and other materiel, and institution of public health measures to limit spread. To be most effective, these measures require international preparation and coordination. The Federal Government will work with the World Health Organization (WHO), the Partnership, and through diplomatic contacts to strengthen these international mechanisms, and we will configure our own Departments and Agencies to deploy personnel and materiel in support of an international response upon the first reports of suspected outbreaks.

We will also press for the establishment of internationally agreed-upon definitions and protocols in support of a containment strategy, including:

• A global epidemiologic standard for triggering an international containment response to a potential pandemic.

• The necessary actions that should be taken by nations in response to a suspected outbreak, including prompt reporting of the outbreak to the WHO Secretariat, and sharing of viral isolates and/or tissue samples.

• The establishment of an international rapid response capability, led by the WHO but with significant contributions of personnel and equipment by the international community, to investigate and respond to the suspected beginning of a pandemic.

• The establishment of national, regional, and international stockpiles of medical and non-medical countermeasures that are pre-positioned for rapid deployment.

Coordinate Public Communication

We recognize that timely, accurate, credible, and coordinated messages will be necessary during a pandemic, and that inconsistent reporting or guidance within and between nations can lead to confusion and a loss of confidence by the public. We will work with the WHO and our international partners to share information as an outbreak proceeds, and to coordinate our response actions as well as the public messaging that accompanies these actions. We will also support the development of targeted and culturally sensitive communications in local languages to help the public in affected countries and countries at risk to understand the threat of influenza with pandemic potential in animals and of human pandemic influenza, the preventive measures that should be taken, and actions necessary in the event of a pandemic.

Assist U.S. Citizens Traveling or Living Abroad

The Federal Government will provide U.S. citizens living and traveling abroad with timely, accurate information on avian influenza, through websites, travel information, and meetings. U.S. Embassies and Consulates will identify local medical capabilities and resources that would be available to U.S. citizens in the event of a "stay in place" response to a pandemic.

Chapter 5 — Transportation and Borders

The containment of an influenza virus with pandemic potential at its origin, whether the outbreak occurs abroad or within the United States, is a critical element of pandemic response efforts. Containment is most effective when approached globally, with all countries striving to achieve common goals. While complete containment might not be successful, a series of containment efforts could slow the spread of a virus to and within the United States, thereby providing valuable time to activate the domestic response.

Our Nation's ports of entry and transportation network are critical elements in our preparation for and response to a potential influenza pandemic. Measures at our borders may provide an opportunity to slow the spread of a pandemic to and within the United States, but are unlikely to prevent it. Moreover, the sheer volume of traffic and the difficulty of developing screening protocols to detect an influenza-like illness pose significant challenges. While we will consider all options to limit the spread of a pandemic virus, we recognize complete border closure would be difficult to enforce, present foreign affairs complications, and have significant negative social and economic consequences.

Measures to limit domestic travel may delay the spread of disease. These restrictions could include a range of options, such as reductions in non-essential travel and, as a last resort, mandatory restrictions. While delaying the spread of the epidemic may provide time for communities to prepare and possibly allow the production and administration of pre-pandemic vaccine and antiviral medications, travel restrictions, per se, are unlikely to reduce the total number of people who become ill or the impact the pandemic will have on any one community. Individual regions would still experience sharp surges in the demand for medical services and the need to meet such demand with local and regional personnel, resources, and capacity. Communities, States, the private sector, and the Federal Government will need to carefully weigh the costs and benefits of transportation measures when developing their response plans, including the effectiveness of an action in slowing the spread of a pandemic, its social and economic consequences, and its operational feasibility.

Border and transportation measures will be most effective in slowing the spread of a pandemic if they are part of a larger comprehensive strategy that incorporates other interventions, such as the adherence to infection control measures (hand hygiene and cough etiquette), social distancing, isolation, vaccination, and treatment with antiviral medications.

Actions to Implement the National Strategy for Pandemic Influenza

Modeling to Inform Transportation and Border Decisions

Models are powerful tools that can be used to inform policy decisions by highlighting the impact of various interventions on the spread of disease. Models can also predict the social and economic ramifications of specific transportation and movement interventions and can inform the assessment of the operational feasibility of these interventions. We will expand our infectious disease modeling capabilities and ensure that mechanisms are in place to share the findings of these models with State and local authorities and the private sector to inform transportation decisions. We will use these models to develop guidance for State and local authorities on interventions that are likely to limit the spread of a pandemic and on protocols for implementation.

Screening Mechanisms and Travel Restrictions

Our ability to limit the spread of a pandemic, target our public health interventions, and limit the unintended consequences of these actions will be greatly enhanced by the widespread availability of cost-effective screening tools for influenza viruses such as rapid diagnostic tests. We will expand our research and development efforts to bring such tools to market as soon as possible.

The Federal Government's plan for responding to and containing pandemic outbreaks focuses on initial source containment and the use of a layered series of actions to limit spread, including traveler screening for influenza at the point of exit from a source country, en route during air travel, and upon arrival at U.S. airports. In order to ensure that international arrivals undergo proper screening protocols and are subject to isolation and quarantine if appropriate, we are likely to limit the number of airports accepting international flights early in a pandemic. Protocols will be developed to implement these policies for air travelers.

As we have done with air travel, we will establish policies to address movement of people across our land and maritime borders and the role, if any, of domestic movement restrictions. These policies and the protocols to support them will be developed in concert with State, local, and tribal stakeholders, the private sector, and our international partners.

Quarantine and Isolation of Travelers

Current Centers for Disease Control and Prevention (CDC) recommendations for managing air passengers who may be infected with an influenza virus with pandemic potential include isolation of ill persons, quarantine of all non-ill travelers (and crew), and targeted treatment and prophylaxis with antiviral medications. The Federal Government will develop criteria and protocols for isolation and quarantine of travelers early in a pandemic, prior to significant spread of the virus in the United States.

Trade and Movement of Cargo

Excluding live animal and animal product cargo, the risk of influenza transmission by cargo is low. (Inanimate ship-borne cargo poses low risk, and routine surfaces are easily decontaminated.) With appropriate protective measures for workers in specific settings, cargo shipments could continue. The development of prevention measures/protocols that provide protection against the infection of workers in specific settings (e.g., those who handle/inspect cargo) would allow cargo traffic to and from the United States to continue, and thus mitigate the economic impact of the pandemic.

Sustaining the Transportation Infrastructure

Sustaining critical transportation services during a pandemic will be crucial to keep communities functioning and emergency supplies and resources flowing. We will make it clear to State, local, tribal, and private sector entities that planning efforts should assess systemic effects such as supply chain impact, just-in-time delivery, warehousing, and logistics, and should support the development of contingency plans to address lack of critical services and delivery of essential commodities, such as chlorine for water purification, gasoline, food, and medical supplies.

Chapter 6 — Protecting Human Health

Protecting human health is the crux of pandemic preparedness. The components of the Strategy, the elements of this Plan, and the projected allocation of resources to preparedness, surveillance, and response activities all reflect the overarching imperative to reduce the morbidity and mortality caused by a pandemic. In order to achieve this objective, we must leverage all instruments of national power and ensure coordinated action by all segments of government and society, while maintaining the rule of law, and other basic societal functions.

The cardinal determinants of the public health response to a pandemic will be its severity, the prompt implementation of local public health interventions, and the availability and efficacy of vaccine and antiviral medications. Decisions about the prioritization and distribution of medical countermeasures; the content of risk communication campaigns; the application of community infection control and public health containment (social distancing) measures; and whether and when to make adjustments in the way care is delivered are interrelated and all fundamentally determined by the ability of the pandemic virus to cause severe morbidity and mortality and the availability and effectiveness of vaccine and antiviral medications.

While a pandemic may strain hundreds of communities simultaneously, each community will experience the pandemic as a local event. In the best of circumstances, patients and health care resources are not easily redistributed; in a pandemic, conditions would make the sharing of resources and burdens even more difficult. The Federal Government is committed to expanding national stockpiles of both vaccines and antiviral medications and will provide these medical countermeasures as well as other available resources and personnel in support of communities experiencing pandemic influenza, but communities should anticipate that in the event of multiple simultaneous outbreaks, there may be insufficient medical resources or personnel to augment local capabilities. Additionally, manufacturers and suppliers are likely to report inventory shortages and supply chains may be disrupted by the effects of a pandemic on critical personnel. State, local, and tribal entities should thus anticipate that all sources of external aid may be compromised during a pandemic.

The systematic application of disease containment measures can significantly reduce disease transmission rates with concomitant reductions in the intensity and velocity of any pandemics that do occur. The goals of disease containment after a pandemic is underway are to delay the spread of disease and the occurrence of outbreaks in U.S. communities, to decrease the clinical attack rate in affected communities, and to distribute the number of cases that do occur over a longer interval, so as to minimize social and economic disruption and to minimize, so far as possible, hospitalization and death. Decisions as to how and when to implement disease containment measures will be made on a community-by-community basis, with the Federal Government providing technical support and guidance to State and local officials on the efficacy of various social distancing measures, the manner in which they can be implemented, and strategies to mitigate unintended consequences.

Government and public health officials must communicate clearly and continuously with the public now and throughout a pandemic. To maintain public confidence and to enlist the support of individuals and families in disease containment efforts, public officials at all levels of government must provide unambiguous and consistent guidance on what individuals can do to protect themselves, how to care for family members at home, when and where to seek medical care, and how to protect others and minimize the risks of disease transmission. The public will respond favorably to messages that acknowledge its concerns, allay anxiety and uncertainty, and provide clear incentives for desirable behavior. The information provided by public health officials should therefore be useful, addressing immediate needs, but it should also help private citizens recognize and understand the degree to which their collective actions will shape the course of a pandemic.

Ensuring access to, and timely payment for, covered services during a pandemic will be critical to maintaining a functional health care infrastructure. It may also be necessary to extend certain waivers or develop incident-specific initiatives or coverage to facilitate access to care. Pandemic influenza response activities may exceed the budgetary resources of responding Federal and State government agencies, requiring compensatory legislative action.

Actions to Implement the National Strategy for Pandemic Influenza

Achieving National Goals for Production and Stockpiling of Vaccine and Antiviral Medications

The Federal Government has established two primary vaccine goals: (1) establishment and maintenance of stockpiles of pre-pandemic vaccine adequate to immunize 20 million persons against influenza strains that present a pandemic threat; and (2) expansion of domestic influenza vaccine manufacturing surge capacity for the production of pandemic vaccines for the entire domestic population within 6 months of a pandemic declaration. The Federal Government has also established two primary goals for stockpiling existing antiviral medications: (1) establishment and maintenance of stockpiles adequate to treat 75 million persons, divided between Federal and State stockpiles; and (2) establishment and maintenance of a Federal stockpile of 6 million treatment courses reserved for domestic containment efforts.

To accomplish these goals, we will expand Federal, and create State, stockpiles of influenza countermeasures, as well as expand domestic vaccine manufacturing capacity. We will make substantial new investments in the advanced development of cell-culture-based influenza vaccine candidates, with a goal of establishing the domestic surge vaccine production capacity to meet our pre-pandemic stockpile and post-pandemic vaccine production goals.

Prioritizing and Distributing Limited Supplies of Vaccine and Antiviral Medications

The Federal Government is developing guidelines to assist State, local, and tribal governments and the private sector in defining groups that should receive priority access to existing limited supplies of vaccine and antiviral medications. Priority recommendations will reflect the pandemic response goals of limiting mortality and severe morbidity; maintaining critical infrastructure and societal function; diminishing economic impacts; and maintaining national security. Priorities for vaccine and antiviral drug use will vary based on pandemic severity as well as the vaccine and drug supply.

The establishment of credible distribution plans for our countermeasures is equally important. We will work with State and tribal entities to develop and exercise influenza countermeasure distribution plans, to include the necessary logistical support of such plans, including security provisions.

Deploying Limited Federal Assets and Resources to Support Local Medical Surge

Given that local and regional surge capacity will be the foundation of a community's medical response, we will expand and enhance our guidance to State, local, and tribal entities on the most effective ways to develop and utilize surge assets. Recognizing that the availability of health and medical personnel represents the most significant barrier to the care of large numbers of patients, we will establish a joint strategy for the deployment of Federal medical providers from across the U.S. Government, and will expand and enhance programs such as the Medical Reserve Corps and the Commissioned Corps of the Public Health Service. We will also ensure that credible plans are in place to rapidly credential, organize, and incorporate volunteer health and medical providers as part of the medical response in areas that are facing workforce shortages.

Establishing Real-Time Clinical Surveillance

In order to manage an outbreak most effectively, it is necessary to establish mechanisms for "real-time" clinical surveillance in domestic acute care settings such as emergency departments, intensive care units, and laboratories to provide local, State, and Federal public health officials with continuous awareness of the profile of illness in communities. We will support local and national efforts to establish this capability by linking hospital and acute care health information systems with local public health departments, and advancing the development of the analytical tools necessary to interpret and act upon these data streams in real time.

Modeling to Inform Decision Making and Public Health Interventions

Given the power of models to inform decision making, we will establish a single interagency hub for infectious disease modeling efforts, and ensure that this effort integrates related modeling efforts (e.g., transportation decisions, border interventions, economic impact). We will also work to ensure that this modeling can be used in real time as information about the characteristics of a pandemic virus and its impact become available. Finally, we will use this capability to inform the development of more advanced guidance for State, local, and tribal entities on social distancing measures that can be employed to limit disease spread through a community.

Chapter 7 — Protecting Animal Health

Influenza viruses that cause severe disease outbreaks in animals, especially birds, are believed to be a likely source for the emergence of a human pandemic influenza virus. The avian influenza type A "H5N1" virus currently found in parts of Asia, Europe, and Africa is of particular concern due to its demonstrated ability to infect both birds and mammals, including humans. Emergence of a pandemic strain could happen outside the United States or within our borders. Once a pandemic strain emerges, infections will predominantly reflect human-to-human transmission, and birds or other animals are unlikely to be a continuing source of significant virus spread in humans.

Irrespective of whether H5N1 leads to a human pandemic, these viruses have the potential to impact the U.S. poultry industry. Some avian influenza viruses cause high mortality in chickens and are referred to as highly pathogenic avian influenza (HPAI) viruses. The economic consequences of an HPAI outbreak in the United States would depend on the size, location, type, and time necessary to eradicate the outbreak. Although such eradication efforts may help to protect human health, they can result in significant costs due to poultry production losses from bird depopulation activities and from quarantine or other movement restrictions placed on birds. But eradication of these viruses also protects the production of U.S. poultry, worth about $29 billion in 2004.

An extensive amount of influenza surveillance is currently conducted in poultry and wild birds in the United States. Commercial poultry operations are monitored for avian influenza through the National Poultry Improvement Plan, and birds moving through the U.S. live bird marketing system are also tested for avian influenza. Wild birds are examined for avian influenza viruses through efforts involving the Federal Government, State wildlife authorities, and universities.

Actions to Implement the National Strategy for Pandemic Influenza

Bolstering Domestic Surveillance

Although substantial surveillance activities are already in place in the United States to detect avian influenza viruses with human pandemic potential in domestic poultry, enhancing surveillance in domestic animals and wildlife will help ensure that reporting of these events will occur as early as possible. Animal populations that are most critical for additional surveillance activities are poultry and wild birds, not only in terms of increased numbers tested but also in the geographic distribution of testing to increase the probability of detection. To fully utilize data collected as part of the national surveillance for influenza viruses with pandemic potential in animal populations, we will establish capabilities for capturing, analyzing, and sharing data.

Expanding the National Veterinary Stockpile

A National Veterinary Stockpile, already established, contains a variety of materiel that would be necessary for a response to an influenza outbreak, including personal protection equipment (PPE), disinfectant, diagnostic reagents, and antiviral medication (for responders). In addition, there are currently 40 million doses of avian influenza vaccine for use in poultry, should an outbreak occur. We will expand this vaccine stockpile to 110 million doses.

Educating Bird Owners

We will expand our multilevel outreach and education campaign called "Biosecurity for the Birds" to provide disease and biosecurity information to poultry producers, especially those with "backyard" production. The program provides guidance to bird owners and producers on preventing introduction of disease and mitigating spread of disease should it be introduced, and encourages producers to report sick birds, thereby increasing surveillance opportunities for avian influenza.

Advancing Our Domestic Outbreak Response Plans

Regardless of where the risk for emergence exists, the Federal Government will be prepared to respond appropriately. The Federal Government has a history of success in working with the poultry industry to eradicate HPAI viruses that have been introduced into U.S. poultry. If an influenza virus with human pandemic potential is introduced into domestic birds or other animals in the United States, despite all international efforts to prevent it, action must be directed to detecting and eradicating the virus as quickly as possible. If it is found in wild birds, we will act to prevent introduction into domestic birds or other susceptible animals.

Enhancing Infrastructure for Animal Health Research and Development

Enhancement of our knowledge of the ecology of influenza viruses, viral evolution, novel influenza strains that emerge in animals, and the determinants of virulence of influenza viruses in animal populations is essential. We will expand our avian influenza research programs to accelerate the development of the tools necessary to detect influenza viruses in the environment, provide immunity to avian populations, and validate disease response strategies.

Chapter 8 — Law Enforcement, Public Safety, and Security

Due to stresses placed upon the health care system and other critical functions, civil disturbances and breakdowns in public order may occur. Likewise, emergency call centers may be overwhelmed with calls for assistance, including requests to transport influenza victims. Local law enforcement agencies may be called upon to enforce movement restrictions or quarantines, thereby diverting resources from traditional law enforcement duties. To add to these challenges, law enforcement and emergency response agencies can also expect to have their uniform and support ranks reduced significantly as a result of the pandemic. Private sector entities responsible for securing critical infrastructure will face similar challenges.

While significant progress has been made since the terrorist attacks of September 11, 2001, in establishing joint investigative protocols and linkages among the key components of public health, emergency management, and law enforcement/emergency response communities, an influenza pandemic will present new challenges, and it is important that all concerned understand their respective roles and the governing legal authorities so that they can coordinate their efforts under a complex set of Federal, State, tribal, and local laws. Joint training and exercises will help prepare for an effective response to a pandemic influenza outbreak.

State and local law enforcement will normally provide the first response pursuant to State and local law. Consistent with State law, the Governor may deploy National Guard as needed to prevent or respond to civil disturbances. When State and local resources prove incapable of an effective response, the Federal Government can assist by providing Federal law enforcement personnel, and by directing the Armed Forces to assist in law enforcement and maintain order when legal prerequisites are met. Logistical and other support assistance can also be provided.

The response to an influenza pandemic could require, if necessary and appropriate, measures such as isolation or quarantine. Isolation is a standard public health practice applied to persons who have a communicable disease. Isolation of pandemic influenza patients prevents transmission of pandemic influenza by separating ill persons from those who have not yet been exposed. Quarantine is a contact management strategy that separates individuals who have been exposed to infection but are not yet ill from others who have not been exposed to the transmissible infection; quarantine may be voluntary or mandatory. The States, which enact quarantine statutes pursuant to their police powers, are primarily responsible for quarantine within their borders. The Federal Government also has statutory authority to order a quarantine to prevent the introduction, transmission, or spread of communicable diseases from foreign countries into the United States or from one State or possession into any other State or possession. Influenza caused by novel or re-emergent influenza viruses that are causing, or have the potential to cause, a pandemic is on the list of specified communicable diseases for which Federal quarantine is available.

Actions to Implement the National Strategy for Pandemic Influenza

Providing Guidance to State and Local Law Enforcement Entities

We will provide State and local law enforcement with the guidance, training, and exercises needed to prepare them to respond during a pandemic influenza outbreak, including how to assist and facilitate containment measures. Similarly, we will provide Governors with specific information concerning the processes for obtaining Federal law enforcement and military assistance.

Supporting Local Law Enforcement Activities

While we rely upon local and State entities to maintain civil order, it is essential that we be prepared to respond in the event of a breakdown of order that cannot be handled at the local or State level. We will ensure that Federal law enforcement agencies and the military have the necessary plans to assist States with law enforcement and related activities in the event that the need arises.

Chapter 9 -— Institutions: Protecting Personnel and Ensuring Continuity of Operations

Unlike many other catastrophic events, an influenza pandemic will not directly affect the physical infrastructure of an organization. While a pandemic will not damage power lines, banks, or computer networks, it has the potential ultimately to threaten all critical infrastructure by its impact on an organization's human resources by removing essential personnel from the workplace for weeks or months. Therefore, it is critical that organizations anticipate the potential impact of an influenza pandemic on personnel and, consequently, the organization's ability to continue essential functions. As part of that planning, organizations will need to ensure that reasonable measures are in place to protect the health of personnel during a pandemic.

The Federal Government recommends that government entities and the private sector plan with the assumption that up to 40 percent of their staff may be absent for periods of about 2 weeks at the height of a pandemic wave, with lower levels of staff absent for a few weeks on either side of the peak. Absenteeism will increase not only because of personal illness or incapacitation but also because employees may be caring for ill family members, under voluntary home quarantine due to an ill household member, minding children dismissed from school, following public health guidance, or simply staying at home out of safety concerns.

Public and private sector entities depend on certain critical infrastructure for their continued operations. Critical infrastructure encompasses those systems and assets that are so vital to the United States that the incapacity or destruction of such systems and assets would have a debilitating impact on security, national economic security, and national public health or safety. Critical infrastructure protection entails all the activities directed at safeguarding indispensable people, systems (especially communications), and physical infrastructure associated with the operations of those critical infrastructure sectors. Over 85 percent of critical infrastructure is owned and operated by the private sector. Therefore, sustaining the operations of critical infrastructure under conditions of pandemic influenza will depend largely on each individual organization's development and implementation of plans for business continuity under conditions of staffing shortages and to protect the health of their workforces.

Infection control measures are critically important for the protection of personnel. The primary strategies for preventing pandemic influenza are the same as those for seasonal influenza: (1) vaccination; (2) early detection and treatment; and (3) the use of infection control measures to prevent transmission. However, when a pandemic begins, a vaccine may not be widely available, and the supply of antiviral drugs may be limited. The ability to limit transmission and delay the spread of the pandemic will therefore rely primarily on the appropriate and thorough application of infection control measures in health care facilities, the workplace, the community, and for individuals at home.

Simple infection control measures may be effective in reducing the transmission of infection. There are two basic categories of intervention: (1) *transmission interventions,* such as the use of facemasks in health care settings and careful attention to cough etiquette and hand hygiene, which might reduce the likelihood that contacts with other people lead to disease transmission; and (2) *contact interventions,* such as substituting teleconferences for face-to-face meetings, the use of other social distancing techniques, and the implementation of liberal leave policies for persons with sick family members, all of which eliminate or reduce the likelihood of contact with infected individuals. Interventions will have different costs and benefits, and be more or less appropriate or feasible, in different settings and for different individuals.

General Provisions

This Plan provides initial guidance for Federal and non-Federal entities, including State, local, and tribal entities, businesses, schools and universities, communities, and NGOs, on the development of their institutional plans and provides initial guidance for individuals and families on ways that they can prepare for a pandemic. This guidance will be expanded and refined over time, in consultation with the above stakeholders.

As part of their planning, organizations will need to ensure that reasonable measures are in place to protect the health of Americans during a pandemic, sustain critical infrastructure, and mitigate impact to the economy and the functioning of society. The collective response of all Americans will be crucial in mitigating the health, social, and economic effects of a pandemic (see *Individual, Family, and Community Response to Pandemic Influenza* between Chapters 5 and 6).

The actions directed in this Plan will be implemented in a manner consistent with applicable law and subject to availability of appropriations. Nothing in this Plan alters, or impedes the ability to carry out, existing authorities or responsibilities of Federal department and agency heads to perform their responsibilities under law and consistent with applicable legal authorities and Presidential guidance.

The actions directed in this plan are intended only to improve the internal management of the executive branch of the Federal Government, and they are not intended to, and do not, create any right or benefit, substantive or procedural, enforceable at law or in equity, against the United States, its departments, agencies, or other entities, its officers or employees, or any other person.

CHAPTER 2 — U.S. GOVERNMENT PLANNING FOR A PANDEMIC

The Pandemic Threat

Influenza viruses have threatened the health of animal and human populations for centuries. Their diversity and propensity for mutation have thwarted our efforts to develop both a universal vaccine and highly effective antiviral drugs. As a result, and despite annual vaccination programs and modern medical technology, influenza in the United States results in approximately 36,000 deaths and 226,000 hospitalizations each year.

A pandemic occurs when a wholly new strain of influenza virus emerges that has the ability to infect and be passed between humans. Because humans have little immunity to the new virus, a worldwide epidemic, or pandemic, can ensue. Three human influenza pandemics occurred in the 20th century, each resulting in illness in approximately 30 percent of the world population and death in 0.2 percent to 2 percent of those infected. Using this historical information and current models of disease transmission, it is projected that a modern pandemic could lead to the deaths of 200,000 to 2 million U.S. citizens.[2]

The animal population serves as a reservoir for new influenza viruses. Scientists believe that avian, or bird, viruses played a role in the last three pandemics. The current concern for a pandemic arises from an unprecedented outbreak of H5N1 influenza in birds. In 1997, the H5N1 influenza virus emerged in poultry in Hong Kong and infected 18 people, 6 of whom died. Since then, the virus has spread across bird populations in Asia, Europe, and Africa resulting in the deaths, through illness and culling, of over 200 million birds. In addition, the virus has shown the ability to infect multiple species, including long-range migratory birds, pigs, cats, and humans. To date, the virus is known to have infected over 200 persons in the Eastern Hemisphere, and resulted in the deaths of more than half of those known to be infected. This mortality rate is due in part to the fact that H5 influenza viruses have not previously circulated in humans, so the population has no background immunity to these viruses. It is impossible to predict whether the H5N1 virus will lead to a pandemic, but history suggests that if it does not, another novel influenza virus will emerge at some point in the future and threaten an unprotected human population.

While a pandemic will lead to a significant toll that is measured in human illness and death, its impact will extend far beyond hospitals, infirmaries, and doctors' offices. Because influenza viruses do not respect geography, age, race, or gender, the impact of a pandemic will be pervasive, removing essential personnel from the workplace for weeks, due to their own illness, illness in a family member, or as a result of public health guidance to limit contact with others. Absenteeism across multiple sectors will threaten the functioning of critical infrastructure providers, the movement of goods and services, and operation of anchor institutions such as schools and universities. This has significant ramifications for the economy, national security, and the basic functioning of society.

The economic repercussions of a pandemic could be significant. The Congressional Budget Office has estimated that a pandemic on the scale of the 1918 outbreak could result in a loss of 5 percent of gross

---

[2] A Potential Influenza Pandemic: Possible Macroeconomic Effects and Policy Issues.
Congressional Budget Office, December 8, 2005

domestic product, or a loss of national income of about $600 billion. These effects will occur through two main channels. A pandemic will affect the economy directly through illness and mortality caused by the disease, and the associated lost output. A pandemic will also generate indirect costs, from actions taken to prevent and control the spread of the virus. Some of these actions will be taken by the government. Others will be taken by institutional leaders and employers, while still others will be the result of uncoordinated individual responses to avoid infection. These latter reactions will reflect public perceptions and fears.

Preparedness for a pandemic requires the establishment of infrastructure and capacity, a process that can take years. For this reason, significant steps must be taken now. This Implementation Plan (Plan) for the *National Strategy for Pandemic Influenza (Strategy)* acknowledges this reality, and makes it clear that every segment of society must prepare for a pandemic and will be a part of the response. The Plan further recognizes that the Federal Government must provide clear criteria and decision tools to inform State, local, tribal, and private sector planning and response actions, and that Federal agencies must be prepared to supplement and support State, local, and tribal efforts where necessary and feasible.

The National Strategy for Pandemic Influenza

Pandemics represent a unique threat to the health and well being of human populations and ultimately to the functioning of society. As products of a complex ecosystem, their timing cannot be predicted and their emergence cannot be controlled. Because novel influenza viruses meet little immunological resistance in the population, their impact is widespread and can be severe, threatening the functioning of all elements of society. The recognition of this potential impact has led governments around the globe to accelerate their planning efforts to combat and prepare for a pandemic. It has also led governments and international health organizations around the globe to call for transparency in reporting of cases of pandemic influenza, scientific cooperation to characterize the virus and develop effective vaccines, and coordinated international plans to stop, slow, or limit the spread of a pandemic virus after it emerges.

In response to this threat, the President announced the *National Strategy for Pandemic Influenza* on November 1, 2005. The *Strategy* provides a high-level overview of the approach that the Federal Government will take to prepare for and respond to a pandemic, and articulates expectations of non-Federal entities to prepare themselves and their communities.

The *Strategy* contains three pillars: (1) preparedness and communication, (2) surveillance and detection, and (3) response and containment. Each pillar describes domestic and international efforts, animal and human health efforts, and efforts that will be undertaken at all levels of government and in communities to prepare for and respond to a pandemic. It describes the manner in which the Federal Government will support preparedness efforts domestically and internationally in regions affected by avian influenza outbreaks, including the establishment of vaccine and antiviral production capacity and stockpiles; mechanisms to ensure timely coordinated messages to the public, whether from Federal, State, local, or tribal entities, or international authorities; establishment of early warning systems that allow us to activate our response mechanisms and the production and administration of vaccine before the arrival of a pandemic to our shores; and coordinated responses domestically and internationally to limit the spread of disease and mitigate disease, suffering and death.

The *Strategy* makes it clear that the Federal Government will use all instruments of national power to address the pandemic threat. However, if efforts to contain the outbreak at its source fail, the resources of the Federal Government will not be sufficient to prevent the spread of a pandemic across the Nation and its resulting impact on communities, workplaces, families, and individuals. An effective response will require the full participation of all levels of government and all segments of society.

Implementation of the *National Strategy*

While the *Strategy* provides an important framework for Federal Government planning for an influenza pandemic, it must be translated to tangible action that fully engages the breadth of the Federal enterprise. This Plan proposes that Federal departments and agencies take specific, coordinated steps to achieve the goals of the *Strategy*. Because preparedness and response activities depend upon entities outside of the Federal Government, it also outlines expectations with respect to non-Federal stakeholders in the United States and abroad. Joint and integrated planning across all levels of government and the private sector is essential to ensure that available national capabilities and authorities produce detailed plans and response actions that are complementary, compatible, and coordinated.

This Plan supports Homeland Security Presidential Directive 8 (HSPD-8) by identifying coordinated preparedness and response actions to combat pandemic influenza. All actions in this Plan emphasize jointness and coordination of effort between and among Federal, State, tribal, and local entities. The purpose of HSPD-8 is to establish "policies to strengthen the preparedness of the United States to prevent and respond to threatened or actual domestic terrorist attacks, major disasters, and other emergencies by requiring a national domestic all-hazards preparedness goal, establishing mechanisms for improved delivery of Federal preparedness assistance to State and local governments, and outlining actions to strengthen preparedness capabilities of Federal, State, and local entities."

Because it is essential for all institutions to develop their own pandemic plans, this Plan provides guidance for non-Federal entities on the development of their institutional plans, including State, local, and tribal entities, businesses, schools and universities, and non-governmental organizations (NGOs). It also provides guidance for individuals and families on ways that they can prepare for a pandemic. Additional resources to support this planning are available at **www.pandemicflu.gov**. Federal agencies are expected to further supplement this Plan with guidance on pandemic planning for their respective stakeholders.

Finally, this Plan describes the series of actions that the Federal Government will take when an influenza virus with pandemic potential is identified in the human population anywhere in the world, recognizing that while we are devoting significant resources to early warning and containment overseas, a pandemic strain of influenza virus could also originate in the United States.

This Plan is divided into chapters that address the breadth of major considerations raised by a pandemic: protecting human health, protecting animal health, international considerations, transportation and borders, security considerations and institutional considerations. The chapters include the following:

• Narrative descriptions of the scope of the challenges and key considerations, followed by the rationales underlying the Federal Government approach;

• The roles and responsibilities of Federal departments and agencies, State, local, and tribal entities, the private sector, and individuals and families;

• A comprehensive set of over 300 actions for Federal departments and agencies to address the pandemic threat, each accompanied by lead and supporting agencies, outcome measures, and timelines for action; and

• Clearly defined expectations for non-Federal stakeholders.

An appendix at the end of this Plan provides a brief description of relevant legal authorities in each chapter, as well as the manner in which the Federal Government will implement the Plan.

While this Plan proposes that departments and agencies to undertake a series of actions in support of the *Strategy*, it does not describe the operational details of how departments will accomplish these objectives. Departmental pandemic plans will provide those details, and will address additional considerations raised during a pandemic, including (1) protection of employees, (2) maintenance of essential functions and services, and (3) the manner in which departments and agencies will communicate messages about pandemic planning and response to their stakeholders. Specific guidance on the development of department plans is included in Chapter 9 and Appendix A.

The proposals contained within this Plan build upon a historic and comprehensive set of actions taken by the Federal Government in 2005 to address the pandemic threat. The actions include the development of a promising human vaccine against the H5N1 avian influenza virus, the submission of a $7.1 billion budget request to support pandemic preparedness, the establishment of the International Partnership on Avian and Pandemic Influenza, and the first Cabinet-level exercise to assess the Federal Government response to a naturally occurring threat.

Necessary Enablers of Pandemic Preparedness

View Pandemic Preparedness as a National Security Issue

A complex balance exists between humans and the microbial world. We are forced to take notice when this balance is disrupted, but antimicrobials and medical therapies usually allow us to restore the steady state to which we have become accustomed, limiting the impact of infectious disease to an individual or a community. Because our public health and medical system is well equipped to deal with the routine challenges presented by the microbes around us, the impact of infectious diseases and the policies and procedures that guide our actions remain largely within the purview of these communities.

The pandemic threat is different. In the event of a pandemic, the transmissibility of influenza viruses, the universal susceptibility of the world's population to viruses that have not previously circulated, and the mobility of human populations mean that every corner of the globe and every element of society are likely to be touched. This has ramifications not only for the health and well being of populations, but for the national and economic security of nations, and the functioning of society. Once this fundamental premise is recognized, the scope and scale of the measures necessary to prepare for a pandemic become apparent.

Promote Connectivity

One of our greatest vulnerabilities is the lack of connectivity between communities responsible for pandemic preparedness. This applies to the coordination of efforts between nations, between the health and non-health communities, between the public health and medical communities, and between the animal and human health communities.

Public Health and Medical Communities

In the United States, the public health community has responsibility for community-wide health promotion and disease prevention and mitigation efforts, and the medical community is largely focused on action at the individual level. Insufficient communication and coordination between these communities represents a vulnerability in our preparedness for an influenza outbreak. During a pandemic, the medical community must have awareness of the ongoing epidemiological analysis and community-wide interventions being recommended by public health leaders, and the public health community must have situational awareness of the evolution of disease that can only come from connectivity to the emergency departments and other acute care settings where patients with influenza are presenting. The inter-pandemic period presents an opportunity to establish and test these relationships.

International Community

Given that viruses do not respect borders, and that one country's actions will have ramifications for the rest of the globe, we should work to align pandemic preparedness and response efforts across nations. The international community should conform to pre-specified standards for disease reporting, scientific cooperation, public health measures to limit disease spread, and the range of related measures that support our objectives of early warning and rapid response. Early adoption of the International Health Regulations by nations represents an important step in this direction, as does the commitment by nations to the principles of the International Partnership on Avian and Pandemic Influenza. The international community must build upon these agreements to establish coordinated national policies, protocols, and procedures to ensure that we have a consistent response across nations upon the emergence of a pandemic virus.

Health and Non-Health Communities

Because the impact of a pandemic will be felt across society, it is essential that all institutions prepare for what would normally be left to the purview of the health and medical communities. This requires a shift in thinking for most governmental and non-governmental entities, particularly businesses, which may not be accustomed to planning around health considerations. While these organizations have a responsibility to plan on behalf of their employees, customers, students, and other stakeholders, it is incumbent upon the health and medical communities to provide guidance on how to accomplish this planning. This can only be accomplished through the establishment of relationships between the health community and agencies across the government and entities across the community.

Animal and Human Health Communities

Animals serve as a limitless reservoir for new human pathogens. While influenza viruses have demonstrated this over centuries, we have also learned this lesson from HIV and the virus responsible for SARS. We must address the barriers between the animal and human health communities that exist at all levels of government, between NGOs, within academia, and in the community. These barriers have impeded international preparedness and response efforts to the ongoing pandemic in birds, have delayed our recognition of threats to human health, and ultimately have contributed to the overall risk of an avian virus adapting itself to the human host. While cooperation is improving between these sectors domestically, we must encourage the same between ministries of agriculture and health in other nations, and require this of the multilateral organizations that represent these communities.

Communicate Risk and Responsibility

Uncertainty during a pandemic will drive many of the outcomes we fear, including panic among the public, unpredictable, and unilateral actions by governments, instability in markets, and potentially devastating impacts on the economy. The need for timely, accurate, credible, and consistent information that is tailored to specific audiences cannot be overstated. This requires coordinated messaging by spokespersons across government, at the local, State, tribal, and Federal levels, and by our international partners. It also requires the designation and training of a cadre of spokespersons within relevant organizations, the ability to provide guidance in the setting of incomplete information, and the acknowledgement that this guidance may change as more information becomes available. Such a capability should be developed before a pandemic, as should the key messages that we know we will have to communicate upon the emergence of a pandemic virus.

As important as it will be to provide clear guidance during a pandemic, it is equally important to communicate expectations and responsibilities of all relevant stakeholders before a pandemic begins. Disease transmission occurs on an individual basis, and the outbreak of an infectious disease represents the summation of innumerable individual actions. Actions taken at the individual level do matter, as do actions by all organizations, irrespective of their size.

The need for individual and organizational participation in pandemic planning is amplified by the fact that governments and the Federal Government in particular, have limited ability to impact the spread of disease at the community level. Moreover, we can predict that the Federal Government will have limited capacity to augment the health and other infrastructure needs of specific communities when the entire Nation is overwhelmed. This reality, and the concomitant requirement for local self-sufficiency, must be communicated to States, communities, organizations, commercial enterprises, and even individuals before a pandemic begins.

Support Multilateral Organizations

A pandemic is a global threat that has the potential to impact every nation. Because an outbreak in any location in the world threatens all nations, it is critically important that the international community coordinate its preparedness and response activities. Nowhere is this more apparent than in our containment planning efforts. This requires international standards for surveillance, transparency, sample sharing, and swift coordinated action upon the recognition of an outbreak. It also requires the presence of credible and independent arbiters of scientific and epidemiologic information as it becomes available.

The World Health Organization (WHO) represents the linchpin of international preparedness and response activities. It is bolstered by other multilateral and bilateral organizations, but during a pandemic we will rely upon it to be a highly visible and credible coordinator of the international response. Given the critical role that it plays, it is essential that the international community support its efforts with resources and personnel, and expand plans to provide emergency increases in capacity when the emergence of a pandemic virus is suspected or confirmed.

As we take action to support the efforts of the WHO, we must draw attention to the need to expand and enhance coordination of international animal health efforts. Given the near certainty that the next pandemic will emerge from an animal reservoir, it is critically important that the multilateral organizations responsible for animal health, particularly the United Nations (UN) Food and Agriculture Organization (FAO), be prepared to assist nations that are in the midst of or threatened by an outbreak of avian influenza.

Merge Preparedness for Natural and Deliberate Threats

While the initial events leading to a deliberate or natural outbreak of infectious disease are dramatically different, the actions necessary to prepare, provide early warning, and respond are nearly identical. We should make this principle explicit in our planning for outbreaks and ensure, to the extent possible, that the mechanisms that we put in place are mutually supportive. This has clear implications for the manner in which the Federal Government directs its biodefense resources, but it similarly places a responsibility upon the public health community to ensure that the infrastructure established at the State, local, and tribal levels to support traditional public health priorities is configured to meet our biodefense requirements.

Advancing Pandemic Preparedness

The U.S. Government has already taken a historic series of actions, domestically and internationally, to address the pandemic threat:

• The *National Strategy for Pandemic Influenza* was announced on November 1, 2005, and provides strategic direction for all Federal departments and agencies, and clearly articulates expectations of non-Federal stakeholders, in pandemic preparedness, surveillance, and response. It also outlines a strategy for establishing domestic vaccine and antiviral medication production and stockpile capacity to protect the population and limit the spread of a pandemic virus in the United States and to provide treatment to those who become ill. The *Strategy* is supported by this Plan and department and agency-specific pandemic plans.

• **An Emergency Budget Request of $7.1 billion to support activities over several years** was submitted to Congress to support the objectives of the *Strategy*. An initial appropriation in FY06 of $3.8 billion has been made to support the budget requirements of the first year of the initiative. While much of the funding is directed toward domestic preparedness and the establishment of countermeasure stockpile and production capacity, over $400 million is directed to bilateral and multilateral international efforts and builds upon the $25 million appropriation of funds in the emergency Tsunami Appropriation Act Supplemental of 2005. Key programs that will be supported by the funds appropriated to date:

  • Expansion of domestic vaccine production capacity to provide greater quantities of this critical medical countermeasure than now is possible. The primary objective, depending upon availability of future appropriations and the responsiveness of the vaccine industry, is for domestic manufacturers to be able to produce enough vaccine for the entire U.S. population within 6 months of the recognition of a human influenza virus with pandemic potential. A supporting objective is to develop and maintain a standing stockpile of vaccine to protect 20 million U.S. citizens against each currently circulating influenza virus (currently avian H5N1 virus) that could become a virus with human pandemic potential.

  • Expansion of stockpiles of antiviral medications to treat more U.S. citizens than current stockpiles will allow. The primary objective, depending upon the availability of future appropriations and global production capacity, is to acquire sufficient drugs to treat 75 million U.S. citizens, or 25 percent of the U.S. population, during an influenza pandemic plus 6 million courses to be directed to containment of initial outbreaks in the United States.

  • Expansion of surveillance capabilities domestically and internationally, in humans and animals, to provide early warning of a pandemic and its arrival to our shores, and to target public health interventions during a pandemic.

  • Investments in the development of risk communication strategies, to ensure that timely, credible, and consistent messages are being provided to the public by all authorities before and during a pandemic.

• Investments in multilateral organizations and on a bilateral basis to expand scientific, public health, surveillance, and response capacity in countries currently affected by the H5N1 avian outbreak.

Enhancing Domestic Preparedness

• **Over $6 billion has been invested in State and local public health and medical preparedness since 2002 for activities that directly support pandemic preparedness.** The development of pandemic plans by States has been a requirement of the Centers for Disease Control and Prevention Cooperative Agreements and the Health Resources and Services Administration Hospital Bioterrorism Preparedness Grants since 2004.

• **Real-time surveillance of disease in communities is being established by the BioSense Real-Time Clinical Connections Program,** in order to provide real-time "situational awareness" to public health officials in communities across the country during a pandemic and to facilitate the targeting of public health interventions. Ten cities were chosen to initiate the program, with a goal of including all 31 BioWatch communities by the end of 2006.

• **The Department of Homeland Security (DHS) has established a National Biosurveillance Integration System** to collect, integrate, and analyze domestic and international all-source information. The system will integrate human disease, agriculture, food, and environmental surveillance systems.

• **A Cabinet-level tabletop exercise of the Federal Government response to a pandemic** was held in December 2005 to identify and address gaps in capabilities and coordination. The exercise was the first of its kind to test the Federal response to any event, natural or deliberate, and highlighted key policy issues that are currently being addressed and resolved. The exercise will lay the foundation for ongoing assessments of Federal preparedness for a pandemic.

• **The Department of Health and Human Services' (HHS) pandemic influenza plan** and guidance for State, local, and tribal preparedness was released on November 2, 2005. It provides comprehensive guidance for States, communities, tribal entities, hospitals, health care providers, and individuals on actions that they should take to prepare for a pandemic.

• **An HHS National meeting of States** was held in Washington, D.C., in December 2005 to provide guidance on the development of State and local pandemic preparedness and response plans. A series of more than 60 local summits on pandemic preparedness, encompassing all 50 States, will be completed in the first half of 2006.

• **The proposed Federal quarantine regulations,** which have been published for public comment, contain enhanced reporting mechanisms and procedures for conducting epidemiologic investigations, and influenza viruses with pandemic potential have been added to the list of quarantinable diseases.

• **A Memorandum of Understanding has been signed by HHS and DHS** to ensure coordination of border screening activities and information sharing for contact tracing during an outbreak of a communicable disease and references operating guidelines specific to H5N1.

Developing, Producing, and Stockpiling Vaccines and Antiviral Medications

• **Human vaccines against the H5N1 avian influenza virus have been developed** in conjunction with manufacturers and are undergoing testing by HHS. Vaccine will be stockpiled to provide an immediately available supply of "pre-pandemic" H5N1 vaccine while a new vaccine tailored to the specific virus that emerges is developed after a pandemic begins.

- **Investments have been made since 2004 to advance cell culture technology for the production of influenza vaccine.**

- **Over 4 million treatment courses of antiviral medications are held in the Strategic National Stockpile (SNS),** with plans to expand to 50 million courses in the SNS, and another 31 million courses in State-based stockpiles, the procurement of which will be subsidized by the Federal Government.

- **Added procedures for comprehensive liability protection for pandemic and epidemic countermeasure manufacturers, distributors, program planners, persons who prescribe, administer, and dispense countermeasures, officials, agents, and employees of each of these entities, and a compensation program** have been put in place through legislation that was introduced and passed in 2005, thereby removing a major impediment to the establishment of a domestic vaccine production base, while ensuring that those who are harmed by a pandemic vaccine receive compensation.

Enhancing International Cooperation, Capacity, and Preparedness

- **The International Partnership on Avian and Pandemic Influenza** was launched by the United States on September 14, 2005, to ensure transparency, scientific cooperation, rapid reporting of cases, donor coordination, and a series of other actions to support global preparedness and response. The Partnership will increase cooperation among participating countries and international organizations including WHO, FAO, and the World Organization for Animal Health to develop global capacity to address an incipient pandemic. The Partnership agreed at its first meeting in Washington, D.C., in October 2005 to elevate pandemic influenza on national agendas, coordinate efforts among donor and affected nations, mobilize and leverage resources globally, and increase transparency in disease reporting and surveillance and building capacity.

- **The United States is working on a bilateral basis to support local, national, and regional efforts to build capacity, increase reporting, ensure scientific cooperation, and enhance overall preparedness.** The United States, Indonesia, and Singapore also agreed to create a model avian influenza-free zone in Indonesia to develop and demonstrate best practices to prevent infection and spread of a pandemic virus in both animals and humans. The Regional Emerging Disease Intervention Center in Singapore, jointly staffed by Singapore and the United States, is conducting training on avian influenza in Southeast Asia and developing the model for the Joint Avian Influenza Demonstration Project. The United States also is working with China to strengthen vaccine development, disease surveillance and rapid response, and pandemic planning through the U.S.-China Joint Initiative on Avian Influenza. Given the challenge of containing an outbreak of a pandemic virus on the North American continent, the United States has also begun discussions with Canada and Mexico to develop an agreed doctrine to respond to and contain a pandemic.

- **Working through existing multilateral frameworks to advance the goals of the Partnership.**

  - WHO: The United States is assisting WHO in the development of a response and containment protocol for consideration and adoption by the World Health Assembly. In addition, the United States is supporting other WHO efforts at improving the detection and response capabilities of other countries and ensuring that all actions are consistent with the International Health Regulations.

• APEC: At the November 2005 Asia Pacific Economic Cooperation (APEC) Summit, the United States supported APEC's Initiative to Prepare For and Mitigate an Influenza Pandemic to strengthen response and preparedness in the region, including through an inventory of regional disaster management capabilities, exercise of regional communications, and an Emerging Infectious Diseases Symposium in Beijing.

• GHSAG: Health Ministers from Canada, France, Germany, Italy, Japan, Mexico, United Kingdom, and the United States cooperate in the Global Health Security Action Group (GHSAG) to refine national pandemic influenza plans, support development of WHO protocols for early containment of influenza, and coordinate on capacity building in developing countries.

• G-8: The United States is encouraging the G-8 to support the development of an avian influenza plan and information packages for affected countries to use in the event of an outbreak, to agree on deployment of WHO stockpiles of antiviral medications and to adhere early to WHO's revised International Health Regulations.

• The United States is engaged with the private sector, including business groups like the APEC Business Advisory Council, the U.S.-Association of Southeast Asian Nations (ASEAN) Council, the American Chamber of Commerce, and the non-governmental community, on the role the private sector can play in preparing for and responding to a pandemic outbreak.

Planning Assumptions

Planning Assumptions for the Implementation Plan

Pandemics are unpredictable. While history offers useful benchmarks, there is no way to know the characteristics of a pandemic virus before it emerges. Nevertheless, we must make assumptions to facilitate planning efforts. Federal planning efforts assume the following:

1. Susceptibility to the pandemic influenza virus will be universal.

2. Efficient and sustained person-to-person transmission signals an imminent pandemic.

3. The clinical disease attack rate will be 30 percent in the overall population during the pandemic. Illness rates will be highest among school-aged children (about 40 percent) and decline with age. Among working adults, an average of 20 percent will become ill during a community outbreak.

4. Some persons will become infected but not develop clinically significant symptoms. Asymptomatic or minimally symptomatic individuals can transmit infection and develop immunity to subsequent infection.

5. While the number of patients seeking medical care cannot be predicted with certainty, in previous pandemics about half of those who became ill sought care. With the availability of effective antiviral medications for treatment, this proportion may be higher in the next pandemic.

6. Rates of serious illness, hospitalization, and deaths will depend on the virulence of the pandemic virus and differ by an order of magnitude between more and less severe scenarios. Risk groups for severe and fatal infection cannot be predicted with certainty but are likely to include infants, the elderly, pregnant women, and persons with chronic or immunosuppressive medical conditions.

7. Rates of absenteeism will depend on the severity of the pandemic. In a severe pandemic, absenteeism attributable to illness, the need to care for ill family members, and fear of infection may reach 40 percent during the peak weeks of a community outbreak, with lower rates of absenteeism during the weeks before and after the peak. Certain public health measures (closing schools, quarantining household contacts of infected individuals, "snow days") are likely to increase rates of absenteeism.

8. The typical incubation period (interval between infection and onset of symptoms) for influenza is approximately 2 days.

9. Persons who become ill may shed virus and can transmit infection for one-half to one day before the onset of illness. Viral shedding and the risk of transmission will be greatest during the first 2 days of illness. Children will play a major role in transmission of infection as their illness rates are likely to be higher, they shed more virus over a longer period of time, and they control their secretions less well.

10. On average, infected persons will transmit infection to approximately two other people.

11. Epidemics will last 6 to 8 weeks in affected communities.

12. Multiple waves (periods during which community outbreaks occur across the country) of illness are likely to occur with each wave lasting 2 to 3 months. Historically, the largest waves have occurred in the fall and winter, but the seasonality of a pandemic cannot be predicted with certainty.

CHAPTER 3 — FEDERAL GOVERNMENT RESPONSE TO A PANDEMIC

While the Implementation Plan (Plan) directs Federal departments and agencies to take action to prepare for a pandemic, it is important for the Federal Government to coordinate closely its efforts to gather relevant data and overall situational awareness in a timely manner from the initial phases of a pandemic until recovery is complete, and to communicate its approach to its international partners, State, local, and tribal entities, critical infrastructure owners and operators, and the public. This section describes the manner in which the Federal Government will coordinate its actions, the specific roles and responsibilities of the various Federal departments and agencies, and the specific actions to be taken at stages before, during, and after the occurrence of the first wave of a pandemic in the United States.

Command, Control, and Coordination of the Federal Response

A pandemic will differ from most natural or manmade disasters in nearly every respect. Unlike events that are discretely bounded in space or time, a pandemic will spread across the globe over the course of months or over a year, possibly in waves, and will affect communities of all sizes and compositions. The impact of a severe pandemic may be more comparable to that of a widespread economic crisis than to a hurricane, earthquake, or act of terrorism. It may present as a particularly severe influenza season, or it may overwhelm the health and medical infrastructure of cities and have secondary and tertiary impacts on the stability of institutions and the economy. These consequences are impossible to predict before a pandemic emerges because the biological characteristics of the virus and the impact of our interventions cannot be known in advance.

Similarly, the role of the Federal Government in a pandemic response will differ in many respects from its role in most other natural or manmade events. The distributed nature of a pandemic, as well as the sheer burden of disease across the Nation, means that the physical and material support States, localities, and tribal entities can expect from the Federal Government will be limited in comparison to the aid it mobilizes for geographically and temporally bounded disasters like earthquakes or hurricanes. Nevertheless, the Federal Government must maintain complete situational awareness and be ready and able to take decisive action to ensure a comprehensive and timely national response to a pandemic. The Federal Government will also bear primary responsibility for certain critical functions, including the support of containment efforts overseas and limitation of the arrival of a pandemic to our shores; provision of clear guidance to State, local, and tribal entities, the private sector and the public on protective measures and responses that should be taken; modifications to the law and regulations to facilitate the national pandemic response; modifications to monetary policy to mitigate the economic impact of a pandemic on communities and the Nation; and many others. The Federal Government will also work to ensure the production and distribution of vaccine and antiviral medications to State, local, and tribal entities, and the acceleration of research, development, testing, and evaluation of vaccines and therapies during the outbreak.

To ensure an effective response, single points of contact within each State and Tribal Nation for the key functional areas of pandemic response will be identified. The Department of Homeland Security (DHS) will solicit from Governors and Tribal Chief Executive Officers a single point of contact within each State and Tribal Nation for overall incident management of pandemic influenza response efforts. The Department of Health and Human Services (HHS) will solicit lead points of contact for public health and medical emergency response activities, and the Department of Agriculture (USDA) will solicit lead points of contact for veterinary response activities. DHS will coordinate the consolidation of these points of contact.

States, localities, and tribal entities across the Nation will each have to address the medical and non-medical impacts of the pandemic with available resources. This means that it is essential for State, local, and tribal entities to have plans in place to support the full spectrum of societal needs over the course of weeks or months, and for the Federal Government to provide clear guidance on the manner in which these needs can be met.

It is important that the Federal Government have a defined mechanism for coordination of its response. *The National Response Plan* (NRP) is the primary mechanism for coordination of the Federal Government response to terrorist attacks, major disasters, and other emergencies, and will form the basis of the Federal pandemic response. It defines Federal departmental responsibilities for sector-specific responses, and provides the structure and mechanisms for effective coordination among Federal, State, local, and tribal entities, the private sector, and non-governmental organizations (NGOs). Pursuant to the NRP and Homeland Security Presidential Directive 5 (HSPD-5), the Secretary of Homeland Security is responsible for coordination of Federal operations and resources, establishment of reporting requirements, and conduct of ongoing communications with Federal, State, local, and tribal governments, the private sector, and NGOs.

A pandemic will present unique challenges to the coordination of the U.S. Government response. First and foremost, the types of support that the Federal Government will provide to the Nation are of a different kind and character than those it traditionally provides to communities damaged by natural disasters. Second, although it may occur in discrete waves in any one locale, the national impact of a pandemic could last for many months. Finally, a pandemic is a sustained public health and medical emergency that will have sustained and profound consequences for the operation of critical infrastructure, the mobility of people and freight, and the global economy. Health and medical considerations will affect foreign policy, international trade and travel, domestic disease containment efforts, continuity of operations (COOP) within the Federal Government, and many other aspects of the Federal response.

Pursuant to the NRP, as the primary agency for, and coordinator for, Emergency Support Function #8 (Public Health and Medical Services), the Secretary of Health and Human Services will lead Federal health and medical response efforts and will be the principal Federal spokesperson for public health issues, coordinating closely with DHS on public messaging pertaining to the pandemic. Pursuant to HSPD-5, as the principal Federal official for domestic incident management, the Secretary of Homeland Security will provide coordination for Federal operations and resources, establish reporting requirements, and conduct ongoing communications with Federal, State, local, and tribal governments, the private sector, and NGOs. In the context of response to a pandemic, the Secretary of Homeland Security will coordinate overall non-medical support and response actions, and ensure necessary support to the Secretary of Health and Human Services' coordination of public health and medical emergency response efforts.

The NRP stipulates mechanisms for coordination of the Federal response, but sustaining these mechanisms for several months to over a year will present unique challenges. Day-to-day situational monitoring will occur through the national operations center, and strategic policy development and coordination on domestic pandemic response issues will be accomplished through an interagency body composed of senior decision makers from across the government and chaired by the White House. These and other considerations applicable to response to a pandemic will be incorporated in the NRP review process and inform recommendations on revisions and improvements to the NRP and associated annexes.

Pursuant to the NRP, policy issues that cannot be resolved at the department level will be addressed through the Homeland Security Council/National Security Council (HSC/NSC)-led policy coordination process.

Roles and Responsibilities

The Federal Government

The *National Response Plan* is the primary mechanism for coordination of the Federal Government response to terrorist attacks, major disasters, and other emergencies, and will form the basis of the Federal pandemic response. While the Secretary of Homeland Security is responsible for overall coordination of Federal response actions for a pandemic, nothing in the NRP alters or impedes the ability of Federal, State, local, or tribal departments and agencies to carry out their specific authorities or perform their responsibilities under all applicable laws, Executive orders, and directives. Individual departments and agencies have responsibilities within the NRP for a pandemic, consistent with what is described below:

The Secretary of Health and Human Services will be responsible for the overall coordination of the public health and medical emergency response during a pandemic, to include coordination of all Federal medical support to communities; provision of guidance on infection control and treatment strategies to State, local, and tribal entities, and the public; maintenance, prioritization, and distribution of countermeasures in the Strategic National Stockpile; ongoing epidemiologic assessment, modeling of the outbreak, and research into the influenza virus, novel countermeasures, and rapid diagnostics.

The Secretary of Homeland Security, will be responsible for coordination of the Federal response as provided by the *National Strategy for Pandemic Influenza (Strategy)*, the Homeland Security Act of 2002, and HSPD-5, and will support the Secretary of Health and Human Services' coordination of overall public health and medical emergency response efforts. The Secretary will be responsible for coordination of the overall response to the pandemic, implementation of policies that facilitate compliance with recommended social distancing measures, the provision of a common operating picture for all departments and agencies of the Federal Government, and ensuring the integrity of the Nation's infrastructure, domestic security, and entry and exit screening for influenza at the borders.

The Secretary of State will be responsible for the coordination of the international response, including ensuring that other nations join us in our efforts to contain or slow the spread of a pandemic virus, helping to limit the adverse impacts on trade and commerce, and coordinating our efforts to assist other nations that are impacted by the pandemic.

The Secretary of Defense will be responsible for protecting American interests at home and abroad. The Secretary of Defense may assist in the support of domestic infrastructure and essential government services or, at the direction of the President and in coordination with the Attorney General, the maintenance of civil order or law enforcement, in accordance with applicable law. The Secretary of Defense will retain command of military forces providing support.

The Secretary of Transportation will be responsible for coordination of the transportation sector and will work to ensure that appropriate coordinated actions are taken by the sector to limit spread of infection while preserving the movement of essential goods and services and limiting the impact of the pandemic on the economy.

The Secretary of Agriculture will be responsible for overall coordination of veterinary response to a domestic animal outbreak of a pandemic virus or virus with pandemic potential and ongoing surveillance for influenza in domestic animals and animal products. The Secretary of Agriculture will also be responsible for ensuring that the Nation's commercial supply of meat, poultry, and egg products are wholesome, not adulterated, and properly labeled and packaged.

The Secretary of the Treasury will be responsible for monitoring and evaluating the economic impacts of the pandemic and will help formulate the economic policy response and advise on the likely economic impacts of containment efforts. The Secretary of the Treasury will also be responsible for preparing policy responses to pandemic-related international economic developments, for example, leading the Federal Government's engagement with the multilateral development banks (MDB) and international financial institutions (IFI), including encouraging MDB and IFI efforts to assist countries to address the impact of pandemic influenza.

The Secretary of Labor will be responsible for promoting the health, safety, and welfare of employees and tracking changes in employment, prices, and other economic measurements.

Other Cabinet heads will retain responsibility for their respective sectors. All departments and agencies will be responsible for developing pandemic plans that (1) provide for the health and safety of their employees; (2) ensure that the department or agency will be able to maintain its essential functions and services in the face of significant and sustained absenteeism; (3) provide clear direction on the manner in which the department will execute its responsibilities in support of the Federal response to a pandemic as described in this Plan; and (4) communicate pandemic preparedness and response guidance to all stakeholders of the department or agency.

Non-Federal Entities

The *Strategy* and this Plan clearly articulate expectations for all stakeholders for pandemic preparedness and response, including international partners, State, local, and tribal entities, the private sector and infrastructure providers, and individuals and families. These expectations can be found under "Roles and Responsibilities" in the subsequent chapters and the "Actions and Expectations" contained at the end of each chapter.

Federal Government Actions during a Pandemic

While the majority of this Plan describes specific actions that will be taken to improve our preparedness, it is important to show how this preparedness will translate to action in the period of time immediately before, during, and after the emergence of a pandemic. The unpredictable nature of a pandemic, the character of the pandemic virus, and the state of our preparedness efforts when a pandemic begins make it difficult to accurately predict all actions that the Federal Government will take during a pandemic. Nevertheless, it is possible to describe what action would be taken if a pandemic begins tomorrow, recognizing that our preparedness and ability to respond will improve with each passing month.

For containment to be effective, the United States and the international community must develop a comprehensive containment strategy that involves commitments of funding, supplies, equipment, training, expertise, personnel, countermeasures (e.g., antiviral medications, vaccine, and personal protective equipment (PPE)), and animal and public health measures in a coordinated, global approach. The success of such an effort, however, will be highly dependent on early notification of influenza cases, in both humans and animals, caused by strains that have pandemic potential. Countries must immediately notify the World Health Organization (WHO) of such infections in humans, and the World Organization for Animal Health (OIE) for infections in animals, and provide timely sharing of samples to allow for an international response to be initiated.

World Health Organization Phases of a Pandemic

It is most appropriate to link our actions to the phases of a pandemic. The WHO has defined six phases, before and during a pandemic, that are linked to the characteristics of a new influenza virus and its spread through the population. This characterization represents a useful starting point for discussion about Federal Government actions.

Inter-Pandemic Period (period of time between pandemics)

Phase 1: No new influenza virus subtypes have been detected in humans. An influenza virus subtype that has caused human infection may be present in animals. If present in animals, the risk of human disease is considered to be low.

Phase 2: No new influenza virus subtypes have been detected in humans. However, a circulating animal influenza virus subtype poses a substantial risk of human disease.

Pandemic Alert Period

Phase 3: Human infection(s) with a new subtype, but no human-to-human spread, or at most rare instances of spread to a close contact.

Phase 4: Small cluster(s) with limited human-to-human transmission but spread is highly localized, suggesting that the virus is not well adapted to humans.

Phase 5: Larger cluster(s) but human-to-human spread still localized, suggesting that the virus is becoming increasingly better adapted to humans, but may not yet be fully transmissible (substantial pandemic risk).

Pandemic Period

Phase 6: Pandemic phase: increased and sustained transmission in general population.

We are currently in WHO Phase 3 of the Pandemic Alert Period. As previously described, significant action is underway to prepare for a pandemic. It is the policy of the Federal Government to accelerate these preparedness efforts prior to WHO Phase 4, then initiate pandemic response actions at Phase 4, when epidemiological evidence of two generations of human-to-human transmission of a new influenza virus is documented anywhere in the world.

Stages of the Federal Government Response

The WHO phases provide succinct statements about the global risk for a pandemic and provide benchmarks against which to measure global response capabilities. In order to describe the Federal Government approach to the pandemic response, however, it is more useful to characterize the stages of an outbreak in terms of the immediate and specific threat a pandemic virus poses to the U.S. population

(See *WHO Global Pandemic Phases and the Stages for Federal Government Response* between Chapters 5 and 6). The following stages provide a framework for Federal Government actions:

Stage 0: New Domestic Animal Outbreak in At-Risk Country

Stage 1: Suspected Human Outbreak Overseas

Stage 2: Confirmed Human Outbreak Overseas

Stage 3: Widespread Human Outbreaks in Multiple Locations Overseas

Stage 4: First Human Case in North America

Stage 5: Spread throughout United States

Stage 6: Recovery and Preparation for Subsequent Waves

The following description of the Federal Government response at each of these stages is divided into objectives, actions, policy decisions, and messaging considerations (see *Stages of Federal Government Response* between Chapters 5 and 6). "Immediate Actions" reflect those agreed-upon measures that would be triggered as each landmark for increasing risk to the U.S. population was passed. "Policy Decisions" reflect issues that would have to be considered by the Federal Government at the time, in the context of the available information about the pandemic and the status of our response. Finally, "Communications and Outreach" describes the high-level objectives of the guidance that is provided to the public; institutions; State, local, and tribal authorities; and our international partners.

This Plan will be updated on a regular basis to reflect ongoing policy decisions, as well as improvements in domestic preparedness (e.g., increases in the size of our domestic stockpile or vaccine production capacity).

The list of decisions and actions is not exhaustive—it is intended to provide a high-level overview of the Federal Government approach to a pandemic response. It should also be recognized that during a pandemic a number of actions and decisions will proceed in the face of incomplete information, or in the setting of a rapidly evolving epidemiologic or societal picture. It will be important to maintain a flexible and nimble response posture throughout the response, and adjust our approach as additional situational information becomes available. Finally, there are a series of crosscutting actions that will occur throughout the response. We will continuously review, reassess, and adjust our strategy as new information or response capabilities become available, in areas such as risk communication to the public, our allocation scheme for countermeasures, and the support provided to different sectors of critical infrastructure and the economy.

While this set of actions and decisions represents the Federal Government approach to the pandemic response, this approach will not be taken in a vacuum. We will ensure that our response is closely coordinated with our international partners, multilateral organizations, and State, local, and tribal entities, and that we provide clear, accurate, credible, and timely information about our response to the public and all other stakeholders on an ongoing basis.

Summary of Federal Government Actions during a Pandemic

Stage 0: New Domestic Animal Outbreak in At-Risk Country (WHO Phase 1, 2, or 3)

A human pandemic influenza virus could emerge outside the United States or within our borders. Because of the potential for an HPAI virus, including the current HPAI H5N1, to become a pandemic strain, many international animal health initiatives are being implemented to assist affected countries with their response to disease outbreaks in poultry. Control of threatening viruses among animals is a critical element of the strategy to reduce the level of human exposure, a key risk factor for infection and, therefore, emergence of a pandemic strain.

Regardless of where the risk exists for emergence of a pandemic strain, we must be prepared to respond appropriately. A robust surveillance system in domestic animals and wildlife is required to ensure detection and identify new outbreaks in previously unaffected countries. Of the two, outbreaks in domestic animals present a relatively higher likelihood of human exposure to influenza virus than do outbreaks in wildlife. Domestic animal infections may also present more opportunity than do wildlife infections for an influenza virus to undergo genetic reassortment and become a human pandemic strain. This means that when an influenza virus with human pandemic potential is introduced into domestic birds or other domestic animals in a previously unaffected country, the infection must be detected and eradicated as quickly as possible. If such a virus is found in wild birds or other wildlife, efforts should be directed at preventing it from being introduced into domestic birds or other susceptible animals.

Perhaps most importantly, surveillance of animals needs to be integrated with human influenza surveillance activities at a national level. It is important for results of animal surveillance to serve as an input that may help target human surveillance efforts, relative to temporal, geographic, or other risk factors, especially when an influenza virus with human pandemic potential is detected in birds or other animals.

A confirmed outbreak in domestic animals of an influenza virus with pandemic potential, especially one that has already shown the ability to cause illness in humans, signals an important opportunity to decrease the risk of a human pandemic. When such an outbreak occurs in a country that is not currently experiencing other outbreaks caused by that strain of influenza virus, there will be a variety of actions that need to be taken to address the situation. It is incumbent upon the international community to take rapid action to ascertain the facts on the ground and provide appropriate assistance to the affected country. The steps taken in this stage will be closely coordinated with our international partners and multilateral organizations such as the United Nations Food and Agriculture Organization (FAO) and the OIE.

Should such an outbreak occur within the United States, appropriate response and coordination activities will be initiated as presented in Chapter 7 — Protecting Animal Health.

Objectives

- Track outbreaks until control/resolution.

- Provide coordination mechanisms, logistical support, and technical guidance.

- Monitor for reoccurrence of disease.

Immediate Actions

• Initiate dialogue with FAO, other relevant international health organizations, and other international partners to ensure complete coordinated support (Department of State (DOS) and USDA).

• Initiate dialogue with affected nation through diplomatic, animal health, and human health channels to ascertain situation, offer scientific, technical, and, potentially, economic and trade assistance, and encourage full and open sharing of information (DOS, HHS, and USDA).

• Prepare to deploy rapid response team including influenza epidemiology, diagnostics, public-health management, and communications, as part of bilateral and multilateral teams to assess situation and requirements for successful animal disease eradication and human disease prevention effort (DOS, USDA, U.S. Agency for International Development (USAID), Department of Defense (DOD), and HHS).

• Prepare to supply testing protocols and deploy reagents and equipment to support diagnostic requirements for both animal and human testing (USDA, HHS, DOD, and DHS).

• Prepare to deploy animal disease response materiel, including PPE (USDA and USAID).

Policy Decisions

• Deployment of countermeasures to affected country as part of the U.S. contribution to an animal disease control and eradication effort.

Communications and Outreach

• All: Advise that the Federal Government, along with international partners, is working to ascertain situation as quickly as possible, and that information will be communicated as it becomes available.

• International: Encourage nations and international animal and public health organizations to engage in rapid, coordinated assessments and coordinated communication of findings.

• Public: Reassure public that disease containment measures have been implemented and indicate that measures are targeted at preventing animal-to-animal and animal-to-human transmission.

Stage 1: Suspected Human Outbreak Overseas (WHO Phase 3)

There are many ways in which suspicious clusters of illness may come to our attention, including through reporting to the WHO, news reporting, clinical results in regional laboratories, or through word of mouth or other informal channels. It is incumbent upon the international community to take rapid action to ascertain the facts on the ground, irrespective of the manner in which the reporting occurs. The steps taken here and at subsequent stages will be closely coordinated with our international partners and multilateral organizations such as the WHO.

With the WHO Secretariat and other partners, countries should agree ahead of time on the core content of basic information packages that will be necessary to give to the public in the event of a pandemic, and, to the greatest extent possible, develop an agreed "script" of common, harmonized messages to broadcast to the public immediately and continuing for at least 36 to 48 hours after a pandemic has potentially begun.

Objectives

• Rapidly investigate and confirm or refute reports of human-to-human transmission.

• Initiate coordination mechanisms and logistical support that will be necessary if outbreak confirmed.

Immediate Actions

• Initiate dialogue with WHO and other relevant international health organizations to ensure complete coordinated support (DOS and HHS).

• Deploy rapid response team including influenza epidemiology, microbiology, public health management, infection control, and communications, as part of bilateral and multilateral teams to assess situation and identify situation-specific requirements for successful containment effort if human-to-human transmission strongly suspected or confirmed (HHS).

• Ensure rapid genetic sequencing of viral isolates is performed, providing U.S. facilities and resources to support sequencing and comparison with existing influenza gene libraries as needed (HHS).

• Activate logistical capability to transport samples to the United States or other key locations (HHS and DOD).

• Prepare to deploy reagents to support surge diagnostic requirements (HHS).

• Amplify laboratory-based and clinical surveillance in region (DOD and HHS).

• Prepare to provide logistical support for deployment of stockpile materiel to region, including identification of necessary equipment, supplies, and personnel (DOD and HHS).

• Activate Assistant Secretary-level task force to track developments in region, coordinate and communicate information flow across interagency, and coordinate response efforts and decisions (DOS, HHS, and DHS).

• Initiate dialogue with potentially affected nations through diplomatic and health channels to ascertain situation, offer scientific, technical, and potentially economic and trade assistance, and encourage full and open sharing of information; initiate dialogue with international partners to ensure complete coordinated support (DOS and HHS).

• Review domestic plans to increase layered protective measures at borders and prepare to implement travel restrictions from affected areas, as appropriate (DHS, HHS, and Department of Transportation (DOT).

Policy Decisions

• Pre-positioning of U.S. contribution to international stockpile assets in region of suspected outbreak.

• Vaccination of selected populations with pre-pandemic vaccine.

Communications and Outreach

• All: Advise that the Federal Government, along with international partners, is working to ascertain situation as quickly as possible, and that information will be communicated as it becomes available.

• International: Encourage nations and international organizations to engage in rapid, coordinated assessments and coordinated communication of findings.

• State/local/tribal entities and Institutions: Review pandemic plans and direct to trusted information sources such as **www.pandemicflu.gov.**

• Public: Reassure public, explain confirmed facts, and direct to trusted information sources such as **www.pandemicflu.gov.**

Stage 2: Confirmed Human Outbreak Overseas (WHO Phase 4 or 5)

We will rely upon the WHO to confirm sustained human-to-human transmission of a novel influenza virus, but it is possible that confirmation will come directly from an affected nation or through our own scientists in the affected region.

Objectives

• Contain the outbreak to the affected region(s) and limit potential for spread to the United States.

• Activate the domestic public health and medical response.

Immediate Actions

• Deploy non-countermeasure components of international stockpile and diagnostic reagents to support outbreak investigation, as well as technical and medical assistance (DOS, HHS, and DOD).

• Rapidly assess conditions and likelihood of international containment or slowing of pandemic spread (HHS, DHS, DOD, and DOS).

• Support international deployment of countermeasures to affected region(s) (see below).

• Work with other countries to implement host country pre-departure screening and initiate U.S. en route and arrival screening at U.S. ports of entry (DOS, DOT, DHS, HHS, and DOD).

• Consider travel or routing restrictions from the affected area and for countries that do not have adequate pre-departure screening (DHS, DOT, DOS, and DOD).

• Implement protocols for cargo handling that allow trade to continue, when possible (DHS, DOD, DOS, and DOT).

• Implement protocols to manage or divert inbound international flights with suspected cases of pandemic influenza and prepare to limit domestic ports of entry to manage increased demand for screening, as needed (DOT, DOS, DHS, HHS, and DOD).

• Activate domestic quarantine stations and ensure coordination at State, local, and tribal level, especially with health care resources (HHS and DHS).

• Declare Incident of National Significance (DHS in coordination with other Federal departments).

• Amplify hospital-based surveillance in all communities (HHS).

• Develop seed for vaccine and prepare to produce monovalent vaccine (HHS).

• Meet with vaccine and pharmaceutical manufacturers to discuss maximal exploitation of production capacity and regulatory modifications to facilitate countermeasure production (HHS).

• Develop, produce, and deploy diagnostic reagents for pandemic virus to Laboratory Response Network (LRN) laboratories (HHS).

• Prepare to provide military bases and installation support to Federal, State, local, and tribal agencies (DOD).

• Evaluate ability of pandemic virus to infect and replicate efficiently in poultry or other animals and take appropriate actions based on the results of the evaluation (USDA).

• Determine whether pre-pandemic vaccine is effective against pandemic strain (HHS).

• Review domestic pandemic plans and prepare for response, placing critical staff on recall and pre-deploying assets where appropriate (All).

Policy Decisions

• Deployment of countermeasures to affected region(s) as part of the U.S. contribution to a containment effort.

• Entry/exit screening criteria, nations/regions involved, protocol for isolation and quarantine of passengers and employees.

• Diversion of annual trivalent vaccine production to monovalent pandemic vaccine when seed virus available.

• Pre-vaccination with or administration of a primer dose of pre-pandemic (unmatched) vaccine for emergency response teams (to be followed by pandemic strain vaccine, when available).

• Revision of prioritization and allocation scheme for pandemic vaccine and antiviral medications, based upon real-time situational analysis of characteristics of the pandemic virus, epidemiological analyses, and the most recent data regarding available stockpiles of countermeasures.

• Deployment of pre-pandemic vaccine to State/tribal entities and to Federal departments and agencies, and initiation of vaccination.

Communications and Outreach

• All: Place all on alert that a high likelihood of a pandemic exists, educate all stakeholders on Federal Government response and containment strategies and expectations for all entities below.

• International: Encourage rapid, coordinated containment effort and coordinated actions to limit from region and to screen passengers.

• State/local/tribal: Place on alert for spread of outbreak to the United States; activate preparedness/response plans and surveillance systems; initiate regular calls with Governors and State/tribal public health and emergency preparedness leaders to provide guidance on preparedness actions necessary and to coordinate messaging.

• Institutions: Make organizations aware of continuity plans and measures to limit infection transmission in workplace; reassure that efforts will be made to limit adverse impact on movement of goods, services and people.

• Public: Prepare public for possibility of a pandemic while providing information about containment efforts, reassure that we have not yet seen cases domestically; review actions that reduce likelihood of influenza exposure and limit influenza transmission.

Stage 3: Widespread Human Outbreaks in Multiple Locations Overseas (WHO Phase 6)

The occurrence of widespread outbreaks suggests that efforts are unlikely to be successful in containing the emerging pandemic. We will focus our efforts on our domestic preparedness posture and response actions and on delaying the onset of epidemics within the United States.

Objectives

• Delay the emergence of pandemic influenza in the U.S. and North American populations.

• Ensure the earliest warning possible of the first case(s) in North America.

• Prepare our domestic containment and response mechanisms.

Immediate Actions

• Re-examine limitation on international travel from affected regions (or regions that do not institute pre-departure screening) and maintain layered screening measures for host country pre-departure, en route, and arrival of U.S.-bound travelers (DOS, DHS, and HHS).

• Prepare "containment stockpile" for deployment to quarantine stations and other locations as appropriate (HHS).

• Maintain heightened hospital-based surveillance in all communities (HHS).

- If not previously available, develop and deploy diagnostic reagents for pandemic virus to all LRN laboratories (HHS).

- Perform real-time modeling and epidemiological analyses to characterize the virus, its speed of spread, and impact on the population to inform recommendations concerning public health interventions and countermeasure prioritization (HHS).

- Deploy antiviral stockpile with appropriate security to State/tribal entities and to Federal departments and agencies, with prioritization and treatment recommendations (HHS).

- Prepare to implement surge plans at Federal medical facilities (HHS, DOD and Department of Veterans Affairs (VA).

- Activate domestic emergency medical personnel plans (HHS and VA).

- If not previously done, divert annual trivalent vaccine production to monovalent pandemic vaccine (HHS).

- Deploy pre-pandemic vaccine to State/tribal entities and to Federal agencies, and initiation of vaccination.

Policy Decisions

- Prioritize efforts for domestic preparedness and response.

Communications and Outreach

- International: Reinforce importance of limiting travel in affected areas and continuing entry/exit screening.

- State/local/tribal: Advise governments to activate pandemic response plans; review influenza case definition and testing protocols used by public health and medical community; announce preliminary conclusions of epidemiologic assessments and modeling; request that State, local, and tribal leadership reach out to critical infrastructure providers to ensure that continuity plans are in place.

- Institutions: Review COOP guidance.

- Public: Review preparedness and countermeasure distribution guidance; advise public to prepare to reduce non-essential domestic travel once epidemic reaches United States.

Stage 4: First Human Case in North America (WHO Phase 6)

We recognize that the development of the first case anywhere in North America represents a significant threat to the entire continent, as for practical purposes it will be impossible to prevent completely the migration of disease across land borders. We also recognize that a pandemic could originate in North America, rather than overseas, in which case our response would begin with the steps below. We will work with Canada and Mexico to delay the spread of the pandemic across North America through aggressive attempts to contain the initial North American outbreaks, recognizing the challenges associated with such an effort.

Objectives

• Contain the first cases on the continent with slowing of first and subsequent pandemic waves of spread.

• Antiviral treatment and prophylaxis.

• Implement the national response.

Immediate Actions

• Deploy "containment stockpile," if available, to any domestic region with confirmed or suspected cases of pandemic influenza, if an epidemiologic link to an affected region exists (HHS).

• Limit non-essential passenger travel in affected areas and institute protective measures/social distancing, and support continued delivery of essential goods and services (DHS, DOT, and HHS).

• Ensure that pandemic plans are activated across all levels of government and in all institutions (HHS and DHS).

• Continue with development of pandemic vaccine (HHS).

• Activate surge plans within Federal health care systems and request that State, local, and tribal entities do the same (HHS and DHS).

• Continue to develop and deploy diagnostic reagents for pandemic virus to all LRN laboratories and other laboratories with capability and expertise in pandemic influenza diagnostic testing (HHS).

• Antiviral treatment and targeted antiviral prophylaxis (HHS).

Policy Decisions

• Revision of prioritization and allocation scheme for pandemic vaccine as appropriate, based upon characteristics of the pandemic virus and available quantities of vaccine.

Communications and Outreach

• All: Communicate up-to-date information on epidemiologic characteristics of virus and outbreak modeling.

• International: Reinforce importance of travel restrictions and entry/exit screening.

• State/local/tribal: Advise State, local, and tribal leadership to implement pandemic response plans; provide guidance on public communication.

• Institutions: Advise institutions to implement continuity plans.

• Public: Review actions that reduce likelihood of influenza exposure and limit influenza transmission; assure public of ability to maintain domestic safety and security; advise public to curtail non-essential travel and prepare for implementation of community disease containment measures as epidemic spreads (See *Individual, Family, and Community Response to Pandemic Influenza* between chapters 5 and 6).

Stage 5: Spread throughout United States (WHO Phase 6)

The emergence of human cases in multiple locations around the country will portend a progressive increase in case load on communities and a resulting impact on all institutions, including those supporting critical infrastructure.

Objectives

• Support community responses to the extent possible to mitigate illness, suffering, and death.

• Preserve the functioning of critical infrastructure and mitigate impact to the economy and functioning of society.

Immediate Actions

• Maintain continuous situational awareness of community needs, triage, and direct Federal support of health and medical systems, infrastructure, and maintenance of civil order as feasible (All).

• Deploy pandemic vaccine, if available, with continuously updated guidance on prioritization and use (HHS).

• Continuously evaluate the epidemiology of the pandemic virus and update recommendations on treatment of patients and protective actions for all sectors on an ongoing basis (HHS and DHS).

• Provide guidance on judicious use of key commodities to reduce the likelihood of shortages (DHS).

Policy Decisions

• Determination of whether (and if so, the form of) Federal intervention is required to support critical infrastructure and the availability of key goods and services (such as food, utilities, and medical supplies and services).

• Determination of when travel restrictions previously enacted can be lifted.

Communications and Outreach

• International: Advise that the United States is executing its plans to assure continuity of society and national defense.

• State/local/tribal entities and Institutions: Advise that Federal Government will continue to provide support, as possible; advise continued implementation of continuity plans, update guidance on epidemiology and successful COOP plans.

- Public: Review actions that reduce likelihood of influenza exposure and limit influenza transmission; provide candid messages about the epidemiology of the virus, the likelihood of contracting influenza and likelihood of severe illness.

Stage 6: Recovery and Preparation for Subsequent Waves (WHO Phase 6 or 5)

While a pandemic may impact the Nation for several months or over a year, a given community can expect to be affected by a pandemic over the course of 6 to 8 weeks. While subsequent waves have been the norm in previous pandemics, it will be important for communities to begin reconstituting themselves as soon as possible in order to mitigate persistent secondary and tertiary impacts of the outbreak, including the adverse economic consequences that are anticipated.

Objectives

- Return all sectors to a pre-pandemic level of functioning as soon as possible.

- Prepare for subsequent waves of pandemic.

Immediate Actions

- Work with private sector, State, local, and tribal entities to prioritize and begin restoring essential services and reviewing plans to maintain continuity of operations in subsequent waves with support of employees that are immunized or have developed immunity (DHS and HHS).

- Redeploy and refit Federal response assets (All).

- Resume essential Federal functions and ensure continuity of operation through subsequent waves (DHS and All).

- Maintain continuous situational awareness of disease in communities, in order to forecast the reduction in illness and reduction in strain on critical infrastructure (HHS and DHS).

- Provide continuously updated information about the epidemiology of the virus, effective treatments, and lessons learned from the first wave, so as to enhance preparedness for subsequent waves (HHS).

- Continue deployment of pandemic vaccine in preparation for subsequent waves (HHS).

- Review lessons learned to develop strategies for subsequent waves (All).

Policy Decisions

- Determination as to whether Federal support is needed for any sector(s) unable to function effectively after the pandemic.

Communications and Outreach

- All: Advise that additional waves of the pandemic may occur and emphasize need to prepare accordingly; communicate key lessons learned to all sectors, and recommend actions to enhance preparedness for subsequent waves.

CHAPTER 4 — INTERNATIONAL EFFORTS

Introduction

Pandemic influenza is a global threat. Given the rapid speed of transmission, the universal susceptibility of human populations, and even a modest degree of lethality, an outbreak of pandemic influenza anywhere poses a risk to populations everywhere. Our international effort to contain and mitigate the effects of an outbreak of pandemic influenza beyond our borders is a central component of our strategy to stop, slow, or limit the spread of infection to the United States.

To meet this important international challenge, all nations and the broader international community must be able to detect and respond rapidly to outbreaks of animal or human influenza with pandemic potential to contain the infection and delay its spread. Many countries, however, do not have sufficient resources or expertise to detect and respond to outbreaks independently. International mechanisms to support effective global surveillance and response, including coordinated provision of accurate and timely information to the public, are also inadequate.

For these reasons, through the International Partnership on Avian and Pandemic Influenza (the Partnership), established by President George W. Bush in September 2005, and other bilateral and multi-lateral international engagement, the Federal Government is heightening awareness of the threat on the part of foreign governments and publics, and promoting development of national and international capacity and commitment to prevent, detect, and limit the spread of animal and human pandemic influenza within and beyond national borders. We are elevating pandemic influenza on national agendas, coordinating efforts among donor and affected nations, mobilizing and leveraging global resources, increasing transparency in global disease reporting and surveillance, and building global public health capacity. The United States is also offering bilateral assistance to strengthen capacity to fight pandemic influenza in the countries at highest risk.

Key Considerations

With the ever-present threat that a newly emerging strain of animal influenza could spark a human pandemic, it is essential that highly pathogenic viruses in animals, wherever they appear, be carefully monitored for changes that could indicate an elevated threat to humans. An outbreak of a novel strain or subtype of influenza capable of sustained and efficient human-to-human transmission, which could occur in the United States or abroad, would spread quickly within an affected community, doubling in size approximately every 3 days. Thorough preparedness, robust surveillance, and strong response on the part of all countries are critically important, as the probability of containing an outbreak of a pandemic virus at its site of origin depends on how quickly a country detects and reports it, shares and tests viral samples, distributes effective countermeasures, and implements public health measures to limit spread.

There are significant challenges to a rapid response to an incipient human pandemic in many countries at risk. The threat of pandemic influenza may not be widely recognized or understood. Many countries at risk lack robust public health and communications infrastructure, pandemic preparedness plans, and proven logistics capability. In many developing countries the livelihood of families is linked to the animals they own, and reporting an outbreak of animal influenza can result in the destruction of a family's animals and, therefore, a threat to their livelihood. Lack of infrastructure and expertise to detect an outbreak in a remote location and quickly transport a sample to a laboratory with appropriate diagnostic capability can impede timely and effective application of countermeasures. Many countries at risk also do not have the veterinary, medical, and non-medical countermeasures, including antiviral medications, to contain a confirmed outbreak.

To promote an effective global response to a pandemic outbreak, donor countries and relevant international health organizations should assist countries that have less capacity and expertise as well as fewer of the necessary resources.

Limited International Capacity

In many of the countries in which the risk of emergence of pandemic influenza is considered to be high, the animal and human health sectors lack the expertise, resources, and infrastructure necessary to effectively detect and contain animal cases and prevent human cases. Recent outbreaks of avian influenza in Asia, Europe, and Africa highlight critical shortcomings in national human and animal disease surveillance and reporting. Early warning and clinical surveillance systems are insufficient to detect changes in an influenza virus that could lead to emergence of a pandemic strain. Key gaps include lack of understanding of the nature of the threat and ways to prevent it, scarcity of well-trained laboratory, epidemiologic, medical, and veterinary staff to provide effective in-country surveillance, and the need for greater commitment and capacity to share data, specimens, and viral isolates rapidly and transparently with national and international animal and human health authorities. International animal and human health mechanisms and resources also need to be strengthened.

Because the risk to public health from an animal influenza virus with human pandemic potential is directly related to the ability to detect and control such viruses in animal populations, the effectiveness of national veterinary services of affected, high-risk, and at-risk countries is critical to minimize human exposure to threatening animal viruses. The objective of controlling or eliminating an animal influenza virus with pandemic potential can only be attained, and then maintained, through concurrent strengthening of national veterinary services. This will require international support for the development of sustainable veterinary services in affected, high-risk, and at-risk countries, and the domestic will of those countries to make such development a priority. Support for development should be based on a unified assessment approach that can be applied in a consistent manner to individual countries to help determine what must be done to create an adequate and sustainable animal health infrastructure.

Likewise, in many countries, limited capacity to detect and control outbreaks of respiratory diseases among humans also adversely impacts on international ability to detect and control the emergence of an influenza pandemic. Countries must give priority to strengthening their public health and respiratory disease case management capacities. The international community must support this prioritization in a consistent and coordinated manner.

As a key part of the U.S. Government's international efforts in support of the *National Strategy for Pandemic Influenza (Strategy)*, under the coordination of the Department of State (DOS) and the U.S. Agency for International Development (USAID), the Department of Health and Human Services (HHS), the Department of Agriculture (USDA), the Department of Homeland Security (DHS), the Department of Transportation (DOT), and the Department of Defense (DOD) are working in cooperation, through complementary strategies, to build capacity in countries at risk to address aspects of avian influenza related to human and animal health.

Preparedness and Planning

Comprehensive preparation including the development and exercise of national and regional plans to respond to a pandemic will facilitate containment efforts and should help mitigate social impacts when containment fails. HHS, DOS, USAID, and USDA are working together to assist priority countries, especially those in which highly pathogenic H5N1 avian influenza is endemic or emerging, to develop, and exercise plans for effective response to a possible extended human pandemic outbreak. We also are supporting public education and risk communication on best practices to prevent and contain animal and human infection.

Surveillance and Response

A country's ability to respond to a human outbreak quickly, requires a broad surveillance network to detect cases of influenza-like illnesses in people, coupled with rapid diagnostic and response capabilities. To help address these challenges, HHS and USAID, in collaboration with DOS, DOD, and international partners, will work together and with the WHO Influenza Network to assist countries at risk, including those that are experiencing outbreaks of H5N1 highly pathogenic avian influenza, to build and improve infrastructure at the central, provincial, and local levels to provide timely notification of suspected human cases of influenza with pandemic potential. Building this capability in countries at risk will facilitate monitoring of disease spread and rapid response to contain influenza outbreaks with pandemic potential. HHS, USAID, DHS, and DOS will support development of rapid response teams, coordinated logistics capability, and new modeling efforts to support containment; increase involvement of the private sector in prevention and control of animal influenza, pandemic planning, and risk management; and improve the ability of the health care sector to control infection and manage cases.

Donor Coordination

To fully address the needs of countries at risk, increased assistance from other countries and international organizations is necessary. In addition, donors must coordinate international assistance resources and activities to avoid duplication of effort and maximize results. DOS, with relevant U.S. Government agencies, is working through the Partnership and other multilateral and bilateral diplomatic contacts to encourage increased, coordinated, international assistance. The United States also will intensify efforts to engage the private sector on the role it can play in preparing for and responding to a pandemic outbreak.

In our bilateral assistance efforts, the United States takes into account assistance pledged by other donors. We target bilateral assistance and expertise to build global veterinary and public health capacity in the countries we believe to be at highest risk, taking into account existing country capacities and needs, and the likelihood that U.S. Government funding will have an impact in a particular country or region given the disease situation, population size, and existing capacities and needs, which vary from country to country. U.S. assistance abroad is intended to protect the health of the American people abroad.

Strengthening International Animal Health Infrastructure

To address needs related to developing sustainable animal health infrastructures in affected, high-risk, or at-risk countries, we will work with the World Organization for Animal Health (OIE), the United Nations (UN) Food and Agriculture Organization (FAO), and other members of the Partnership to develop a unified and consistent approach for such infrastructure development in all countries. The approach will include an assessment of needs for the reduction of animal influenza with human pandemic potential in countries where it exists, and of needs that individual countries may have in making the building of their national veterinary services capacity a domestic priority. Potential options for funding to meet those needs will also be identified. The ultimate goal will be to implement a program through the OIE and FAO and other partners to develop stronger international coordination and support for the animal health response to the current H5N1 avian influenza outbreak in Asia, Europe, and Africa, and for prevention and containment of any future animal disease outbreaks of international concern or consequence.

Key Elements of Effective International Response and Containment

To contain an outbreak of influenza with pandemic potential or delay its spread, a coordinated response by the international community in support of national efforts is key. Many affected countries or regions will require international assistance to detect cases early and respond quickly and effectively to prevent spread. Instituting countermeasures to prevent or slow the spread of infection, including exit and entry screening, restrictions on movement across borders, and rapid deployment of international stocks of antiviral medications, requires international preparation and coordination to be most effective. The U.S. Government is working with WHO, the Partnership, and through diplomatic contacts to strengthen international mechanisms to respond to an outbreak of influenza with pandemic potential, including finalization of WHO's doctrine of international response and containment which lays out the responsibilities of the international community and countries with human outbreaks, and includes provisions to develop and deploy critical resources needed to contain the virus. The U.S. Government considers the following to be key elements of an international response effort.

Agreed Epidemiological "Trigger" for International Response and Containment

While WHO has stated that the first potential signal of early pandemic activity cannot be known in advance and precise "triggering" activity cannot be fully developed ahead of time, WHO also has stated that containment will be strongly considered in the following circumstances:

- Moderate-to-severe respiratory illness (or deaths) in three or more health care workers who have no known exposure other than contact with ill patients, and laboratory confirmation of infection (novel influenza virus) in at least one of these workers.

- Moderate-to-severe respiratory illness (or deaths) in 5 to 10 persons with evidence of human-to-human transmission in at least some, and laboratory confirmation of infection (novel influenza virus) in more than two of these persons.

- Compelling evidence that more than one generation of human-to-human transmission of the virus has occurred.

- Isolation of a novel (influenza) virus combining avian and human genetic material or a virus with an increased number of mutations not seen in avian isolates from one or more persons with moderate-to-severe respiratory illness (acute onset), supported by epidemiological evidence that transmission patterns have changed.

The WHO also has stated that containment will not be attempted in any of the following circumstances:

- Laboratory studies fail to confirm infection caused by a novel influenza virus.

- The number or geographical distribution of affected persons is so large at time of detection that it renders containment impracticable for logistic reasons (i.e., the number of persons requiring prophylactic administration of antiviral drugs exceeds available supplies, or the size of the affected community makes it impossible to ensure adequate supplies of food and shelter, and the provision of medical care and emergency services during a containment operation).

- More than 4 to 6 weeks have passed since detection of the initial cluster, thus decreasing the likelihood that containment would be successful.

The feasibility of rapid containment will further depend on the number of contacts of the initial cases and the ability of the government authorities and international teams to ensure basic infrastructure and essential services to the affected population. Such services include shelter, power, water, sanitation, food, security, and communications with the outside world.

With disease confirmation, the WHO Director-General would announce a human outbreak of an influenza virus with pandemic potential, after consultation with experts from HHS and scientists from other governments. As outlined above, the basis for announcing a human outbreak of pandemic potential would consider a number of factors, including the number of individuals affected, the rapidity of spread, and the virulence of the disease. An outbreak of an influenza virus with pandemic potential is considered a Public Health Emergency of International Concern under the revised International Health Regulations, adopted by the World Health Assembly in May 2005.

Rapid, Transparent Reporting and Sharing of Samples

Countries should immediately take certain actions in response to a suspected outbreak, including prompt reporting of the outbreak to the WHO Secretariat, sharing of viral isolates and/or tissue samples with WHO-designated laboratories for confirmation and vaccine development, activation of national response plans in an effort to contain the outbreak, implementation of public health measures including prophylaxis, vaccination, and social distancing measures (e.g., school closures, snow days, quarantines) in the affected area, epidemiological investigation to identify additional cases and pinpoint the source of the infection, and implementation of screening of passengers. The United States will work with the international community to develop capacity and resources to encourage these actions by countries and regions affected by human outbreaks.

Rapid Response Teams

The international community should develop international Rapid Response Teams to investigate and respond to the suspected beginning of a pandemic. The United States is identifying experts to commit to the teams and encouraging other countries with significant veterinary and public health capacity to do the same. The international community should encourage and assist the WHO Secretariat, the FAO, and the OIE to organize, train, equip, exercise, and deploy these teams.

Stockpiles of Countermeasures

Medical and non-medical countermeasures should be stockpiled and pre-positioned for rapid deployment to help ensure that countries affected by an outbreak of pandemic influenza can launch an effective effort to contain the incipient pandemic. The WHO Secretariat has called for the establishment of an international stockpile of medical countermeasures and the development of an agreed international plan to allocate and deploy them in the event of a pandemic outbreak. WHO is now working with health experts to determine the size, composition, and locations of stockpiles needed for a rapid and effective response and to develop a doctrine of deployment. The U.S. Government has identified medical countermeasures it is prepared to commit for deployment to the international stockpile when needed, and is urging other countries to do the same. We also are supporting international efforts to stockpile non-medical countermeasures, both goods and services, to support containment of animal or human influenza outbreaks with pandemic potential, including transportation of personnel and materiel, personal protective equipment, screening and isolation equipment, disinfectants, temporary shelters, and technical and logistical resources needed to implement an effective containment response.

Logistical Support for an International Response

The international community needs to develop a plan and to identify resources to rapidly transport personnel, supplies and other materiel to support an international containment response, including in geographically remote or underdeveloped locations. The U.S. Government is determining its capabilities in this regard, and will encourage the international community to explore the logistical needs for a coordinated international response and how to address them.

Surveillance to Limit Spread

Early outbreak detection with continued surveillance of travelers and institution of appropriate measures, including social distancing, isolation of infected individuals, quarantine of suspected cases, or treatment with antiviral medications can help delay or limit the spread of a virus once a case occurs. Well-coordinated international implementation of entry and exit restrictions is an important component of an effective global response to contain cases and prevent a pandemic. All countries should prepare to implement steps to limit spread, including local, regional, and national entry and exit restrictions based on veterinary and health monitoring, screening and surveillance for humans, animals, and animal products, and information sharing and cooperation to manage borders. Recognizing the significant costs to implementing border restrictions and the need for international coordination to achieve maximum efficacy, the U.S. Government is examining which surveillance steps will be most effective in limiting spread, including pre-departure exit screening for travelers from affected areas, a reduction of the number of entry and exit points to the United States for international travelers, disease surveillance and entry screening at U.S. borders, and exit screening for travelers leaving the United States in the event of a case occurring here. The international community should provide technical assistance and support personnel to countries that need it to implement screening quickly and effectively. We will endeavor to establish agreements and arrangements with our international partners to ensure the international community takes coordinated action on screening, that such measures are tailored as narrowly as possible to be consistent with efficacy, and that they are lifted quickly when their utility has ended.

Development of Vaccines and Rapid Diagnostics

Vaccines when they become available will be a major means of controlling the spread of a pandemic and reducing associated mortality and morbidity. The vaccine industry, however, faces many risks and uncertainties, including unpredictable market demand and pricing, liability and intellectual property considerations, and regulatory and tax issues. As a result, global and domestic vaccine research and manufacturing capacity is limited. Strong public/private partnerships are needed among government, academia, and industry globally as well as nationally to build vaccine production capacity to levels necessary to address a pandemic and establish a reliable vaccine supply. In addition to its efforts to increase domestic vaccine production capacity, the United States is working through several programs to provide direct and indirect support to multinational vaccine manufacturers, foreign academic institutions, and foreign governments to increase global vaccine production capacity. HHS is supporting advanced development of cell-based influenza vaccines, the evaluation of new H5N1 vaccine candidates, and development of global capacity to produce large quantities of pre-pandemic vaccine (i.e., a vaccine against human infection with the strain of influenza A (H5N1) that is currently circulating among poultry) on a commercial scale through the award of contracts to U.S. and international companies. HHS also is supporting development of H5N1 vaccines in Vietnam and other countries at risk, and beginning discussions with health officials in Southeast Asia concerning possible joint clinical evaluation of avian influenza vaccines in human subjects. HHS also will continue to support development of pandemic influenza vaccines at eligible international as well as domestic research institutions. HHS, USDA, and the Department of the Interior (DOI) are supporting additional efforts to sequence influenza viruses from wild birds, live bird markets, and pigs in Asia and North America, with plans to expand surveillance and collection sites in the future.

The development of rapid diagnostic tests and the distribution of diagnostic reagents and tests are also critical components of pandemic influenza preparedness. USDA has developed and applied a real-time diagnostic protocol to analyze influenza in animal specimens and is assisting countries to adopt and apply this protocol in support of surveillance and response programs for avian influenza among animals. The HHS Centers for Disease Control and Prevention (CDC) and the private sector have developed high-throughput rapid diagnostic kits that can provide results in 4 hours and will undergo field testing by U.S. and Southeast Asian scientists and public health officials to ascertain the utility and robustness of these products in real-time scenarios for detection and reporting of influenza and other viruses in humans and animals.

Effective Public Communication

Public audiences in affected countries and countries at risk will require targeted communications in local languages to understand the threat of influenza with pandemic potential in animals and of human pandemic influenza, the preventive measures that should be taken now, and what actions must be taken if a pandemic occurs. The WHO Secretariat requires the resources to develop and implement international media and risk communications strategies. The Federal Government is pursuing a two-track approach. HHS, USAID, USDA, DOD, and DOS are implementing coordinated, complementary communication plans to reach their respective constituencies with focused and consistent messages. In addition, the Federal Government is working with the WHO Secretariat to coordinate U.S. Government messages with those of other countries so the public receives the same message from their governments, WHO, and U.S. public health authorities. In addition to executing a comprehensive risk communication strategy in the United States, HHS also is working with health officials overseas to develop effective local language health-based messages for the foreign audiences. USAID and USDA are targeting behavior change communications to poultry farmers and the general public in affected regions and DOS is implementing broad-based domestic and international communications plans that inform U.S. and foreign audiences about international initiatives and plans to address the threat of avian and pandemic influenza.

Assistance to United States Citizens Traveling or Living Abroad

The Federal Government will provide U.S. citizens living and traveling abroad with timely, accurate information on avian influenza, through websites, travel information, and meetings. U.S. Embassies and Consulates in countries in which a virus with pandemic potential has been found in wild and/or domestic birds, or where human cases have occurred, will use town hall meetings and their local warden system information networks to disseminate information and enable U.S. citizens to make informed decisions. U.S. Embassies and Consulates are also working to identify local medical capabilities and resources that would be available to Americans in the event of a "stay in place" response to a pandemic, noting WHO and HHS advice that the close physical proximity entailed by air travel poses a particular risk of human-to-human transmission. The Federal Government's ability to provide consular assistance to U.S. citizens who are living and traveling abroad in the event of a pandemic may be limited because travel into, out of, or within a country may not be possible, safe, or medically advisable.

Assistance to the United States

We will develop policies to request, accept, and utilize foreign aid, both material and personnel, quickly in the event that a pandemic outbreak first occurs in the United States, or elsewhere in North America or the Western Hemisphere.

Roles and Responsibilities

The responsibility for preparing for, detecting, and responding to an outbreak of influenza with pandemic potential is global. An outbreak anywhere is a threat to populations everywhere. All nations and relevant international organizations have a responsibility to prepare to respond immediately and leverage all resources, domestic and international, to contain human or animal cases, wherever they may occur. In the event of an outbreak, the government of the affected nation has an obligation to report it immediately to appropriate international organizations (e.g., WHO, OIE) and share epidemiological data and samples with relevant international organizations. In addition, the Federal Government, States, tribal entities, and localities, private sector entities with activities overseas, and international health organizations all have key roles to play in fighting pandemic influenza.

The Federal Government

The Federal Government will encourage engagement by other governments, relevant international organizations, and the private sector to strengthen international capacity and commitment to prepare for, detect, and respond to animal or human outbreaks of influenza with pandemic potential.

Department of State: DOS leads the Federal Government's international engagement, bilateral and multilateral, to promote development of global capacity to address an influenza pandemic. With technical support from HHS and USDA, DOS also leads coordination of the Federal Government's international efforts to prepare for and respond to a pandemic, including the interagency process to identify countries requiring U.S. assistance, identify priority activities, and ensure Federal Government assistance reflects those priorities. DOS is also the coordinating agency for the International Coordination Support Annex to the *National Response Plan* (NRP), with assistance provided by other Federal agencies. DOS is responsible for providing consular services to American citizens who are traveling or residing abroad, including endeavoring to inform American citizens abroad where they can obtain up-to-date information and pandemic risk level assessments to enable them to make informed decisions and take appropriate personal protective measures. DOS sets policies for Federal employees who are working abroad under Chief of Mission authority, including in the event of a pandemic.

In carrying out these responsibilities, DOS works closely with other Federal departments and agencies that bring critical expertise to bear and play a key role in our international prevention and containment efforts, including through engagement with their counterparts in foreign governments and with relevant international organizations. Overseas, in particular, Federal Government departments and agencies cooperate under the authority of the Chief of Mission to bring their respective expertise and resources to bear in a coordinated Federal Government effort.

U.S. Agency for International Development: USAID leads on international disaster response, the development of health capacity abroad, including public health capacity, the training of non-health professionals, and operational coordination for the provision of U.S. international health and development assistance. USAID plays a critical role in bridging between the human and animal health sectors to ensure a comprehensive and cross-sectoral international response to the threat of avian influenza. With technical guidance from HHS and USDA respectively, USAID will work closely with WHO and FAO to ensure strong coordination and standardization of efforts to prepare for, identify, and respond to outbreaks of influenza with pandemic potential in either animal or human populations. In addition, working through non-governmental organizations (NGOs) and the private sector, USAID will expand capacities for the early detection of outbreaks, and support behavior change communications and public efforts in affected countries. A key part of these efforts will be to provide direct financial and commodity support to country-level rapid response teams to ensure timely and effective containment of influenza outbreaks in humans and animals.

Department of Health and Human Services: HHS's primary international responsibilities are those actions required to protect the health of all Americans, in cooperation with the Secretariat of the WHO and other technical partners, including leading Federal Government efforts in the surveillance and detection of influenza outbreaks overseas; supporting rapid containment of localized outbreaks of novel human influenza viruses where and when containment is feasible; leading Federal Government participation in international collaboration on research into human influenza, including zoonotic varieties; providing training to foreign health professionals in how to recognize and treat influenza; providing training and guidance to national and local public health authorities in foreign nations on the use, timing, and sequencing of community infection control measures; and implementing any necessary travel restrictions. HHS's international roles and responsibilities are further defined in the International Coordination Support Annex to the NRP. HHS also will work with USAID in developing local-language campaigns overseas to communicate information related to pandemic influenza, and in supporting the U.S. Government's participation in international efforts to stockpile countermeasures against possible influenza pandemics, and offer our international partners recommendations related to the use, distribution, and allocation of such countermeasures. HHS is the lead Federal Government technical agency for interactions within the Global Health Security Action Initiative, manages the development of a North American Pandemic Influenza Plan under the Security and Prosperity Partnership of North America, and supports DOS in diplomatic and scientific efforts undertaken under the umbrella of the International Partnership on Avian and Pandemic Influenza.

Department of Agriculture: USDA leads the Federal Government's participation in international collaboration on animal health research, risk analyses, transboundary movement of animals and animal products, governance of international agricultural organizations (e.g., FAO, OIE), and delivery of veterinary and agricultural expertise to other countries. USDA personnel at U.S. missions throughout the world collect information, facilitate policy dialogue, and encourage host countries' cooperation with the United States and compliance with international standards on matters concerning animal health. USDA conducts agricultural research and technical and policy outreach with its established public (e.g., land-grant universities) and private stakeholders, strategically coordinating with international, domestic, and other Federal Government participants. USDA analyzes the short- and long-term economic impact of influenza outbreaks among animals, as well as the impact of a potential pandemic on the agricultural sector, while pursuing prevention and control strategies to support international agricultural systems and commerce.

Department of Homeland Security: DHS coordinates overall Federal domestic incident management in accordance with the NRP and supports implementation of the International Coordination Support

Annex to the NRP. With respect to the U.S. Government's international efforts to fight pandemic influenza, DHS supports DOS as the coordinating agency for the international component of an incident under the NRP. DHS, in coordination with DOT, will engage the international transportation industry via the various industry associations and groups. DHS, in collaboration with DOS and HHS, leads the effort to engage foreign entities in sharing passenger manifest information on travelers exposed to pandemic influenza. DHS supports DOS, DOT, and HHS efforts with foreign governments to screen and limit travel to the United States of travelers exposed to pandemic influenza.

Department of Transportation: DOT will support DOS efforts to coordinate with other Federal Government participants on international pandemic response. DOT will collaborate with DHS to implement transportation and border measures, conduct outreach with its public and private stakeholders, and provide emergency management and guidance for civil transportation resources and systems. In its role in the global transportation network, DOT will support international efforts by marshaling transportation planning and emergency support activities.

Department of Defense: DOD supports DOS in international engagement to promote global capacity to address an influenza pandemic consistent with its national security mission. DOD is responsible for the protection of its forces, including providing up-to-date information and pandemic risk-level assessments to enable DOD forces abroad to make informed decisions and take appropriate personal protective measures. The first priority of DOD support, in the event of a pandemic, will be to provide sufficient personnel, equipment, facilities, materials, and pharmaceuticals to care for DOD forces, civilian personnel, dependents, and beneficiaries to protect and preserve the operational effectiveness of our forces throughout the globe. DOD sets policies for deployed military forces working abroad in the Geographic Combatant Commander's area of responsibility and under the commander's command authority, consistent with the responsibilities outlined in the Unified Command Plan. DOD, in conjunction with DOS and HHS, will utilize its existing research centers to strengthen recipient nation capability for surveillance, early detection, and rapid response to animal and human avian influenza.

Department of the Treasury: Treasury assists in analyzing potential economic impacts and monitoring and preparing policy responses to pandemic-related international economic developments. Treasury also leads the U.S. Government's engagement with the multilateral development banks (MDB) and international financial institutions (IFI), including encouraging MDB and IFI efforts to assist countries to address the impact of pandemic influenza.

Department of Commerce: DOC facilitates the expedited interagency review for any export licenses needed for items necessary for overseas shipment in response to an avian influenza pandemic. DOC coordinates, as needed, with HHS/CDC to expedite export licenses of strains, test kits/equipment, and technology to specified destinations in order to allow rapid identification of strains, and provide on ground support to contain/mitigate a pandemic to support development of scientific and epidemiological expertise in affected regions to ensure early recognition of changes in pattern of outbreak.

State, Local, and Tribal Entities

State, local, and tribal authorities ensure that foreign diplomatic and consular personnel in the United States are kept informed of developments relevant to their rights and responsibilities under international and domestic law and that they can perform their authorized functions, including functions of consular protection and assistance. In the event of a pandemic, personal inviolability and other privileges and immunities need to be taken into account when protective measures such as quarantine are being considered, and it will be important that States, localities, and tribal entities afford consular communication and access to non-official foreign nationals who may be quarantined. State, local, and tribal entities, especially those along a U.S. border, should work with DOS on these matters and more generally in pandemic preparedness planning, including engaging with foreign countries and the broader international community on measures to prevent and contain pandemic influenza. The interaction between U.S. States/Tribal Nations and their Canadian and Mexican counterparts, under DOS coordination, will be crucial during implementation of the North American Pandemic Influenza Plan under the Security and Prosperity Partnership.

The Private Sector and Critical Infrastructure Entities

The U.S. Government works with the private sector to leverage its presence and resources overseas to prepare for, detect, and respond to a pandemic.

Individuals and Families

Private Americans who are living or traveling abroad should make personal plans relating to their medical care, ability to address a "stay-in-place" response, and the possibility that international movement will be restricted for public health reasons.

International Partners

Three international organizations play key roles with respect to preparing for, detecting, and containing an outbreak of animal or pandemic influenza. The WHO Secretariat and its Regional Offices and the WHO Influenza Network help build international public health capacity, encourage and assist countries to develop and exercise pandemic preparedness plans, and set international public health standards. The WHO leadership coordinates the international response to an outbreak of pandemic influenza, including through its Global Outbreak Alert and Response Network (GOARN), consistent with the revised International Health Regulations (IHRs) as adopted by the World Health Assembly in May 2005 for entry into force in June 2007, which will govern the obligations of WHO member states to report public health emergencies of international concern to the WHO Secretariat and describe steps countries may take to limit international movement of travelers, conveyances, or cargo to prevent the spread of disease. The OIE and the FAO share the lead on animal health and work with the United States and other nations to detect, respond to, and contain outbreaks of influenza with pandemic potential in animals. The Senior UN System Coordinator for Avian and Human Influenza, appointed by the UN Secretary General in September 2005, will coordinate the efforts of WHO and the full range of UN organizations that may be tapped in the fight against pandemic influenza.

MDBs are preparing to provide loans and technical assistance to help borrowing member countries assess the potential economic impact of and develop action plans to respond to an influenza pandemic. The Asian Development Bank has approved a line of credit and approved grants to fight infectious diseases in Asia, including avian influenza, and has conducted initial economic analysis on the impact that a wider avian influenza outbreak could have on the regional economy. The World Bank has opened a line of credit to fight an influenza pandemic and is establishing a unit to track donor financial commitments and spending.

Actions and Expectations

4.1. Pillar One: Preparedness and Communication

Preparedness is key to an effective effort to contain an outbreak of influenza with pandemic potential at home or abroad. The United States will work to improve the international community's capacity and the commitment to take coordinated, effective action to contain an outbreak at its site of origin if possible and if not, to slow or limit its spread; to provide and coordinate assistance to nations that lack the capacity to detect independently and respond to an outbreak of animal or human influenza with pandemic potential; to develop and exercise pandemic response plans; to increase medical, veterinary, and scientific capacity and national and international supplies of countermeasures; and to communicate clearly and effectively with all stakeholders before and during a pandemic. These international activities will benefit or advance the health of the American people.

a. Planning for a Pandemic

4.1.1. Support the development and exercising of avian and pandemic response plans.

4.1.1.1. DOS, in coordination with HHS, USAID, DOD, and DOT, shall work with the Partnership, the Senior UN System Coordinator for Avian and Human Influenza, other international organizations (e.g., WHO, World Bank, OIE, FAO) and through bilateral and multilateral initiatives to encourage countries, particularly those at highest risk, to develop and exercise national and regional avian and pandemic response plans within 12 months. Measure of performance: 90 percent of high-risk countries have response plans and plans to test them.

4.1.1.2. USDA, USAID, and HHS shall use epidemiological data to expand support for animal disease and pandemic prevention and preparedness efforts, including provision of technical assistance to veterinarians and other agricultural scientists and policymakers, in high-risk countries within 12 months. Measure of performance: all high-risk and affected countries have in place (1) national task forces meeting regularly with representation from both human and animal health sectors, government ministries, businesses, and NGOs; (2) national plans, based on scientifically valid information, developed, tested, and implemented for containing influenza in animals with human pandemic potential and for responding to a human pandemic.

4.1.1.3. DOD, in coordination with DOS and other appropriate Federal agencies, host nations and regional alliance military partners, shall, within 18 months: (1) conduct bilateral and multilateral assessments of the avian and pandemic preparedness and response plans of the militaries in partner nations or regional alliances such as NATO focused on preparing for and mitigating the effects of an outbreak on assigned mission accomplishment; (2) develop solutions for identified national and regional military gaps; and (3) develop and execute bilateral and multilateral military-to-military influenza exercises to validate preparedness and response plans. Measure of performance: all countries with endemic avian influenza engaged by U.S. efforts; initial assessment and identification of exercise timeline for the military of each key partner nation completed.

4.1.2.   Expand in-country and abroad, medical, veterinary, and scientific capacity to respond to an outbreak.

4.1.2.1.   DOS shall ensure strong U.S. Government engagement in and follow-up on bilateral and multilateral initiatives to build cooperation and capacity to fight pandemic influenza internationally, including the Asia-Pacific Economic Cooperation (APEC) initiatives (inventory of resources and regional expertise to fight pandemic influenza, a region-wide tabletop exercise, a Symposium on Emerging Infectious Diseases to be held in Beijing in April 2006 and the Regional Emerging Disease Intervention (REDI) Center in Singapore), the U.S.-China Joint Initiative on Avian Influenza, and the U.S.-Indonesia-Singapore Joint Avian Influenza Demonstration Project; and shall develop a strategy to expand the number of countries fully cooperating with U.S. and/or international technical agencies in the fight against pandemic influenza, within 6 months. Measure of performance: finalized action plans that outline goals to be achieved and timeframes in which they will be achieved.

4.1.2.2.   HHS shall staff the REDI Center in Singapore within 3 months. Measure of performance: U.S. Government staff provided to REDI Center.

4.1.2.3.   USDA, working with USAID and the Partnership, shall support the FAO and OIE to implement an instrument to assess priority countries' veterinary infrastructure for prevention, surveillance, and control of animal influenza and increase veterinary rapid response capacity by supporting national capacities for animal surveillance, diagnostics, training, and containment in at-risk countries, within 9 months. Measure of performance: per the OIE's Performance, Vision and Strategy Instrument, assessment tools exercised and results communicated to the Partnership, and priority countries are developing, or have in place, an infrastructure capable of supporting their national prevention and response plans for avian or other animal influenza.

4.1.2.4.   USDA, in coordination with DOS, USAID, the OIE, and other members of the Partnership, shall support FAO to enhance the rapid detection and reporting of, response to, and control or eradication of outbreaks of avian influenza, within 12 months. Measure of performance: an international program is established and providing functional support to priority countries with rapid detection and reporting of, response to, and control or eradication of outbreaks of avian influenza, as appropriate to the country's specific situation.

4.1.2.5.   HHS, in coordination with USAID, shall increase rapid response capacity within those countries at highest risk of human exposure to animal influenza by supporting national and local government capacities for human surveillance, diagnostics, and medical care, and by supporting training and equipping of rapid response and case investigation teams for human outbreaks., within 9 months. Measure of performance: trained, deployable rapid response teams exist in countries with the highest risk of human exposure.

4.1.2.6.   DOD, in coordination with DOS, host nations, and regional alliance military partners, shall assist in developing priority country military infection control and case management capability through training programs, within 18 months. Measure of performance: training programs carried out in all priority countries with increased military infection control and case management capability.

4.1.2.7.   Treasury shall encourage and support MDB programs to improve health surveillance systems, strengthen priority countries' response to outbreaks, and boost health systems' readiness, consistent with legislative voting requirements, within 12 months. Measure of performance: projects that fit relevant MDB criteria approved in at least 50 percent of priority countries.

4.1.3.   Educate people in priority countries about high-risk practices that increase the likelihood of virus transmission from animals and between humans.

4.1.3.1.   USAID, HHS, and USDA shall conduct educational programs focused on communications and social marketing campaigns in local languages to increase public awareness of risks of transmission of influenza between animals and humans, within 12 months. Measure of performance: clear and consistent messages tested in affected countries, with information communicated via a variety of media have reached broad audiences, including health care providers, veterinarians, and animal health workers, primary and secondary level educators, villagers in high-risk and affected areas, poultry industry workers, and vendors in open air markets.

4.1.3.2.   HHS and USAID shall work with the WHO Secretariat and other multilateral organizations, existing bilateral programs and private sector partners to develop community- and hospital-based health prevention, promotion, and education activities in priority countries countries within 12 months. Measure of performance: 75 percent of priority countries are reached with mass media and community outreach programs that promote AI awareness and behavior change.

b. Communicating Expectations and Responsibilities

4.1.4.   Work to ensure clear, effective, and coordinated risk communication, domestically and internationally, before and during a pandemic. This includes identifying credible spokespersons at all levels of government to effectively coordinate and communicate helpful, informative, and consistent messages in a timely manner.

4.1.4.1.   DOS and HHS, in coordination with other agencies, shall ensure that the top political leadership of all affected countries understands the need for clear, effective coordinated public information strategies before and during an outbreak of avian or pandemic influenza within 12 months. Measure of performance: 50 percent of priority countries that developed outbreak communication strategies consistent with the WHO September 2004 Report detailing best practices for communicating with the public during an outbreak.

4.1.4.2.   DOS and HHS, in coordination with other agencies, shall implement programs within 3 months to inform U.S. citizens, including businesses, NGO personnel, DOD personnel, and military family members residing and traveling abroad, where they may obtain accurate, timely information, including risk level assessments, to enable them to make informed decisions and take appropriate personal measures. Measure of performance: majority of registered U.S. citizens abroad have access to accurate and current information on influenza.

4.1.4.3.   DOS and HHS shall ensure that adequate guidance is provided to Federal, State, tribal, and local authorities regarding the inviolability of diplomatic personnel and facilities and shall work with such authorities to develop methods of obtaining voluntary cooperation from the foreign diplomatic community within the United States consistent with U.S. Government treaty obligations within 6 months. Measure of performance: briefing materials and an action plan in place for engaging with relevant Federal, State, tribal, and local authorities.

4.1.4.4.   USAID, USDA, and HHS shall work with the WHO Secretariat, FAO, OIE, and other donor countries within 12 months to implement a communications program to support government authorities and private and multilateral organizations in at-risk countries in improving their national communications systems with the goal of promoting behaviors that will minimize human exposure and prevent further spread of influenza in animal populations. Measure of performance: 50 percent of priority countries have improved national avian influenza communications.

4.1.4.5.   USAID, in coordination with DOS, HHS, and USDA, shall develop and disseminate influenza information to priority countries through international broadcasting channels, including international U.S. Government mechanisms such as Voice of America and Radio Free Asia (radio, television, shortwave, Internet), and share lessons learned and key messages from communications campaigns, within 12 months. Measure of performance: local language briefing materials and training programs developed and distributed via WHO and FAO channels.

c. Producing and Stockpiling Vaccines, Antiviral Medications, and Medical Material

4.1.5.   Encourage nations to develop production capacity and stockpiles to support their response needs, to include pooling of efforts to create regional capacity.

4.1.5.1.   DOS, in coordination with other agencies, shall use the Partnership and bilateral and multilateral diplomatic contacts on a continuing basis to encourage nations to increase international production capacity and stockpiles of safe and effective human vaccines, antiviral medications, and medical material within 12 months. Measure of performance: increase by 50 percent the number of priority countries that have plans to increase production capacity and/or stockpiles.

4.1.5.2.   HHS and USAID shall work to coordinate and set up emergency stockpiles of protective equipment and essential commodities other than vaccine and antiviral medications for responding to animal or human outbreaks within 9 months. Measure of performance: essential commodities procured and available for deployment within 24 hours.

4.1.5.3.   HHS shall provide technical expertise, information, and guidelines for stock-piling and use of pandemic influenza vaccines within 6 months. Measure of performance: all priority countries and partner organizations have received relevant information on influenza vaccines and application strategies.

4.1.5.4.   USDA and USAID, in cooperation with FAO and OIE, shall provide technical expertise, information and guidelines for stockpiling and use of animal vaccines, especially to avian influenza affected countries and those countries at highest risk, within 6 months. Measure of performance: all priority countries and relevant international organizations have received information on animal vaccines' efficacy and application strategies to guide country-specific decisions about preparedness options

4.1.6.   Facilitate appropriate coordination of efforts across the vaccine manufacturing sector.

4.1.6.1.   DOS, in coordination with HHS and other agencies, shall continue to work through the Partnership and other bilateral and multilateral venues to build international cooperation and encourage countries and regional organizations to develop diagnostic, research and vaccine manufacturing capacity within 24 months. Measure of performance: global diagnostic and research capacity increased significantly compared to 24 months earlier; significant investments made to expand international vaccine manufacturing capacity.

4.1.6.2.   HHS, in coordination with the WHO Secretariat, shall establish at least six new sites for Collaborative Clinical Research on Emerging Infectious Diseases to conduct collaborative clinical research on the diagnostics, therapeutics, and natural history of avian influenza and other human emerging infectious diseases. In addition, within 18 months it will provide in-country support for one or more partner countries for human avian influenza clinical trials. Measure of performance: cooperative programs established in six new sites, to include the initiation of research protocols and design of clinical trials.

4.1.6.3.   USDA shall generate new information on avian vaccine efficacy and production technologies and disseminate to international organizations, animal vaccine manufacturers, and countries at highest risk within 6 months. Measure of performance: information disseminated to priority entities.

d. Establishing Distribution Plans for Vaccines and Antiviral Medications

4.1.7.   Develop credible countermeasure distribution mechanisms for vaccine and antiviral agents prior to and during a pandemic.

4.1.7.1.   DOS shall work with HHS and USAID, in collaboration with the WHO Secretariat, to coordinate the U.S. Government contribution to an international stockpile of antiviral medications and other medical countermeasures, including international countermeasure distribution plans and mechanisms and agreed prioritization of allocation, within 6 months. Measure of performance: release of proposed doctrine of deployment and concept of operations for an international stockpile.

4.1.7.2.   The Department of Justice (DOJ) and DOS, in coordination with HHS, shall consider whether the U.S. Government, in order to benefit from the protections of the Defense Appropriations Act, should seek to negotiate liability-limiting treaties or arrangements covering U.S. contributions to an international stock-pile of vaccine and other medical countermeasures, within 6 months. Measure of performance: review initiated and decision rendered.

4.1.7.3.   USDA, in collaboration with FAO and OIE, shall develop and provide best-prac-tice guidelines and technical expertise to countries that express interest in obtaining aid in the implementation of a national animal vaccination program, within 4 months. Measure of performance: interested countries receive guide-lines and other assistance within 3 months of their request.

e. Advancing Scientific Knowledge and Accelerating Development

4.1.8.   Ensure that there is maximal sharing of scientific information about influenza viruses between governments, scientific entities, and the private sector.

4.1.8.1.   HHS shall support the Los Alamos H5 Sequence Database and the Institute for Genomic Research (TIGR), for the purpose of sharing avian H5N1 influenza sequences with the scientific community within 24 months. Measure of performance: completed H5 sequences entered into both the Los Alamos data-base and GenBank and annotated.

4.1.8.2.   HHS shall enhance a regional influenza genome reference laboratory in Singapore within 9 months. Measure of performance: capacity to sequence complete influenza virus genome established in Singapore; all reported novel animal influenza samples sequenced and made available on public databases.

4.1.8.3.   USDA and USAID shall work with international organizations, governments, and scientific entities to disseminate and exchange information to bolster and apply avian influenza prevention and response plans in priority countries, within 12 months. Measure of performance: 50 percent of priority countries have national epizootic prevention and response plans based upon pragmatic, comprehensive, and scientifically valid information.

4.1.8.4.   HHS and DOD, in coordination with DOS, shall enhance open source informa-tion sharing efforts with international organizations and agencies to facilitate the characterization of genetic sequences of circulating strains of novel influenza viruses within 12 months. Measure of performance: publication of all reported novel influenza viruses which are sequenced.

4.2. Pillar Two: Surveillance and Detection

To increase the probability of containing a virus with pandemic potential that originates outside the United States or delaying its spread as long as possible as we activate protective measures at home, we will need early recognition of the problem. We will work to ensure effective surveil-lance, rapid detection, and transparent reporting of outbreaks internationally by strengthening scientific and epidemiological expertise abroad; enhancing laboratory capacity and diagnostic capabilities; and establishing international mechanisms and commitment to ensure transparent and rapid reporting. We will develop, enhance, and encourage early implementation of international screening and monitoring mechanisms to limit the spread of viruses with pandemic potential.

a. Ensuring Rapid Reporting of Outbreaks

4.2.1. **Work through the International Partnership on Avian and Pandemic Influenza, as well as through other political and diplomatic channels such as the United Nations and the Asia-Pacific Economic Cooperation forum, to ensure transparency, scientific cooperation, and rapid reporting of avian and human influenza cases.**

4.2.1.1. DOS, in coordination with other agencies, shall work on a continuing basis through the Partnership and through bilateral and multilateral diplomatic contacts to promote transparency, scientific cooperation, and rapid reporting of avian and human influenza cases by other nations within 12 months. Measure of performance: all high-risk countries actively cooperating in improving capacity for transparent, rapid reporting of outbreaks.

4.2.1.2. HHS, in coordination with DOS, shall pursue bilateral agreements with key affected countries on health cooperation including transparency, sample and data sharing, and development of rapid response protocols; and develop and train in-country rapid response teams to quickly assess and report on possible outbreaks of avian and human influenza, within 12 months. Measure of performance: agreements established with Vietnam, Cambodia, and Laos, 100 teams throughout Asia, including China, Thailand, and Indonesia, trained and available to respond to outbreaks.

4.2.1.3. HHS shall place long-term staff at key WHO offices and in select affected and high-risk countries to provide coordination of HHS-sponsored activities and to serve as liaisons with HHS within 9 months. Measure of performance: placement of staff and increased coordination with the WHO Secretariat and Regional Offices.

4.2.1.4. HHS shall, to the extent feasible, negotiate agreements with established networks of laboratories around the world to enhance its ability to perform laboratory analysis of human and animal virus isolates and to train in-country government staff on influenza-related surveillance and laboratory diagnostics, within 6 months. Measure of performance: completed, negotiated agreement, and financing mechanism with at least one laboratory network outside the United States.

4.2.1.5. HHS shall support the WHO Secretariat to enhance the early detection, identification and reporting of infectious disease outbreaks through the WHO's Influenza Network and Global Outbreak and Alert Response Network (GOARN) within 12 months. Measure of performance: expansion of the network to regions not currently part of the network.

4.2.1.6.   USAID, in coordination with USDA, shall initiate a pilot program to evaluate strategies for farmer compensation and shall engage and leverage the private sector and other donors to increase the availability of key commodities, compensation, financing and technical support for the control of avian influenza, within 6 months. Measure of performance: a model compensation program measured in value of goods and services available for compensation is developed.

4.2.1.7.   USAID, HHS, USDA, and DOS shall support NGOs, FAO, OIE, WHO, the Office of the Senior UN System Coordinator for Avian and Human Influenza, and host governments to expand the scope, accuracy, and transparency of human and animal surveillance systems and to streamline and strengthen official protocols for reporting avian influenza cases, within 6 months. Measure of performance: 75 percent of priority countries have established early warning networks, international case definitions, and standards for laboratory diagnostics of human and animal samples.

4.2.2.   Support the development of the proper scientific and epidemiologic expertise in affected regions to ensure early recognition of changes in the pattern of avian or human outbreaks.

4.2.2.1.   HHS and USDA, in collaboration with one or more established networks of laboratories around the world, including the WHO Influenza Network, shall train staff from priority countries' Ministries of Health and Agriculture, to conduct surveillance and perform epidemiologic analyses on influenza-susceptible species and manage and report results of findings, within 12 months. Measure of performance: 75 percent of priority countries have access to multi-year epidemiology and surveillance training programs.

4.2.2.2.   HHS and USDA shall increase support of scientists tracking potential emergent influenza strains through disease and virologic surveillance in susceptible animal species in priority countries within 9 months. Measure of performance: surveillance for emergent influenza strains expanded in priority countries.

4.2.2.3.   HHS, in coordination with DOD, shall provide support to Naval Medical Research Unit (NAMRU) 2 in Jakarta, Indonesia and Phnom Penh, Cambodia, the Armed Forces Research Institute of Medical Sciences in Bangkok, Thailand, and NAMRU-3 in Cairo, Egypt to expand and expedite geographic surveillance of human populations at-risk for H5N1 infections in those and neighboring countries through training, enhanced surveillance, and enhancement of the Early Warning Outbreak Recognition System, within 12 months. Measure of performance: reagents and technical assistance provided to countries in the network to improve and expand surveillance of H5N1 and number of specimens tested by real-time processing.

4.2.2.4.   HHS shall enhance surveillance and response to high priority infectious disease, including influenza with pandemic potential, by training physicians and public health workers in disease surveillance, applied epidemiology and outbreak response at its GDD Response Centers in Thailand and China and at the U.S.-China Collaborative Program on Emerging and Re-Emerging Infectious

Diseases, within 12 months. Measure of performance: 50 physicians and public health workers living in priority countries receive training in disease surveillance applied epidemiology and outbreak response.

4.2.2.5.   DOD shall develop active and passive systems for inpatient and outpatient disease surveillance at its institutions worldwide, with an emphasis on index case and cluster identification, and develop mechanisms for utilizing DOD epidemiological investigation experts in international support efforts, to include validation of systems/tools and improved outpatient/inpatient surveillance capabilities, within 18 months. Measure of performance: monitoring system and program to utilize epidemiological investigation experts internationally are in place.

4.2.2.6.   DOD shall monitor the health of military forces worldwide (CONUS and OCONUS bases, deployed operational forces, exercises, units, etc.), and in coordination with DOS, coordinate with allied, coalition, and host nation public health communities to investigate and respond to confirmed infectious disease outbreaks on DOD installations, within 18 months. Measure of performance: medical surveillance "watchboard" reports show results of routine monitoring, number of validated outbreaks, and results of interventions.

4.2.2.7.   DOD, in coordination with DOS and with the cooperation of the host nation, shall assist with influenza surveillance of host nation populations in accordance with existing treaties and international agreements, within 24 months. Measure of performance: medical surveillance "watchboard" expanded to include host nations.

4.2.3.   Support the development and sustainment of sufficient U.S. and host nation laboratory capacity and diagnostic reagents in affected regions and domestically, to provide rapid confirmation of cases in animals or humans.

4.2.3.1.   HHS shall develop and implement laboratory diagnostics training programs in basic laboratory techniques related to influenza sample preparation and diagnostics in priority countries within 9 months. Measure of performance: 25 laboratory scientists trained in influenza sample preparation and diagnostics.

4.2.3.2.   HHS in collaboration with one or more established networks of laboratories, including the WHO Influenza Network, shall train staff from priority countries on influenza-related laboratory diagnostics, within 12 months. Measure of performance: 100 percent of priority countries have training programs established.

4.2.3.3.   HHS, in cooperation with the WHO Secretariat and other donor countries, shall expand an existing specimen transport fund that enables developing countries to transport influenza samples to WHO regional reference laboratories and collaborating centers, within 6 months. Measure of performance: 100 percent of priority countries funded for sending influenza samples to WHO regional reference laboratories.

4.2.3.4.   HHS shall invest in the development and evaluation of more accurate rapid diagnostics for influenza to enhance the ability of the global healthcare community to rapidly diagnose influenza, within 18 months. Measure of performance: new grants and contracts issued to researchers to develop and evaluate new diagnostics.

4.2.3.5.   HHS and USAID shall work with the WHO Secretariat and private sector partners, through existing bilateral agreements, to provide support for human health diagnostic laboratories by developing and giving assistance in implementing rapid international laboratory diagnostics protocols and standards in priority countries, within 12 months. Measure of performance: 75 percent of priority countries have improved human diagnostic laboratory capacity.

4.2.3.6.   USDA and USAID shall work with FAO and OIE to provide technical support for animal health diagnostic laboratories by developing and implementing international laboratory diagnostic protocols, standards, and infrastructure in priority countries that can rapidly screen avian influenza specimens from susceptible animal populations, within 12 months. Measure of performance: 75 percent of priority countries have improved animal diagnostic laboratory capacity.

4.2.3.7.   USDA and USAID shall provide technical expertise to help priority countries develop their cadre of veterinary diagnostic technicians to screen avian influenza specimens from wild and domestic bird populations, and other susceptible animals, rapidly and in a manner that adheres to international standards for proficiency and safety, within 12 months. Measure of performance: all priority countries have access to laboratories that are able to screen avian influenza specimens and confirm diagnoses in a manner that supports effective control of cases of avian influenza.

4.2.3.8.   DOD, in coordination with HHS, shall develop and refine its overseas virologic and bacteriologic surveillance infrastructure through Global Emerging Infections Surveillance and Response System (GEIS) and the DOD network of overseas labs, including fully developing and implementing seasonal influenza laboratory surveillance and an animal/vector surveillance plan linked with WHO pandemic phases, within 18 months. Measure of performance: animal/vector surveillance plan and DOD overseas virologic surveillance network developed and functional.

4.2.3.9.   DOD, in coordination with HHS, shall prioritize international DOD laboratory research efforts to develop, refine, and validate diagnostic methods to rapidly identify pathogens, within 18 months. Measure of performance: completion of prioritized research plan, resources identified, and tasks assigned across DOD medical research facilities.

4.2.3.10.   DOD shall work with priority nations' military forces to assess existing laboratory capacity, rapid response teams, and portable field assay testing equipment, and fund essential commodities and training necessary to achieve an effective national military diagnostic capability, within 18 months. Measure of performance: assessments completed, proposals accepted, and funding made available to priority countries.

b. Using Surveillance to Limit Spread

4.2.4. Develop mechanisms to rapidly share information on travelers who may be carrying or may have been exposed to a pandemic strain of influenza, for the purposes of contact tracing and outbreak investigation.

4.2.4.1. HHS and USAID shall, in coordination with regional and international multi-lateral organizations, develop village-based alert and response surveillance systems for human cases of influenza in priority countries, within 18 months. Measure of performance: 75 percent of all priority countries have established a village alert and response system for human influenza.

4.2.4.2. DOD shall incorporate international public health reporting requirements for exposed or ill military international travelers into the Geographic Combatant Commanders' pandemic influenza plans within 18 months. Measure of performance: reporting requirements incorporated into Geographic Combatant Commanders' pandemic influenza plans.

4.2.5. Develop and exercise mechanisms to provide active and passive surveillance during an outbreak, both within and beyond our borders.

4.2.5.1. HHS and USAID shall develop, in coordination with the WHO Secretariat and other donor countries, rapid response protocols for use in responding quickly to credible reports of human-to-human transmission that may indicate the beginnings of an influenza pandemic, within 12 months. Measure of performance: adoption of protocols by WHO and other stakeholders.

4.2.5.2. HHS, in coordination with DOS and other agencies participating in the Security and Prosperity Partnership, shall pursue cooperative agreements on pandemic influenza with Canada and Mexico to create and implement a North American early warning surveillance and response system in order to prevent the spread of infectious disease across the borders, within 9 months. Measure of performance: implementation of early warning surveillance and response system.

4.2.5.3. USDA and USAID shall provide technical expertise to priority countries in order to expand the scope and accuracy of systematic surveillance of avian influenza cases, within 12 months. Measure of performance: 75 percent of priority countries have expanded animal surveillance capabilities.

4.2.6. Expand and enhance mechanisms for screening and monitoring animals that may harbor viruses with pandemic potential.

4.2.6.1. DHS, USDA, DOI, and USAID, in collaboration with priority countries, NGOs, WHO, FAO, OIE, and the private sector shall support priority country animal health activities, including development of regulations and enforcement capacities that conform to OIE standards for transboundary movement of animals, development of effective biosecurity measures for commercial and domestic animal operations and markets, and identification and confirmation of infected animals, within 12 months. Measure of performance: 50 percent of priority countries have implemented animal health activities as defined above.

4.2.7.   Develop screening and monitoring mechanisms and agreements to appropriately control the movement and shipping of potentially contaminated products to and from affected regions if necessary, and to protect unaffected populations.

4.2.7.1.   DOS, in coordination with DOT, DHS, HHS, and U.S. Trade Representative (USTR), shall collaborate with WHO, the International Civil Aviation Organization (ICAO), and the International Maritime Organization (IMO) to assess and revise, as necessary and feasible, existing international agreements and regulations governing the movement and shipping of potentially infectious products, in order to ensure that international agreements are both adequate and legally sufficient to prevent the spread of infectious disease, within 12 months. Measure of performance: international regulations reviewed and revised.

4.2.7.2.   USDA shall provide technical assistance to priority countries to increase safety of animal products by identifying potentially contaminated animal products, developing screening protocols, regulations, and enforcement capacities that conform to OIE avian influenza standards for transboundary movement of animal products, within 36 months. Measure of performance: all priority countries have protocols and regulations in place or in process.

4.2.8.   Share guidance with international partners on best practices to prevent the spread of influenza, including within hospitals and clinical settings.

4.2.8.1.   HHS and USAID shall develop community- and hospital-based infection control and prevention, health promotion, and education activities in local languages in priority countries within 9 months. Measure of performance: local language health promotion campaigns and improved hospital-based infection control activities established in all Southeast Asian priority countries.

4.3. Pillar Three: Response and Containment

The United States is working now with other nations and relevant international organizations to detect and contain outbreaks of animal influenza with pandemic potential with the aim of preventing its spread to humans. We will work to ensure nations and relevant international organizations agree as soon as possible on a doctrine of international response and containment to implement in the event of a human outbreak. Once health authorities signal sustained, efficient human transmission of a virus with pandemic potential overseas, we will encourage rigorous implementation of the agreed doctrine for international containment and response and offer technical expertise and assistance as needed. Critical to this effort will be the timely implementation of a coordinated and accurate international public awareness campaign to define the facts and establish realistic expectations. We will monitor economic and social effects of a pandemic and employ appropriate measures to limit their impact on global stability and security.

a. Containing Outbreaks

4.3.1. **Work to develop a coalition of strong partners to coordinate actions to limit the spread of a virus with pandemic potential beyond the location where it is first recognized abroad in order to protect U.S. interests.**

4.3.1.1. DOS, in coordination with HHS, USDA, USAID, and DOD, shall coordinate the development and implementation of U.S. capability to respond rapidly to assess and contain outbreaks of avian influenza with pandemic potential abroad, including coordination of the development, training and exercise of U.S. rapid response teams; and coordination of U.S. support for development, training and exercise of, and U.S. participation in, international support teams. Measure of performance: agreed operating procedures and operational support for U.S. rapid response, and for U.S. participation in international rapid response efforts, are developed and function effectively.

4.3.1.2. DOS, in coordination with HHS, shall work with WHO and the international community to secure agreement (e.g., through a resolution at the World Health Assembly in May 2006) on an international containment strategy to be activated in the event of a human outbreak, including an accepted definition of a "triggering event" and an agreed doctrine for coordinated international action, responsibilities of nations, and steps they will take, within 4 months. Measure of performance: international agreement on a response and containment strategy.

4.3.1.3. HHS, in coordination with DOS, and the WHO Secretariat, and USDA, USAID, DOD, as appropriate, shall rapidly deploy disease surveillance and control teams to investigate possible human outbreaks through WHO's GOARN network, as required. Measure of performance: teams deployed to suspected outbreaks within 48 hours of investigation request.

4.3.1.4. DOS, in coordination with HHS, and the WHO Secretariat, and USDA, USAID, DOD, as appropriate, shall coordinate United States participation in the implementation of the international response and containment strategy (e.g., assigning experts to the WHO outbreak teams and providing assistance and advice to ministries of health on local public health interventions, ongoing disease surveillance, and use of antiviral medications and vaccines if they are available). Measure of performance: teams deployed to suspected outbreaks within 48 hours of investigation request.

4.3.1.5. USDA and USAID, in coordination with DOS, HHS, and DOD, and in collaboration with relevant international organizations, shall support operational deployment of rapid response teams and provide technical expertise and technology to support avian influenza assessment and response teams in priority countries as required. Measure of performance: all priority countries have rapid access to avian influenza assessment and response teams; deployment assistance provided in each instance and documented in a log of technical assistance rendered.

4.3.1.6. DOS shall lead U.S. Government engagement with the international community's effort to develop a coordinated plan for avian influenza assistance (funds, materiel, and personnel) to streamline national assistance efforts within 12 months. Measure of performance: commitments from countries on funds, personnel, and materiel they will contribute to an integrated and prioritized international prevention, preparedness, and response effort.

4.3.1.7. DOS, in coordination with and drawing on the expertise of USAID, HHS, and DOD, shall work with the international community to develop, within 12 months, a coordinated, integrated, and prioritized distribution plan for pandemic influenza assistance that details a strategy for (1) strategic lift of WHO stockpiles and response teams; (2) theater distribution to high-risk countries; (3) in-country coordination to key distribution areas; and (4) establishment of internal mechanisms within each country for distribution to urban, rural, and remote populations. Measure of performance: commitments by countries that specify their ability to support distribution, and specify the personnel and material for such support.

4.3.1.8. DOS, in coordination with HHS, USDA, USAID, and DHS, and in collaboration with WHO, FAO, OIE, the World Bank and regional institutions such as APEC, the Association of Southeast Asian Nations and the European Community, shall work to improve public affairs coordination and establish a set of agreed upon operating principles among these international organizations and the United States that describe the actions and expectations of the public affairs strategies of these entities that would be implemented in the event of a pandemic, within 6 months. Measure of performance: list of key public affairs contacts developed, planning documents shared, and coordinated public affairs strategy developed.

4.3.1.9. DOS and DOC, in collaboration with NGOs and private sector groups representing business with activities abroad, shall develop and disseminate checklists of key activities to prepare for and respond to a pandemic, within 6 months. Measure of performance: checklists developed and disseminated.

4.3.2. Where appropriate, use governmental authorities to limit movement of people, goods, and services into and out of areas where an outbreak occurs.

4.3.2.1. DOS, in coordination with DHS, HHS, DOD, and DOT, and in collaboration with foreign counterparts, shall support the implementation of pre-existing passenger screening protocols in the event of an outbreak of pandemic influenza. Measure of performance: protocols implemented within 48 hours of notification of an outbreak of pandemic influenza.

4.3.2.2. DOD, in coordination with DOS, HHS, DOT, and DHS, shall limit official DOD military travel between affected areas and the United States. Measure of performance: DOD identifies military facilities in the United States and OCONUS that will serve as the points of entry for all official travelers from affected areas, within 6 months.

b. Leveraging International Medical and Health Surge Capacity

4.3.3. **Activate plans to distribute medical countermeasures, including non-medical equipment and other material, internationally.**

4.3.3.1. DOS, in coordination with HHS, USAID, USDA, and DOD, shall work with the Partnership to assist in the prompt and effective delivery of countermeasures to affected countries consistent with U.S. law and regulation and the agreed upon doctrine for international action to respond to and contain an outbreak of influenza with pandemic potential. Measure of performance: necessary countermeasures delivered to an affected area within 48 hours of agreement to meet request.

4.3.4. **Address barriers to the flow of public health, medical, and veterinary personnel across international borders to meet local shortfalls in public health, medical, and veterinary capacity.**

4.3.4.1. DOS in collaboration with the Partnership and WHO shall negotiate international instruments and/or arrangements to facilitate the flow of rapid response teams and other public health, medical, and veterinary personnel across international borders, within 12 months. Measure of performance: negotiated agreements for facilitating deployment of rapid response teams deployed across international borders using instruments and/or arrangements as detailed above, within 48 hours of request.

4.3.4.2. DHS shall assist in the expeditious movement of public health, medical, and veterinary officials, equipment, supplies, and biological samples for testing through U.S. ports of entry/departure. Measure of performance: delivery of persons, equipment, and samples involved in the detection of and response to outbreaks of avian or pandemic influenza within 48 hours of decision to deploy.

c. Sustaining Infrastructure, Essential Services, and the Economy

4.3.5. **Analyze the potential economic and social impact of a pandemic on the stability and security of the international community and identify means to address it.**

4.3.5.1. DOS shall organize an interagency group to analyze the potential economic and social impact of a pandemic on the stability and security of the international community, within 3 months. Measure of performance: issues identified and policy recommendations prepared.

4.3.5.2. Treasury shall urge the IMF to enhance its surveillance of priority countries and regions, including further assessment of the macroeconomic and financial vulnerability to an influenza pandemic, within 3 months. Measure of performance: updated, expanded IMF analysis of the potential impact of an influenza pandemic on priority countries and regions, as defined above.

4.3.5.3. Treasury, in collaboration with the IMF and the multilateral development banks, shall take the lead on dialogue with creditor countries to ensure that financial assistance to affected economies is provided on terms consistent with the goals of restoring economic activity and maximizing economic growth (within existing international financial agreements), within 6 months. Measure of performance: official financing strategies in place that are consistent with the goals above.

d. Ensuring Effective Risk Communication

4.3.6. **Ensure that timely, clear, coordinated messages are delivered to the American public from trained spokespersons at all levels of government and assist the governments of affected nations to do the same.**

4.3.6.1.   DOS, in coordination with HHS, USAID, USDA, DOD, and DHS, shall lead an interagency public diplomacy group to develop a coordinated, integrated, and prioritized plan to communicate U.S. foreign policy objectives relating to our international engagement on avian and pandemic influenza to key stakeholders (e.g., the American people, the foreign public, NGOs, international businesses), within 3 months. Measure of performance: number and range of target audiences reached with core public affairs and public diplomacy messages, and impact of these messages on public responses to avian and pandemic influenza.

4.3.6.2.   DOS, in coordination with HHS, shall provide at least monthly updates to its foreign counterparts, through diplomatic channels and U.S. Government websites, regarding changes to national policy or regulations that may result from an outbreak, and shall coordinate posting of such information to U.S. Government websites (e.g., **www.pandemicflu.gov**). Measure of performance: foreign governments and key stakeholders receive authoritative and regular information on U.S. Government avian influenza policy.

4.3.6.3.   USDA, in coordination with DHS, USTR, and DOS, shall ensure that clear and coordinated messages are provided to international trading partners regarding animal disease outbreak response activities in the United States. Measure of performance: within 24 hours of an outbreak, appropriate messages will be shared with key animal/animal product trading partners.

CHAPTER 5 — TRANSPORTATION AND BORDERS

Introduction

Our Nation's 317 official ports of entry and vast transportation network are critical elements in our preparation for and response to a potential influenza pandemic. Our border measures might provide an opportunity to slow the spread of a pandemic to the United States, but are unlikely to prevent it. The sheer volume of traffic and the difficulty of developing screening protocols to detect an influenza-like illness pose significant challenges. On a typical day, about 1.1 million passengers and pedestrians cross our borders, as do approximately 64,000 truck, rail, and sea containers, 2,600 aircraft, and 365,000 vehicles.

Our transportation system regularly delivers essential commodities to communities, and — in emergencies — rapidly moves critical supplies, emergency workers, and needed resources into affected areas. This vast and complex system moves billions of people and trillions of dollars worth of goods each year. Each of the six major transportation modes (i.e., aviation, rail, highway, maritime, pipeline, and mass transit) has unique characteristics, operating models, responsibilities, and stakeholders. As a decentralized network, the transportation sector is predominantly owned and operated by State and local governments and the private sector. Decisions made by State and local entities and the private sector can have cascading impacts across the transportation sector. Effective transportation management during a pandemic will require planning and close coordination across the sector — at the national, State, and local levels — and with those who depend on it.

Our ability to help maintain infrastructure services, mitigate adverse economic impacts, and sustain societal needs will hinge in part on our ability to make effective international and domestic transportation decisions. While the overall pandemic response will be driven by disease characteristics and the status of domestic preparation, transportation and border decisions should also be based on the effectiveness of an action in slowing the spread of a pandemic and related health benefits; its social and economic consequences; its international implications; and its operational feasibility.

Key Considerations

Goals of Transportation and Border Measures

The *National Strategy for Pandemic Influenza (Strategy)* guides our preparedness and response to an influenza pandemic, with the intent of (1) stopping, slowing, or otherwise limiting the spread of a pandemic to the United States, (2) limiting the domestic spread of a pandemic and mitigating disease, suffering, and death, and (3) sustaining infrastructure and mitigating impact to the economy and the functioning of society. Transportation and border measures, when combined with other social distancing and public health measures, can help support these goals.

The containment of an influenza virus with pandemic potential at its origin — whether the outbreak occurs abroad or within the United States — is a critical element of pandemic response efforts. Containment is most effective when approached globally, with all countries striving to achieve common goals. Even if such efforts prove unsuccessful, delaying the spread of disease could provide the Federal Government with valuable time to activate the domestic response. The Secretariat of the World Health

Organization (WHO) has established guidelines to support the control of spread of a pandemic virus across and within borders.[3] These guidelines provide a useful starting point for the development of U.S. Government national policy and could be modified and extended where necessary. The specifics of how a novel influenza virus will enter the United States and how the epidemic will actually unfold are unknown, and therefore, implementation of U.S. Government response must remain flexible and adaptable to a pandemic as it unfolds. To the extent possible and in accordance with treaties or other binding agreements, the United States will seek to coordinate containment measures with global organizations and partners.

Building on the International Efforts set forth in Chapter 4, this chapter identifies actions to address a number of key policy issues, including developing a cohesive, integrated U.S. border entry and exit strategy for aviation, maritime, and land border ports of entry, and a strategy to guide domestic efforts to delay the spread of disease. Within this policy framework, the Federal Government will develop a toolkit of options that can be used by individuals, within communities and States, and across the Nation. This toolkit will require significant, collaborative planning with States, communities, and the private sector to develop a range of scalable options, the protocols to implement them, and the trigger points that define thresholds to implement and remove measures. It will be critical to quantify, to the extent possible, the costs and benefits of these options, as many of the options will have significant second- and third-order effects.

Deciding which measures to use at which points in the lifecycle of a pandemic will require complex decisions that carefully weigh costs and benefits to evaluate which options best serve the public. Key factors that affect decision making include the ability to delay the pandemic and the resulting health benefits, the associated social and economic consequences, and the operational feasibility to implement transportation or border measures.

Ability to Delay a Pandemic and Resulting Health Benefits

There are many public health interventions and social distancing measures that can help limit international spread, reduce spread within nations and local populations, and reduce an individual's risk for infection.[4] Transportation and border measures are two of many social distancing measures that can reduce transmission by limiting the proximity of individuals and reducing interaction within and across social networks. Modeling indicates that these measures are most effective when used in combination with other social distancing and public health measures, such as school closures, canceling large public gatherings, and limiting work group interaction.

Research is underway to better understand the effects of movement restrictions and their interactions with other social distancing measures in delaying a pandemic. Current models suggest that highly restrictive border measures could delay a pandemic by a few weeks. However, given the economic and societal impacts of these measures, recent recommendations from WHO encourage countries to focus their efforts to contain spread of a pandemic at national and community levels rather than at international borders. Based on a review of prior pandemics, including quarantines enacted during the 1918 pandemic as well as the 2003 SARS and influenza outbreak, WHO recommendations for border-related measures focus on providing information to international travelers, screening travelers departing countries with transmissible human infection, and limiting travel to affected areas. The

---

[3] World Health Organization. WHO global influenza preparedness plan: the role of WHO and recommendations for national measures before and during pandemics. November 2005.

[4] World Health Organization. Non-pharmaceutical interventions for pandemic influenza, international measures. 2006. Emerging Infection Diseases, Vol. 12, No. 1, Jan 2006.

recommendations for national and community measures during a pandemic focus on delaying spread and reducing effects through population–based measures.[5] If the pandemic becomes severe, WHO recommends countries encourage social distancing measures and defer non-essential domestic travel to affected areas. As part of our pandemic planning efforts, guidance and protocols for border and domestic transportation measures will be developed that can be tailored, in the event of a pandemic, based on our level of domestic preparedness and real-time epidemiological disease characteristics, including transmission pattern, pandemic stage, and illness severity and extent.

Depending on the length, delay can provide valuable time to implement pandemic preparedness measures that have been planned in advance.[6] A delay in spread may also allow the administration of pre-pandemic vaccine, assessment of disease epidemiology, and mobilization of resources for screening and diagnosis. It should be noted that current estimates are that it will take approximately 5 months to develop, produce, and distribute a pandemic vaccine after the declaration of a pandemic and isolation of the pandemic virus. While delay may reduce peak overall demand on the health care system, this will not necessarily translate to benefits at the community level. It is unlikely that communities will be able to shift scarce resources that will be needed locally once the pandemic reaches their area. Unlike a hurricane or other localized disaster, national capacity will not be easily distributed across communities and States. Scarce resources, such as personnel and ventilators, will be needed to meet local demand, and it is unlikely that transporting large numbers of infected patients out of medically overwhelmed areas would be a viable option (see Chapter 6 - Protecting Human Health).

Further work will be done to better understand the potential delay that can be obtained through transportation and border measures, how these measures work in concert with other public health and social distancing measures, and the resulting health benefits.

Social and Economic Consequences

The transportation system and the choices it offers support the social, economic, and business needs of communities. Travel is a critical part of our daily routine, with Americans taking an average of 1.1 billion trips per day, or about four trips for every person in the United States each day.[7] A pandemic will require curtailment in travel and dramatically change our travel priorities, choices, and decisions, resulting in significant social and economic consequences.

By carefully examining the public's reliance on travel, existing travel patterns, and anticipated changes in travel during a pandemic, communities and States can develop a range of travel options that help delay spread of the pandemic, but also minimize social and economic consequences. For example, travel options can range from provision of travel information, voluntary advisories with health warnings, selective restrictions that limit certain types of travel, advance notification followed by a defined period of restriction, and mandatory measures under extreme circumstances.

At the onset of a pandemic, the public will almost certainly automatically limit vacation travel, and this would be recommended by public health authorities. It is anticipated that significant portions of business travel would be curtailed as well, with only essential travel continuing (related to overall pandemic response, sustaining critical infrastructure, and sustaining essential business functions). The purpose of

---

[5] World Health Organization. Non-pharmaceutical interventions for pandemic influenza, national and community measures. 2006. Emerging Infection Diseases, Vol. 12, No. 1, Jan 2006.

[6] World Health Organization. WHO global influenza preparedness plan: the role of WHO and recommendations for national measures before and during pandemics. November 2005.

[7] U.S. Department of Transportation, Bureau of Transportation Statistics, Federal Highway Administration, National Household Travel Survey data, CD-ROM, February 2004.

long-distance travel will also change. Initially, there may be a small surge in trips as people who are out of town return home. During an evolving pandemic it would not be surprising to expect family members to attempt to return home, as well as travel to assist other family members in need, such as elderly parents, ill family members, or others requiring special assistance.

In addition, it is presumed that the public will change daily travel patterns based on what they perceive will reduce their personal risk and the risk to their families and friends. Communities might see a surge in local travel as people gather groceries and other items similar to patterns before large snow storms where the public expects limitations in local travel for short durations. The planned length of travel curtailment is a significant factor that will help families and communities prepare for potential restrictions.

Clear messages regarding travel, risk of transmission, and specific travel recommendations for each stage of a pandemic will be important during a pandemic, and even more critical to guide preparedness efforts. There is a wide range of options that can be used to reduce overall travel, such as provision of travel information, voluntary advisories with health warnings, selective restrictions that limit certain types of travel, advance notification followed by a defined period of restriction, and mandatory measures that would prohibit all travel under extreme circumstances.

As travel restriction policies are evaluated, it will be critical to include the societal consequences of restrictions on individuals, families, and communities. Economic consequences vary widely based on transportation and border actions, but are discussed more under the following section.

Significant planning will be needed at local, State, and national levels to increase the Nation's preparedness, including joint planning to identify the range of transportation options and the supporting policies to facilitate safe transportation of food, fuel, and other critical supplies to affected communities, to help delay the spread with minimal societal and economic consequences.

Operational Feasibility

Effective transportation and border decisions must also consider operational feasibility, which includes evaluating how travel or trade measures could affect all relevant aspects of the transportation system and carefully weighing competing interests, views, and goals. Such an approach considers the complex, interconnected relationships of a decentralized network where small changes can strategically change travel and trade patterns or unknowingly transfer risk and/or create a secondary layer of challenges. For example, closure of a community to reduce spread would also sever that community from "just-in-time" deliveries to restock grocery stores, pharmacies, and could impede incoming emergency teams and or supplies for the medical and emergency response efforts underway. Even strong messages to reduce non-essential travel voluntarily, if not fully explained and accompanied by clear guidelines of how transport workers can reduce personal risk, could significantly reduce the movement of essential goods and availability of emergency transportation services. Transportation providers will be concerned about protecting their employees, risks to travelers and goods, and the potential impact on facilities and vehicles.

An operational approach gives full consideration to linkages, tradeoffs, or impacts on other transportation entities, facilities, systems, or users. Moreover, this approach considers non-health issues, such as manpower, market factors, how the transportation system operates, and the potential to transfer risk across the network. For example, mandatory restrictions in air travel could potentially transfer travel to other modes, such as rail or personal vehicles. The redundancies of the transportation network can make restrictions challenging to implement. However, a robust planning effort with the public, communities, and transportation providers and stakeholders can develop options based on a joint understanding of risk, the natural changes in travel patterns, advance notice to aid preparedness, and, in extreme circumstances, mandatory restrictions to safeguard communities.

Curtailment and changes in border and transportation operations will be essential during a pandemic response and to a certain extent will likely occur spontaneously. Transportation professionals and planners will be a valuable resource to assist with the pre-pandemic planning that anticipates theses changes and help communities and public health professionals identify how to achieve public health goals related to travel and trade at the time of a pandemic. This demands inclusive decision making with all parties involved both during pre-pandemic planning and at the earliest stages of the process, when issues and potential problems are first defined.

Circumstances and Impacts of Complete Border Closure

Any nation, including the United States, has the sovereign right to control, and if necessary, close its borders. However, in the event of a pandemic, a border closure would likely delay but not stop the spread of influenza to the United States, and would have significant negative social, economic, and foreign policy consequences. Other less drastic measures could potentially be layered to provide similar benefits without the substantial negative consequences of a complete border closure. The discussion below addresses U.S. border closure, as well as the potential that foreign countries may close their borders in response to a pandemic influenza outbreak in the United States.

In the absence of any border or travel restrictions, cases of pandemic influenza would likely arrive in the United States within 1 to 2 months after the virus first emergence elsewhere in the world. Current models suggest that highly restrictive border measures might delay the peak of pandemic by a few weeks. Depending on the length of delay, national preparedness may be enhanced as previously described.

An outbreak of pandemic influenza abroad might result in other countries closing their borders and generate calls for similar action in the United States. Outbreaks in Canada or Mexico might further increase pressure to close U.S. borders. Conversely, an outbreak within the United States might result in other countries closing their borders to the United States to delay spread. This could have a significant impact on overseas commerce, military missions, and the movement of American citizens.

A United States border closure would have a devastating economic impact, interrupt delivery of essential services, and would disrupt substantial cross-border commerce, resulting in hardship at manufacturing and production plants that rely on export markets and just-in-time delivery. United States international trade was almost $2.3 trillion in 2004,[8] with $599 billion in international air freight alone.[9] Given the importance of maritime trade to the U.S. economy,[10] any significant disruptions to trade at our seaports will have immediate and significant economic impacts. During the 2002 West Coast dock shutdown, the economic loss was estimated at $140 million per day.[11] A complete closure of U.S. borders to international travel and trade would be unprecedented.

---

[8] U.S. Dept. of Commerce, U.S. Census Bureau, Foreign Trade Division, *U.S. Exports of Merchandise and U.S. Imports of Merchandise*, March 2005.

[9] Based on U.S. Dept. of Commerce, U.S. Census Bureau, Foreign Trade Division, *U.S. Exports of Merchandise and U.S. Imports of Merchandise*, March 2005.

[10] Ships are the primary mode of transportation for world trade. Ships carry more than 95 percent of the U.S.' non-North American trade by weight and 75 percent by value, and 80 percent of the foreign oil imported by the U.S. Waterborne cargo contributes about 7.5 percent to the U.S. gross domestic product. In addition to its economic significance, the marine transportation system is vital for national security. The Departments of Defense and Transportation have designated 17 U.S. seaports as strategic because they are necessary for use by DOD in the event of a major military deployment. Thirteen of these ports are commercial seaports.

[11] Calculated from Patrick L. Anderson and Ilhan K. Geckil, *Flash Estimate: Impact of West Coast Shutdown*, Anderson Economic Group (October 15, 2002).

Modeling suggests that border closure would not decrease the total number of illnesses or deaths. Moreover, when the Nation's economic needs require the re-opening of the border, there could be widespread public confusion about the safety of people, freight, and travel. Nevertheless, our level of preparedness when a pandemic strikes and the uncertainties about the characteristics of a pandemic virus requires us to plan for this possibility. The section below describes potential alternatives and later sections identify additional research to explore the effectiveness and economic consequences of these options.

Alternatives to Complete Border Closure and Other Containment Options

There are alternatives to complete border closure that may be effective in delaying the onset of a pandemic in the United States and can help minimize the risk of infection among travelers coming to the United States. These include targeted traveler restrictions to help contain the pandemic at its source, and implementation of layered, risk-based measures, including pre-departure, en route, and arrival screening and/or quarantine. While we should take measures to protect travelers and limit their ability to transmit disease, there is little benefit to trade restriction if there are adequate measures in place to limit exposure to infected individuals and potentially contaminated surfaces. Irrespective of the combination of interventions selected, our efforts should be taken collaboratively with other nations, although unilateral efforts may be necessary in extreme circumstances.

Travelers

The United States will work with the international community to implement targeted passenger travel restrictions (see Chapter 4 - International Efforts). As part of the preparedness effort, the United States will engage WHO and foreign governments to determine how countries with human outbreaks can support containment and help slow global spread of a pandemic. For example, pre-negotiated arrangements and partnerships with other countries could encourage all countries with outbreaks to rapidly restrict non-essential travel for all modes of transportation (e.g., air, vessel, and land travel) in return for technical and other forms of assistance. In addition, the United States could deny entry of travelers, or place conditions on the return of travelers from countries with outbreaks and other countries that have not instituted acceptable pre-departure screening, prohibit entry of travelers from the affected area, or continue to accept travelers with appropriate conditions from countries with outbreaks. Additional options would be considered for U.S. citizens planning to return home from affected areas, such as a voluntary quarantine to monitor for illness through one incubation period prior to departure. This could reduce risk of transmission for the United States, and help identify persons in need of medical care.

Individual screening, for influenza-like illness and risk factors for infection with a pandemic strain, of all persons entering the United States will help minimize the risk of transmission. However, such screening is challenged by a lack of sensitivity (e.g., asymptomatic infected individuals may not be detected) and specificity (e.g., many individuals with influenza-like illness will not be infected with a pandemic strain). The typical incubation period for influenza is 2 days and infected persons with influenza may be contagious for 24 hours prior to the onset of symptoms. Since some asymptomatic travelers, who are incubating influenza, may become symptomatic en route, overall screening effectiveness can be improved by adopting layered pre-departure, en route, and arrival screening measures. The policy of layered screening measures would apply to all U.S.-bound travelers from affected areas, but the characteristics of the outbreak, including the rapidity of spread, may make it necessary to implement this screening at all international airports from which U.S.-bound passengers originate. In addition, development of rapid diagnostic tests can dramatically change our ability to screen effectively.

- **Pre-departure Measures:** Effective host country health screening of all individuals prior to departure may reduce the risk of infected travelers exposing fellow travelers, aircraft and vessel crews, and others upon arrival. This is consistent with the WHO Global Influenza Preparedness Plan and with the newly revised International Health Regulations. Screening could be performed for signs of illness (e.g., temperature scanning) and for risk factors (e.g., contacts, travel history). A clear description of signs of illness and risk factors for infection with pandemic influenza will be critical to develop effective screening protocols. Significant additional personnel and resources will be needed to strengthen in-country pre-departure screening capacity, particularly in countries that are heavily affected by a pandemic. The number of infected persons traveling to the United States could also be reduced by isolating potentially exposed individuals for one incubation period prior to international travel. The need to develop pre-departure measures and identify the necessary staffing resources will apply equally to the United States when pandemic transmission occurs domestically.

- **En Route Measures:** Given the short incubation period of influenza, and the length of some international flights, one can assume that some travelers with influenza will develop their first symptoms during their journey. The training of flight and vessel crews to detect and manage ill travelers can decrease risk for others on the conveyance and permit assessment and treatment upon landing. When combined with pre-departure exit screening, this strategy would detect those who developed signs of illness while en route. Response would include moving ill persons away from other travelers, if possible, placing a surgical mask on the ill person, and emphasizing the importance of hygiene measures, such as hand washing. If a mask is not available, covering coughs and sneezes with a tissue or cloth that is disposed after use will also decrease risk. By regulation, the master of ship or commander of an aircraft destined for a U.S. port is required to report the presence of any ill persons (as defined in the regulation) or deaths on board to the nearest quarantine station at which the ship or aircraft will arrive. In its proposed rule, the Centers for Disease Control and Prevention (CDC) has proposed expanding the definition of ill persons to include additional illness criteria indicative of the presence of a quarantinable disease, such as pandemic influenza.

- **Arrival Measures:** Arrival screening may serve as an important additional layer if we cannot ensure the adequacy and effectiveness of other containment measures. It can also identify individuals who became ill during travel. Arrival screening can be imposed as a precautionary measure, irrespective of other containment measures. Travelers with influenza-like illness should be isolated and undergo diagnostic testing; other travelers may potentially be quarantined until definitive testing is complete. When developed, rapid diagnostic testing could greatly increase effectiveness of screening. These arrival procedures also provide an opportunity to educate travelers to increase their awareness of influenza symptoms and the need for seeking medical care and immediate home quarantine when compatible symptoms arise. It must be recognized that arrival screening will place additional demands on CDC Quarantine Station personnel and Customs and Border Protection officers and agents. It is critical that local quarantine plans leverage available Federal, State, and local assets to implement effective screening, quarantine, and isolation, and provide expanded access to medical treatment. Capacity could also be addressed by examining the costs and benefits of potentially funneling inbound international flights to a subset of U.S. airports. Preliminary research indicates that potentially 96 percent of all inbound international flights arrive at 30 U.S. airports.[12] Additional work will be needed to explore and evaluate options with airlines, airports, and local authorities and public health professionals.

Cargo and Trade Goods

This risk of influenza transmission by cargo or trade goods, excluding live avian or animal cargo, is low. With effective protective measures for workers in specific settings, cargo shipments could continue. Because viable influenza virus may remain on surfaces for up to 48 hours, ship-borne cargo poses the lowest risk of virus transmission. Risk of transmission by or to the vessel's crew could be eliminated by confining them to the vessel and utilizing strict transmission prevention protocols with port personnel during loading/off loading operations. Given the greater speed of international air transport, additional measures may be needed for worker protection and, in some cases, to disinfect and/or isolate air cargo from a country with an outbreak.

Land Borders

Our approach to slowing the introduction of pandemic influenza through land borders will emphasize continental rather than national containment, and will respect our treaty commitments and other arrangements with Canada and Mexico. Our planning efforts with Canada and Mexico will include discussions of each country's efforts to support global containment, plans to implement travel restrictions, and commitments for rigorous screening at arrivals. Should the disease appear in Canada or Mexico, land borders would become the greatest point of vulnerability due to the high volume and nature of land border crossing. Specific measures used at land borders will depend on the temporal and geographic spread of disease and will require more intensive modeling to explore their potential effectiveness.

Unique challenges along our land borders will require significant outreach with the Canadian and Mexican governments and other stakeholders. On-time delivery of goods and workers being prevented from going to their jobs would create major challenges at land border locations, and could potentially affect the U.S. economy. On the northern border, the major manufacturing industries (e.g., automotive) would likely be adversely affected by restrictions or slow-downs at the border. On the southern border, textile and agriculture product importation could be impaired. In addition, there are a significant number of day workers that transit across the border. Therefore, planning should consider a range of alternatives, from approaches that permit the cross border flow of critical goods to complete border closure. Potentially infected illegal aliens attempting to cross between our ports of entry present another challenge and could create facility challenges related to quarantine.

Maintaining operational control of our Nation's borders is an essential function of the Department of Homeland Security (DHS). The presence of pandemic influenza in Central America or Mexico may trigger a mass migration. DHS would need to manage a large increase of additional attempted illegal entrants during a 2-month period. This spike will likely increase during a period when DHS resources are stretched due to employee absenteeism.

---

[12] U.S. Department of Transportation, Research and Innovative Technology Administration, Bureau of Transportation Statistics, T100 SEGMENT data, year-end second quarter 2005. (Note: includes all scheduled flights, as well as most charter, military, and private international flights).

Complexity of Transportation Decisions in Emergencies

The complexities of the transportation system and its relationship with public safety, productivity, health, and the national economy require that its assets be managed wisely during any emergency. During some training exercises, emergency transportation decisions have been made without full appreciation of the resulting consequences, including serious economic implications.

Managing transportation decisions in a pandemic will require extraordinary cooperation between the varied and diverse elements of the sector. In many cases, decision makers will be simultaneously managing complex and competing interests. State and local governments, acting within their authorities, may impose restrictions or closures of transportation systems without consulting or coordinating with Federal entities. This can be in the form of State/county border closures or closure of transit systems, ports, or airports. This could have considerable impact on efforts to move patients, responders, medical personnel, critical pharmaceuticals, and essential supplies. A key role for the Federal Government will be to provide clear criteria to guide and inform State and local actions and to conduct outreach with State, community, and tribal entities to communicate a cohesive national strategy for maintaining movement of essential critical goods and services, while encouraging limitation of non-essential transportation. Closing State or local borders is highly unlikely to be cost-effective, may create significant shortages in essential commodities, and is not preferred (see also Chapter 9 - Institutions: Protecting Personnel and Ensuring Continuity of Operations).

Sustaining Critical Transportation Services

Sustaining critical services during a pandemic will be crucial to keep communities functioning and emergency supplies and resources flowing. Planning efforts need to assess systemic effects (i.e., supply chain impact, just-in-time delivery, warehousing, and logistics) and support the development of contingency plans to address lack of critical services and delivery of essential commodities, such as chlorine for water purification, gasoline, food, and medical supplies.

Due to expected high absenteeism, transportation services may be limited. Interstate movement will become increasingly constrained as the pandemic peaks and local travel restrictions may increase. Passenger transportation will likely decrease as the public opts not to travel due to possible exposure. This will likely begin in international aviation, cruise ships, and highway border crossings. Once cases are present in the United States, this decrease in passenger travel will occur domestically in private automobile, aviation, mass transit, passenger rail, and motor coach travel. However, there may also be a small surge of movement into affected areas as individuals try to return home or help stranded or ill relatives. Others may attempt to temporarily relocate to less populated areas in an attempt to reduce the likelihood of infection. At the beginning of the pandemic, there will also be requests to move emergency workers, equipment, and resources. As the disease spreads to multiple urban areas, emergency transportation of supplies and personnel could decrease because resources will be needed locally.

There is a need to examine critical junctures where the increase in demand for essential commodities and emergency services intersect with a large reduction in workforce due to absenteeism. Identifying these junctures will enable the sector to focus preparedness efforts on areas of the transportation system that will be under the greatest strain during a pandemic.

Emergency Transportation Services

A pandemic outbreak in the United States will result in the activation of the *National Response Plan* (NRP) and Emergency Support Function #1 - Transportation (ESF #1) to coordinate Federal support for emergency transportation services. Activation under pandemic conditions will be considerably more challenging, with many urban areas simultaneously affected for a sustained period of time, as opposed to historically localized and short-duration activations following natural disasters.

Management of a pandemic response during NRP activation will be driven by decisions at the State and local level. Transportation response in such an emergency will be vital, with the Federal role focusing on coordination and communication across the sector, in addition to its emergency transportation services under the NRP. Balancing the demands of a pandemic in the NRP context with existing resources and maintaining response capacity for other disasters or terrorist incidents will be a priority focus.

Another key area is patient movement, which is coordinated primarily by Emergency Support Function #8 - Public Health and Medical Services (ESF #8). It is unlikely that patient movement will be similar in scope and resource requirements to the patient evacuation that has occurred during major hurricanes. Patient movement is discussed in greater detail under Chapter 6 - Protecting Human Health.

Transportation and Border Preparedness

An influenza pandemic poses significant challenges that must be addressed in the border and transportation planning process. All private sector, State and local entity, and Federal Government plans need to address the following four key areas: (1) maintaining situational awareness; (2) rapidly containing cases or initial outbreaks; (3) sustaining critical transportation and border services; and (4) recovery of the transportation system.

Maintaining Situational Awareness

Due to the complexity of transportation and border decisions and the dynamic effect of local decisions on the national network, it will be essential to enhance and maintain situational awareness across the sector. Plans should address:

- Ensuring adequate information sharing, analysis, and coordination among the private sector, State and local governments, the Federal Government, and international partners.

- Providing updates on the status of the transportation system, including operations and closures across the country.

- Maintaining awareness of public health measures under consideration that may have transportation implications, such as vaccine/antiviral distribution, need for food, and other essential services during quarantines, school closures, "snow days," travel restrictions, or other measures for social distancing.

- Establishing clear notification protocols to keep the private sector, State, local, and tribal governments, and the Federal Government informed of the pandemic threat, including early warning signs and potential cases.

Department of Homeland Security: DHS is responsible for ensuring integrity of the Nation's infrastructure, domestic security, providing support to entry and exit screening for pandemic influenza at the borders, facilitating coordination for the overall response to a pandemic, and the provision of a common operating picture for all departments and agencies of the Federal Government. DHS is also responsible for securing the Nation's borders and facilitating legitimate trade and travel through U.S. ports of entry.

DHS supports coordination of the NRP, which is the primary mechanism for coordination of the Federal Government response to Incidents of National Significance, and will form the basis of the Federal pandemic response. The NRP provides an organizing framework for coordinating a variety of support areas, including transportation, mass care, and public affairs, which are led by other Federal departments (see Chapter 3 for more detail). DHS will collaborate with other departments on transportation and border decisions, including the ability to control the spread of a pandemic (Department of Health and Human Services (HHS), Department of Agriculture (USDA), Department of Transportation (DOT), and Department of the Interior (DOI)), understand social and economic consequences (Department of Commerce (DOC), DOT, Department of the Treasury (Treasury), Department of State (DOS), HHS, USDA, DHS components, DOI, and key stakeholders), international and domestic implications (DOS, DOT, DOC, DHS components, and key stakeholders), and to obtain the economic and operational feasibility of actions (DOT, DOC, DHS components, and key stakeholders).

Department of Health and Human Services: HHS's primary responsibilities are to protect the health of all U.S. citizens and provide essential human services. With respect to transportation and borders, HHS will be involved in entry and exit screening and, in consultation with Department of Labor (DOL), protecting the health of transportation and border workers who are implementing measures to limit spread. HHS will support rapid containment of localized outbreaks domestically. HHS will provide recommendations to State, local, tribal, and private sector entities on the ability of transportation restrictions to limit the spread of a pandemic, patient movement, and plans for traveler screening, isolation, and quarantine at ports of entry. In addition, HHS and USDA are responsible for the exclusion and seizure of infectious animals or animal products. HHS exercises this authority with respect to human health, while USDA exercises this authority with respect to animal health.

Department of Transportation: DOT will implement priorities to maintain essential functions of the national transportation system, and provide emergency management and guidance for civil transportation resources and systems. In its role in the global transportation network, DOT will conduct outreach with its established public and private stakeholders — strategically coordinating with international, domestic, and other Federal Government participants, consistent with its responsibilities under the NRP in support of DHS. DOT will consider the short- and long-term economic impacts of a pandemic on the transportation sector in order to develop strategies that might prevent disruption of transportation services.

Department of Defense: DOD's primary responsibilities are those actions required to protect DOD forces, maintain operational readiness, and sustain critical military missions. DOD will increase its readiness to sustain critical DOD services to support the NRP and elements of the U.S. Government's international response. DOD can provide additional support to the extent that DOD's National Security readiness is not compromised.

When directed by the Secretary of Defense in accordance with law, DOD will collaborate with DOS and DOT in building international partnerships and enhancing their transportation capability. Once an outbreak occurs, DOD may play a role, consistent with existing agreements and legal authorities, in implementation of movement controls, controlling movement into and out of areas/borders with affected populations, and assisting in the transportation/movement of rapid response teams, medical countermeasures (antiviral medications and vaccines, if available), and logistical support materials to infected and at-risk populations according to established plan and guidelines when other public or private sector assets are not available.

Department of State: DOS will facilitate international cooperation and coordination and keep foreign governments, international businesses and organizations, and the public informed of U.S. policies and measures affecting travel and transportation. DOS will also communicate travel risk information to U.S. citizens residing and traveling abroad so as to allow them to make informed decisions and plans. In the event of U.S. Government-sponsored evacuations, DOS will provide appropriate assistance to U.S. citizens overseas.

Department of Agriculture: USDA is responsible for protecting the Nation's livestock, including poultry, from exotic or foreign animal diseases, such as highly pathogenic avian influenza. With respect to transportation and borders, USDA will determine, based on the country of origin and other factors, which articles, live animals, or animal products have the potential for introducing or spreading an exotic disease and will establish restrictions or exclusions on their importation into, and/or movements within, the United States. If live animals are not excluded from importation, USDA determines which live animals must undergo USDA-supervised quarantine and health examination prior to final entry into the United States.

Department of the Interior: DOI is responsible for permitting and inspection of wildlife and wildlife products in trade into and out of the United States. With respect to transportation and borders, DOI will work in partnership with DHS, USDA, and DOS to enforce and publicize wildlife border controls and, if appropriate, utilize its own permitting authorities to restrict the import or export of wild birds.

Department of Labor: DOL's primary responsibilities are those actions required to protect the health and safety of workers, including communication of information related to pandemic influenza to workers and employers, and other relevant activities.

State, Local, and Tribal Entities

State and community pandemic preparedness plans should address key transportation issues and outline social distancing measures and strategies to mitigate consequences. States will face challenges in availability of essential commodities, demands for services that exceed capacity, and public pressure to restrict transportation in ways that may hinder economic sustainment and delivery of emergency services and supplies.

State, local, and tribal entities should develop and exercise pandemic influenza plans that address transportation's role in maintaining State and community functions, including delivery of essential services, containment strategies, providing critical services to citizens, support for public health measures, and other key regional or local issues. State and local governments should involve transportation and health professionals to identify transportation options, consequences, and implications. Transportation and border plans should be integrated as part of a comprehensive State plan that addresses the full range of pandemic preparedness (i.e., public health, animal health, protecting institutions, and law enforcement, public safety, and security). States will also need to coordinate closely with neighboring States/regions and the Federal Government to assess the interdependencies of local, State, and national decisions on the viability of the sector.

The Private Sector and Critical Infrastructure Entities

The private sector will play an integral role in preparedness before a pandemic begins and should be part of the national response. As they prepare, respond, sustain, and recover from a pandemic, transportation owners/operators will strive to maintain as close to normal operations as possible within the constraints of a pandemic.

The private sector should develop pandemic influenza plans that identify challenges and outline strategies to sustain core transportation and border functions and mitigate economic consequences. Entities should engage the full spectrum of preparedness planning to maintain essential services as close to normal operations as possible within the constraints of a pandemic.

Individuals and Families

It is important for U.S. citizens to recognize and understand the degree to which their actions will govern the course of a pandemic. The success or failure of border and transportation measures are ultimately dependent upon the acts of individuals, and the collective response of 300 million U.S. citizens will significantly influence the shape of the pandemic and its medical, social, and economic outcomes (see *Individual, Family, and Community Response to Pandemic Influenza* between Chapters 5 and 6). Individuals will, in general, respond to a pandemic and to public health interventions in ways that they perceive to be congruent with their interests and their instinct for self-preservation, and border and transportation authorities should tailor their risk communication campaigns and interventions accordingly. This will directly affect the willingness of the public to participate in travel-related screening and support voluntary domestic and international travel limitations.

International Partners

The response to a pandemic will be a global one, necessitating action by international organizations and governments. DOT and DHS have relationships with many international organizations, governments, and the private sector due to the global nature of today's economy. In close coordination with DOS, DOT and DHS will leverage their international relationships to assist in ensuring the continued movement of goods, services, and people (see Chapter 4 — International Efforts).

Actions and Expectations

5.1. Pillar One: Preparedness and Communication

This section provides an overview of planning expectations across the transportation and border sector (i.e., the private sector, State and local entities, and the Federal Government) and a detailed discussion of actions the Federal Government will take to support preparedness. Effective planning for a pandemic will require the development of plans, procedures, policies, and training to prepare for, respond to, and recover from a pandemic.

a. Planning for a Pandemic

5.1.1.   Develop Federal implementation plans to support the *National Strategy for Pandemic Influenza*, to include all components of the U.S. Government and to address the full range of consequences of a pandemic.

5.1.1.1.   DHS and DOT shall establish an interagency transportation and border preparedness working group, including DOS, HHS, USDA, DOD, DOL, and DOC as core members, to develop planning assumptions for the transportation and border sectors, coordinate preparedness activities by mode, review products and their distribution, and develop a coordinated outreach plan for stakeholders, within 6 months. Measure of performance: interagency working group established, planning assumptions developed, preparedness priorities and timelines established by mode, and outreach plan for stakeholders in place.

5.1.1.2.   HHS and DHS, in coordination with the National Economic Council (NEC), DOD, DOC, U.S. Trade Representative (USTR), DOT, DOS, USDA, Treasury, and key transportation and border stakeholders, shall establish an interagency modeling group to examine the effects of transportation and border decisions on delaying spread of a pandemic, and the associated health benefits, the societal and economic consequences, and the international implications, within 6 months. Measure of performance: interagency working group established, planning assumptions developed, priorities established, and recommendations made on which models are best suited to address priorities.

5.1.1.3.   DHS and DOT, in coordination with DOD, HHS, USDA, Department of Justice (DOJ), and DOS, shall assess their ability to maintain critical Federal transportation and border services (e.g., sustain National Air Space, secure the borders) during a pandemic, revise contingency plans, and conduct exercises, within 12 months. Measure of performance: revised contingency plans in place at specified Federal agencies that respond to both international and domestic outbreaks and at least two interagency exercises carried out to test the plans.

5.1.1.4.   DHS and DOT, in coordination with DOD, HHS, USDA, USTR, DOL, and DOS, shall develop detailed operational plans and protocols to respond to potential pandemic-related scenarios, including inbound aircraft/vessel/land border traffic with suspected case of pandemic influenza, international outbreak, multiple domestic outbreaks, and potential mass migration, within 12 months. Measure of performance: coordinated Federal operational plans that identify actions, authorities, and trigger points for decision making and are validated by interagency exercises.

5.1.1.5.   DOD, in coordination with DHS, DOT, DOJ, and DOS, shall conduct an assessment of military support related to transportation and borders that may be requested during a pandemic and develop a comprehensive contingency plan for Defense Support to Civil Authorities, within 18 months. Measure of performance: Defense Support to Civil Authorities plan in place that addresses emergency transportation and border support.

5.1.1.6.   DOT, in coordination with DHS, DOD, DOJ, HHS, DOL, and USDA, shall assess the Federal Government's ability to provide emergency transportation support during a pandemic under NRP ESF #1 and develop a contingency plan, within 18 months. Measure of performance: completed contingency plan that includes options for increasing transportation capacity, the potential need for military support, improved shipment tracking, potential need for security and/or waivers for critical shipments, incorporation of decontamination and workforce protection guidelines, and other critical issues.

5.1.2. **Continue to work with States, localities, and tribal entities to establish and exercise pandemic response plans.**

5.1.2.1.   DHS and HHS, in coordination with DOT and USDA, shall review existing grants or Federal funding that could be used to support transportation and border-related pandemic planning, within 4 months. Measure of performance: all State, local, and tribal governments are in receipt of, or have access to, guidance for grant applications.

5.1.2.2.   DOT, in coordination with DHS, HHS, and transportation stakeholders, shall convene a series of forums with governors and mayors to discuss transportation and border challenges that may occur in a pandemic, share approaches, and develop a planning strategy to ensure a coordinated national response, within 12 months. Measure of performance: strategy for coordinated transportation and border planning is developed and forums initiated.

5.1.2.3.   DOT and DHS, in coordination with HHS, USDA, and transportation stakeholders, shall develop planning guidance and materials for State, local, and tribal governments, including scenarios that highlight transportation and border challenges and responses to overcome those challenges, and an overview of transportation roles and responsibilities under the NRP, within 12 months. Measure of performance: State, local, and tribal governments have received or have access to tailored guidance and planning materials.

5.1.2.4.   State, community, and tribal entities, in coordination with neighboring States and communities, the private sector, transportation providers, and health professionals, should develop transportation contingency plans that identify a range of options to respond to different stages of a pandemic, including support for public health containment strategies, maintaining State and community functions, transportation restriction options and consequences, delivery of essential goods and services, and other key regional or local issues, within 18 months.

5.1.2.5.   DHS and DOT, in coordination with DOD and States, shall develop a range of options to cope with potential shortages of commodities and demand for essential services, such as building reserves of essential goods, within 20 months. Measure of performance: options developed and available for State, local, and tribal governments to refine and incorporate in contingency plans.

5.1.3. **Continue to work with States, localities, and tribal entities to integrate non-health sectors, including the private sector and critical infrastructure entities, in these planning efforts.**

5.1.3.1.   DHS, in coordination with DOT, HHS, and USDA, shall conduct tabletop discussions and other outreach with private sector transportation and border entities to provide background on the scope of a pandemic, to assess current preparedness, and jointly develop a planning guide, within 8 months. Measure of performance: private sector transportation and border entities have coordinated Federal guidance to support pandemic planning, including a planning guide that addresses unique border and transportation challenges by mode., within 8 months. Measure of performance: private sector transportation and border entities have coordinated Federal guidance to support pandemic planning, including a planning guide that addresses unique border and transportation challenges by mode.

5.1.3.2.   DHS, in coordination with DOT, HHS, DOC, Treasury, and USDA, shall work with the private sector to identify strategies to minimize the economic consequences and potential shortages of essential goods (e.g., food, fuel, medical supplies) and services during a pandemic, within 12 months. Measure of performance: the private sector has strategies that can be incorporated into contingency plans to mitigate consequences of potential shortages of essential goods and services.

5.1.3.3.   Private sector transportation and border entities, in coordination with States and customers, should develop pandemic influenza plans that identify challenges and outline strategies to sustain core functions, essential services, and mitigate economic consequences, within 16 months.

b. Communicating Expectations and Responsibilities

5.1.4.   Provide guidance to the private sector and critical infrastructure entities on their role in the pandemic response, and considerations necessary to maintain essential services and operations despite significant and sustained worker absenteeism.

5.1.4.1.   HHS, in coordination with DHS, DOT, and DOL, shall establish workforce protection guidelines and develop targeted educational materials addressing the risk of contracting pandemic influenza for transportation and border workers, within 6 months. Measure of performance: guidelines and materials developed that meet the diverse needs of border and transportation workers (e.g., customs officers or agents, air traffic controllers, train conductors, dock workers, flight attendants, transit workers, ship crews, and interstate truckers).

5.1.4.2.   DHS, in coordination with DOT, DOL, Office of Personnel Management (OPM), and DOS, shall disseminate workforce protection information to stakeholders, conduct outreach with stakeholders, and implement a comprehensive program for all Federal transportation and border staff within 12 months. Measure of performance: 100 percent of workforce has or has access to information on pandemic influenza risk and appropriate protective measures.

5.1.4.3.   HHS, in coordination with DHS, DOT, DOD, Environmental Protection Agency (EPA), and transportation and border stakeholders, shall develop and disseminate decontamination guidelines and timeframes for transportation and border assets and facilities (e.g., airframes, emergency medical services transport vehicles, trains, trucks, stations, port of entry detention facilities) specific to pandemic influenza, within 12 months. Measure of performance: decontamination guidelines developed and disseminated through existing DOT and DHS channels.

5.2. Pillar Two: Surveillance and Detection

Early warning of a pandemic is critical to being able to rapidly employ resources to contain the spread of the virus. An effective detection system will save lives by allowing us to activate our response plans before the arrival of a pandemic virus in the United States. DHS will work closely with DOT, HHS, USDA, and DOS to develop and be prepared to implement screening protocols to enhance pre-departure, en route, and arrival screening at the U.S. border (land, air, and sea) for potentially infected travelers, animals, and other cargo.

a. Ensuring Rapid Reporting of Outbreaks

5.2.1. **Advance mechanisms for "real-time" clinical surveillance in domestic acute care settings such as emergency departments, intensive care units, and laboratories to provide local, State, and Federal public health officials with continuous awareness of the profile of illness in communities, and leverage all Federal medical capabilities, both domestic and international, in support of this objective.**

5.2.1.1. HHS and USDA, in coordination with DHS, DOT, DOS, DOD, DOI, and State, local, and international stakeholders, shall review existing transportation and border notification protocols to ensure timely information sharing in cases of quarantinable disease, within 6 months. Measure of performance: coordinated, clear interagency notification protocols disseminated and available for transportation and border stakeholders.

5.2.2. **Develop and deploy rapid diagnostics with greater sensitivity and reproducibility to allow onsite diagnosis of pandemic strains of influenza at home and abroad, in humans, to facilitate early warning, outbreak control, and targeting of antiviral therapy.**

5.2.2.1. DHS, in coordination with HHS and DOD, shall deploy human influenza rapid diagnostic tests with greater sensitivity and specificity at borders and ports of entry to allow real-time health screening, within 12 months of development of tests. Measure of performance: diagnostic tests, if found to be useful, are deployed; testing is integrated into screening protocols to improve screening at the 20-30 most critical ports of entry.

b. Using Surveillance to Limit Spread

5.2.3. **Develop mechanisms to rapidly share information on travelers who may be carrying or may have been exposed to a pandemic strain of influenza, for the purposes of contact tracing and outbreak investigation.**

5.2.3.1. DHS, in coordination with HHS, DOT, DOS, and DOD, shall work closely with domestic and international air carriers and cruise lines to develop and implement protocols (in accordance with U.S. privacy law) to retrieve and rapidly share information on travelers who may be carrying or may have been exposed to a pandemic strain of influenza, within 6 months. Measure of performance: aviation and maritime protocols implemented and information on potentially infected travelers available to appropriate authorities.

5.2.4. Develop and exercise mechanisms to provide active and passive surveillance during an outbreak, both within and beyond our borders.

5.2.4.1. HHS, in coordination with DHS, DOT, DOS, DOC, and DOJ, shall develop policy recommendations for aviation, land border, and maritime entry and exit protocols and/or screening and review the need for domestic response protocols or screening within 6 months. Measure of performance: policy recommendations for response protocols and/or screening.

5.2.4.2. HHS, DHS, and DOT, in coordination with DOS, DOC, Treasury, and USDA, shall develop policy guidelines for international and domestic travel restrictions during a pandemic based on the ability to delay the spread of disease and the resulting health benefits, associated economic impacts, international implications, and operational feasibility, within 8 months. Measure of performance: interagency travel curtailment policy guidelines developed that address both voluntary and mandatory travel restrictions.

5.2.4.3. DOS, in coordination DHS, DOT, and HHS, in consultation with aviation, maritime, and tourism industry stakeholders as appropriate, and working with international partners and through international organizations as appropriate, shall promote the establishment of arrangements through which countries would: (1) voluntarily limit travel if affected by outbreaks of pandemic influenza; and (2) establish pre-departure screening protocols for persons with influenza-like illness, within 16 months. Measure of performance: arrangements for screening protocols are negotiated.

5.2.4.4. DOS and HHS, in coordination with DHS, DOT, and transportation and border stakeholders, shall assess and revise procedures to issue travel information and advisories related to pandemic influenza, within 12 months. Measure of performance: improved interagency coordination and timely dissemination of travel information to stakeholders and travelers.

5.2.4.5. DOT and DHS, in coordination with HHS, DOD, DOS, airlines/air space users, the cruise line industry, and appropriate State and local health authorities, shall develop protocols[13] to manage and/or divert inbound international flights and vessels with suspected cases of pandemic influenza that identify roles, actions, relevant authorities, and events that trigger response, within 12 months. Measure of performance: interagency response protocols for inbound flights completed and disseminated to appropriate entities.

---

[13] Protocols will be revised as new rapid diagnostic tests become available.   [14] Protocols will be revised as new rapid diagnostic tests become available.

5.2.4.6. HHS, in coordination with DHS, DOT, DOS, DOD, air carriers/air space users, the cruise line industry, and appropriate State and local health authorities, shall develop en route protocols for crewmembers onboard aircraft and vessels to identify and respond to travelers who become ill en route and to make timely notification to Federal agencies, health care providers, and other relevant authorities, within 12 months. Measure of performance: protocols developed and disseminated to air carriers/air space users and cruise line industry.

5.2.4.7. DHS, DOT, and HHS, in coordination with transportation and border stakeholders, and appropriate State and local health authorities, shall develop aviation, land border, and maritime entry and exit protocols and/or screening protocols,[14] and education materials for non-medical, front-line screeners and officers to identify potentially infected persons or cargo, within 10 months. Measure of performance: protocols and training materials developed and disseminated.

5.2.4.8. DHS and HHS, in coordination with DOT, DOJ, and appropriate State and local health authorities, shall develop detection, diagnosis, quarantine, isolation, EMS transport, reporting, and enforcement protocols and education materials for travelers, and undocumented aliens apprehended at and between Ports of Entry, who have signs or symptoms of pandemic influenza or who may have been exposed to influenza, within 10 months. Measure of performance: protocols developed and distributed to all ports of entry.

5.2.4.9. DHS, in coordination with DOS, HHS, Treasury, and the travel and trade industry, shall tailor existing automated screening programs and extended border programs to increase scrutiny of travelers and cargo based on potential risk factors (e.g., shipment from or traveling through areas with pandemic outbreaks) within 6 months. Measure of performance: enhanced risk-based screening protocols implemented.

5.2.4.10. HHS, DHS, and DOT, in coordination with DOS, State, community and tribal entities, and the private sector, shall develop a public education campaign on pandemic influenza for travelers, which raises general awareness prior to a pandemic and includes messages for use during an outbreak, within 15 months. Measure of performance: public education campaign developed on how a pandemic could affect travel, the importance of reducing non-essential travel, and potential screening measures and transportation and border messages developed based on pandemic stages.

5.2.5. Develop screening and monitoring mechanisms and agreements to appropriately control travel and shipping of potentially infected products to and from affected regions if necessary, and to protect unaffected populations.

5.2.5.1. HHS and DHS, in coordination with DOS, DOT, DOD, DOL, and international and domestic stakeholders, shall develop vessel, aircraft, and truck cargo protocols to support safe loading and unloading of cargo while preventing transmission of influenza to crew or shore-side personnel, within 12 months.

Measure of performance: protocols disseminated to minimize influenza spread between vessel, aircraft, and truck operators/crews and shore-side personnel.

5.2.5.2. USDA, in coordination with DHS, DOI, and HHS, shall review the process for withdrawing permits for importation of live avian species or products and identify ways to increase timeliness, improve detection of high-risk importers, and increase outreach to importers and their distributors, within 6 months. Measure of performance: revised process for withdrawing permits of high-risk importers.

5.2.5.3. USDA, in coordination with DOI, DHS, shall enhance protocols at air, land, and sea ports of entry to identify and contain animals, animal products, and/or cargo that may harbor viruses with pandemic potential and review procedures to quickly impose restrictions, within 6 months. Measure of performance: risk-based protocols established and in use.

5.2.5.4. USDA, in coordination with DHS, shall review the protocols, procedures, and capacity at animal quarantine centers to meet the requirements outlined in Part 93 of Title 9 of the Code of Federal Regulations, within 4 months. Measure of performance: procedures in place to respond effectively and efficiently to the arrival of potentially infected avian species, including provisions for adequate quarantine surge capacity.

5.2.5.5. USDA, in coordination with DHS, DOJ, and DOI, shall enhance risk management and anti-smuggling activities to prevent the unlawful entry of prohibited animals, animal products, wildlife, and agricultural commodities that may harbor influenza viruses with pandemic potential, and expand efforts to investigate illegal commodities, block illegal importers, and increase scrutiny of shipments from known offenders, within 9 months. Measure of performance: plan developed to decrease smuggling and further distribution of prohibited agricultural commodities and products with influenza risk.

5.2.5.6. USDA, DHS, and DOI, in coordination with DOS, HHS, and DOC, shall conduct outreach and expand education campaigns for the public, agricultural stakeholders, wildlife trade community, and cargo and animal importers/exporters on import and export regulations and influenza disease risks, within 12 months. Measure of performance: 100 percent of key stakeholders are aware of current import and export regulations and penalties for non-compliance.

5.3. Pillar Three: Response and Containment

As the threat of a pandemic increases, the United States will implement incremental, risk-based measures at ports of entry and require similar pre-departure measures at select foreign points of embarkation. Regardless of where an outbreak occurs, the U.S. Government will use its authorities and resources to support rapid containment – whether working with international partners to contain overseas outbreaks or supporting State, local, or private sector efforts to contain domestic outbreaks. DHS should work with DOS, DOT, HHS, Treasury, and USDA to implement risk-based measures to slow the spread of a pandemic, minimize social and economic consequences both internationally and domestically, and ensure operational feasibility. Following is a range of options that will be considered and the agency or agencies responsible for implementation (see also Chapter 4 — International Efforts).

In support of DHS, DOT serves as the coordinator and primary agency for ESF #1. This support function is designed to provide transportation support to assist in domestic incident management and coordinate the recovery, restoration, and safety/security of the transportation sector. Under the NRP, other support agencies include USDA, DOC, DOD, Department of Energy (DOE), DHS, DOI, DOJ, DOS, General Services Administration (GSA), and the U.S. Postal Service.

a. Containing Outbreaks

5.3.1. **Encourage all levels of government, domestically and globally, to take appropriate and lawful action to contain an outbreak within the borders of their community, province, state, or nation.**

5.3.1.1. DOS and DHS, in coordination with DOT, DOC, HHS, Treasury, and USDA, shall work with foreign counterparts to limit or restrict travel from affected regions to the United States, as appropriate, and notify host government(s) and the traveling public. Measure of performance: measures imposed within 24 hours of the decision to do so, after appropriate notifications made.

5.3.1.2. DOS, in coordination with DOT, HHS, DHS, DOD, air carriers, and cruise lines, shall work with host countries to implement agreed upon pre-departure screening based on disease characteristics and availability of rapid detection methods and equipment. Measure of performance: screening protocols agreed upon and put in place in countries within 24 hours of an outbreak.

5.3.1.3. DOS, in coordination with HHS, DHS, and DOT, shall offer transportation-related technical assistance to countries with outbreaks. Measure of performance: countries with outbreaks receive U.S. offer of technical support within 36 hours of an outbreak.

5.3.1.4. DHS, in coordination with DOS, USDA and DOI, shall provide countries with guidance to increase scrutiny of cargo and other imported items through existing programs, such as the Container Security Initiative, and impose country-based restrictions or item-specific embargoes. Measure of performance: guidance, which may include information on restrictions, is provided for increased scrutiny of cargo and other imported items, within 24 hours upon notification of an outbreak

5.3.1.5. DHS, in coordination with DOT, HHS, DOS, DOD, USDA, appropriate State and local authorities, air carriers/air space users, airports, cruise lines, and seaports, shall implement screening protocols at U.S. ports of entry based on disease characteristics and availability of rapid detection methods and equipment. Measure of performance: screening implemented within 48 hours upon notification of an outbreak.

5.3.1.6.   DHS, in coordination with DOT, HHS, USDA, DOD, appropriate State, and local authorities, air carriers and airports, shall consider implementing response or screening protocols at domestic airports and other transport modes as appropriate, based on disease characteristics and availability of rapid detection methods and equipment. Measure of performance: screening protocols in place within 24 hours of directive to do so.

5.3.2.   Where appropriate, use governmental authorities to limit non-essential movement of people, goods, and services into and out of areas where an outbreak occurs.

5.3.2.1.   DHS, DOS, and HHS, in coordination with DOT and USDA, shall issue travel advisories/public announcements for areas where outbreaks have occurred and ensure adequate coordination with appropriate transportation and border stakeholders. Measure of performance: coordinated announcements and warnings developed within 24 hours of becoming aware of an outbreak and timely updates provided as required.

5.3.2.2.   DHS and DOT, in coordination with DOS and Treasury, and international and domestic stakeholders, shall consider activating plans, consistent with international law, to selectively limit or deny entry to U.S. airspace, U.S. territorial seas (12 nautical miles offshore), and ports of entry, including airports, seaports, and land borders and/or restrict domestic transportation, based on risk, public health benefits, and economic impacts. Measure of performance: measures implemented within 6 hours of decision to do so.

5.3.2.3.   DHS, in coordination with USDA, DOS, DOC, DOI, and shippers, shall rapidly implement and enforce cargo restrictions for export or import of potentially contaminated cargo, including embargo of live birds, and notify international partners/shippers. Measure of performance: measures implemented within 6 hours of decision to do so

b. Sustaining Infrastructure, Essential Services, and the Economy

5.3.3.   Encourage the development of coordination mechanisms across American industries to support the above activities during a pandemic.

5.3.3.1.   HHS and USDA, in coordination with DHS, DOT, DOS, and DOI, shall provide emergency notifications of probable or confirmed cases and/or outbreaks to key international, Federal, State, local, and tribal transportation and border stakeholders through existing networks. Measure of performance: emergency notifications occur within 24 hours or less of events of probable or confirmed cases or outbreaks.

5.3.3.2.   DHS and DOT, in coordination with DOS, shall gather information from the private sector, international, State, local, and tribal entities, and transportation associations to assess and report the status of the transportation sector. Measure of performance: decision makers have current and accurate information on the status of the transportation sector.

5.3.4. Provide guidance to activate contingency plans to ensure that personnel are protected, that the delivery of essential goods and services is maintained, and that sectors remain functional despite significant and sustained worker absenteeism.

5.3.4.1. DHS and DOT shall notify border and transportation stakeholders and provide recommendations to implement contingency plans and/or use authorities to restrict movement based on ability to limit spread, economic and societal consequences, international considerations, and operational feasibility. Measure of performance: border and transportation stakeholders receive notification and recommendations within no more than 24 hours (depending on urgency) of an outbreak or significant development that may warrant a change in stakeholder actions or protective measures.

5.3.4.2. DHS and DOT shall consider activating contingency plans as needed to ensure availability of Federal personnel at more critical facilities and higher volume crossings or hubs. Measure of performance: Federal services sustained at high-priority/high-volume facilities.

5.3.4.3. DHS, if needed, will implement contingency plans to maintain border control during a period of pandemic influenza induced mass migration. Measure of performance: contingency plan activated within 24 hours of notification.

5.3.4.4. DHS and DOT, in coordination with USDA, DOI, DOC, and DOS, shall consult with the domestic and international travel industry (e.g., carriers, hospitality industry, and travel agents) and freight transportation partners to discuss travel and border options under consideration and assess potential economic and international ramifications prior to implementation. Measure of performance: initial stakeholder contacts and solicitation for inputs conducted within 48 hours of an outbreak and re-established if additional countries affected.

5.3.4.5. DOT shall issue safety-related waivers as needed, to facilitate efficient movement of goods and people during an emergency, balancing the need to expedite services with safety, and States should consider waiving state-specific regulatory requirements, such as size and weight limits and convoy registration. Measure of performance: all regulatory waivers as needed balance need to expedite services with safety.

5.3.4.6. DOJ and DHS shall protect targeted shipments of critical supplies and facilities by providing limited Federal security forces under Emergency Support Function #13 - Public Safety and Security (ESF #13) of the NRP, as needed. Measure of performance: all appropriate Federal, State, local, and tribal requests for Federal law enforcement and security assistance met via activation of ESF #13 of the NRP. (See also Chapter 8 - Law Enforcement, Public Safety, and Security.)

5.3.4.7. DHS, in coordination with DOS, DOT, DOD, and the Merchant Marine, shall work with major commercial shipping fleets and the international community to ensure continuation of maritime transport and commerce, including activation of plans, as needed, to provide emergency medical support to crews of vessels that are not capable of safe navigation. Measure of performance: maritime transportation capacity meets demand and vessel mishaps remain proportional to number of ship movements.

5.3.4.8.   DOD, in coordination with DHS and DOS, shall identify those domestic and foreign airports and seaports that are considered strategic junctures for major military deployments and evaluate whether additional risk-based protective measures are needed, within 18 months. Measure of performance: identification of critical air and seaports and evaluation of additional risk-based procedures, completed.

5.3.5.   Determine the spectrum of infrastructure-sustainment activities that the U.S. military and other government entities may be able to support during a pandemic, contingent upon primary mission requirements, and develop mechanisms to activate them.

5.3.5.1.   DOT, in coordination with DHS and other ESF #1 support agencies, shall monitor and report the status of the transportation sector, assess impacts, and coordinate Federal and civil transportation services in support of Federal agencies and State, local, and tribal entities (see Chapter 6 — Protecting Human Health, for information on patient movement (ESF #8)). Measure of performance: when ESF #1 is activated, regular reports provided, impacts assessed, and services coordinated as needed.

5.3.5.2.   DOT, in coordination with DHS and other ESF #1 support agencies, shall coordinate emergency transportation services to support domestic incident management, including transport of Federal emergency teams, equipment, and Federal Incident Response supplies. Measure of performance: all appropriate Federal, State, local, and tribal requests for transportation services provided on time via ESF #1 of the NRP.

5.3.5.3.   DOT, in coordination with DHS, State, local, and tribal governments, and the private sector, shall monitor system closures, assess effects on the transportation system, and implement contingency plans. Measure of performance: timely reports transmitted to DHS and other appropriate entities, containing relevant, current, and accurate information on the status of the transportation sector and impacts resulting from the pandemic; when appropriate, contingency plans implemented within no more than 24 hours of a report of a transportation sector impact or issue.

5.3.5.4.   DOT, in support of DHS and in coordination with other ESF #1 support agencies, shall work closely with the private sector and State, local, and tribal entities to restore the transportation system, including decontamination and re-prioritization of essential commodity shipments. Measure of performance: backlogs or shortages of essential commodities and goods quickly eliminated, returning production and consumption to pre-pandemic levels.

5.3.5.5.   DOD, when directed by Secretary of Defense and in accordance with law, shall monitor and report the status of the military transportation system and those military assets that may be requested to protect the borders, assess impacts (to include operational impacts), and coordinate military services in support of

Federal agencies and State, local, and tribal entities. Measure of performance: when DOD activated, regular reports provided, impacts assessed, and services coordinated as needed.

5.3.5.6. DOT and DHS, in coordination with NEC, Treasury, DOC, HHS, DOS, and the interagency modeling group, shall assess the economic, safety, and security related effects of the pandemic on the transportation sector, including movement restrictions, closures, and quarantine, and develop strategies to support long-term recovery of the sector, within 6 months of the end of a pandemic. Measure of performance: economic and other assessments completed and strategies implemented to support long-term recovery of the sector.

c. Ensuring Effective Risk Communication

5.3.6. Ensure that timely, clear, coordinated messages are delivered to the American public from trained spokespersons at all levels of government and assist the governments of affected nations to do the same.

5.3.6.1. DOT and DHS, in coordination with HHS, DOS, and DOC, shall conduct media and stakeholder outreach to restore public confidence in travel. Measure of performance: outreach delivered and traveling public resumes use of the transportation system at or near pre-pandemic levels.

5.3.6.2. DHS and DOT, in coordination with DOS, DOD, HHS, USDA, DOI, and State, local, and tribal governments, shall provide the public and business community with relevant travel information, including shipping advisories, restrictions, and potential closing of domestic and international transportation hubs. Measure of performance: timely, consistent, and accurate traveler information provided to the media, public, and business community.

WHO Global Pandemic Phases and the Stages for Federal Government Response

WHO Phases		Federal Government Response Stages	
INTER-PANDEMIC PERIOD			
1	No new influenza virus subtypes have been detected in humans. An influenza virus subtype that has caused human infection may be present in animals. If present in animals, the risk of human disease is considered to be low.	**0**	New domestic animal outbreak in at–risk country
2	No new influenza virus subtypes have been detected in humans. However, a circulating animal influenza virus subtype poses a substantial risk of human disease.		
PANDEMIC ALERT PERIOD			
3	Human infection(s) with a new subtype, but no human-to-human spread, or at most rare instances of spread to a close contact.	**0**	New domestic animal outbreak in at–risk country
		1	Suspected human outbreak overseas
4	Small cluster(s) with limited human-to-human transmission but spread is highly localized, suggesting that the virus is not well adapted to humans.	**2**	Confirmed human outbreak overseas
5	Larger cluster(s) but human-to-human spread still localized, suggesting that the virus is becoming increasingly better adapted to humans, but may not yet be fully transmissible (substantial pandemic risk).		
PANDEMIC PERIOD			
6	Pandemic phase: increased and sustained transmission in general population.	**3**	Widespread human outbreaks in multiple locations overseas
		4	First human case in North America
		5	Spread throughout United States
		6	Recovery and preparation for subsequent waves

PANDEMIC INFLUENZA

Stages of Federal Government Response

STAGE 0

New Domestic Animal Outbreak in At–Risk Country

GOALS

Provide coordination, support, technical guidance

Track outbreaks to resolution

Monitor for reoccurrence of disease

ACTIONS

Support coordinated international response

Prepare to deploy rapid response team and materiel

Offer technical assistance, encourage information sharing

POLICY DECISIONS

Deployment of countermeasures

WHO Phase 1 or 2
Inter-Pandemic Period

STAGE 1

Suspected Human Outbreak Overseas

GOALS

Rapidly investigate and confirm or refute

Coordination and logistical support

ACTIONS

Initiate dialogue with WHO

Deploy rapid response team

Amplify lab-based and clinical surveillance to region

Prepare to implement screening and/or travel restrictions from affected area

POLICY DECISIONS

Pre-positioning of U.S. contribution to international stockpile assets

Use of pre-pandemic vaccine

WHO Phase 3
Pandemic Alert Period

STAGE 2

Confirmed Human Outbreak Overseas

GOALS

Contain outbreak and limit potential for spread

Activate domestic medical response

ACTIONS

Declare Incident of National Significance

Support international deployment of countermeasures

Implement layered screening measures; activate domestic quarantine stations

Prepare to limit domestic ports of entry

Prepare to produce monovalent vaccine

POLICY DECISIONS

Contribution to countermeasures for affected region

Entry/exit screening criteria; isolation/quarantine protocols

Diversion of trivalent vaccine production to monovalent

Revise prioritization and allocation of pandemic vaccine and antiviral medications

WHO Phase 4 or 5
Pandemic Alert Period

STAGE 3

Widespread Outbreaks Overseas

GOALS

Delay emergence in North America

Ensure earliest warning of first case(s)

Prepare domestic containment and response mechanisms

ACTIONS

Activate domestic emergency medical personnel plans

Maintain layered screening measures at borders

Deploy pre-pandemic vaccine and antiviral stockpiles; divert to monovalent vaccine production

Real-time modeling; heighten hospital-based surveillance

Prepare to implement surge plans at Federal medical facilities

POLICY DECISIONS

Prioritize efforts for domestic preparedness and response

STAGE 4

First Human Case in North America

GOALS

Contain first cases in North America

Antiviral treatment and prophylaxis

Implement national response

ACTIONS

Ensure pandemic plans activated across all levels

Limit non-essential domestic travel

Deploy diagnostic reagents for pandemic virus to all laboratories

Continue development of pandemic vaccine

Antiviral treatment and targeted antiviral prophylaxis

POLICY DECISIONS

Revision of prioritization and allocation scheme for pandemic vaccine

STAGE 5

Spread throughout United States

GOALS

Support community response

Preserve critical infrastructure

Mitigate illness, suffering, and death

Mitigate impact to economy and society

ACTIONS

Maintain overall situational awareness

Evaluate epidemiology; provide guidance on community measures

Deploy vaccine if available; prioritization guidance

Sustain critical infrastructure, support health and medical systems, maintain civil order

Provide guidance on use of key commodities

POLICY DECISIONS

Federal support of critical infrastructure and availability of key goods and services

Lifting of travel restrictions

HO Phase 6
lemic Period

Individual, Family, and Community Response to Pandemic Influenza

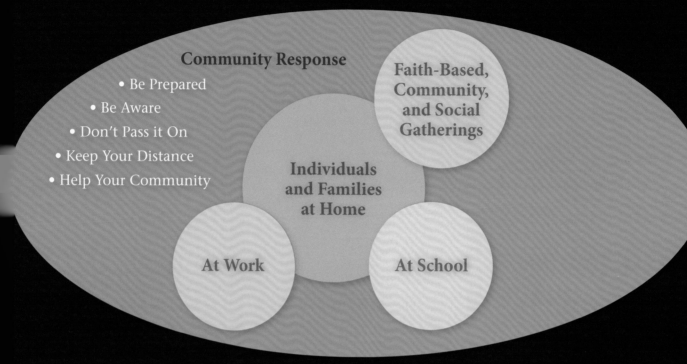

Community Response
- Be Prepared
- Be Aware
- Don't Pass it On
- Keep Your Distance
- Help Your Community

Faith-Based, Community, and Social Gatherings

Individuals and Families at Home

At Work

At School

Response	Individuals and Families	At School	At Work	Faith-Based, Community, and Social Gatherings
Be Prepared	Review Individuals and Families Planning Checklist www.pandemicflu.gov	Review School Planning Checklists www.pandemicflu.gov	Review Business Planning Checklist www.pandemicflu.gov	Review Faith-Based and Community Organizations Preparedness Checklist www.pandemicflu.gov
Be Aware	Identify trusted sources for information; stay informed about availability/use of anti-viral medications/vaccine	Review school pandemic plan; follow pandemic communication to students, faculty, and families	Review business pandemic plan; follow pandemic communication to employees and families	Stay abreast of community public health guidance on the advisability of large public gatherings and travel
Don't Pass it On	If you are ill--stay home; practice hand hygiene/cough etiquette; model behavior for your children; consider voluntary home quarantine if anyone ill in household	If you are ill--stay home; practice hand hygiene/cough etiquette; ensure sufficient infection control supplies	If you are ill--stay home; practice hand hygiene/cough etiquette; ensure sufficient infection control supplies	If you are ill--stay home; practice hand hygiene/cough etiquette; modify rites and religious practices that might facilitate influenza spread
Keep Your Distance	Avoid crowded social environments; limit non-essential travel	Prepare for possible school closures; plan home learning activities and exercises; consider childcare needs	Modify face-to-face contact; flexible worksite (telework); flexible work hours (stagger shifts); snow days	Cancel or modify activities, services, or rituals; follow community health social distancing recommendations
Help Your Community	Volunteer with local groups to prepare and assist with emergency response; get involved with your community as it prepares	Contribute to the local health department's operational plan for surge capacity of health care (if schools designated as contingency hospitals)	Identify assets and services your business could contribute to the community response to a pandemic	Provide social support services and help spread useful information, provide comfort, and encourage calm

CHAPTER 6 — PROTECTING HUMAN HEALTH

Introduction

Protecting human health is the crux of pandemic preparedness, and the goals and pillars of the *National Strategy for Pandemic Influenza (Strategy)* reflect this. If we fail to protect human health, we are likely to fail in our secondary goals of preserving societal function and mitigating the social and economic consequences of a pandemic. Consequently, the components of the Strategy, the elements of this Implementation Plan (Plan), and the projected allocation of resources to preparedness, surveillance, and response activities all reflect the overarching imperative to reduce the morbidity and mortality caused by a pandemic. In order to achieve this objective, we must leverage all instruments of national power and ensure coordinated action by all segments of government and society, while maintaining constitutional government, law and order, and other basic societal functions.

The emergence of an easily transmissible novel strain of influenza into a human population anywhere poses a threat to societies everywhere. Influenza does not respect geographic or political boundaries. When pandemic strains emerge they sweep through communities and nations with frightening velocity. The three pandemics of the 20th century each encircled the globe, sparing few if any communities, within months of their emergence into human populations. The cumulative and concentrated mortality of a pandemic can be appalling. The 1918 pandemic, for example, killed more people in 6 months than acquired immunodeficiency syndrome (AIDS) has killed in the last 25 years and more than were killed in all of World War I. The primary strategy for protecting human health, therefore, must be prevention of emergence of a pandemic strain from animal reservoirs, if possible, or rapid containment of a human outbreak at the source, if emergence does occur. Federal Government efforts to prepare for and to support prevention and containment strategies are described throughout this document.

Protecting human health in the setting of a pandemic will require: (1) effective domestic and international surveillance for, and prompt response to, influenza outbreaks in both humans and animals; (2) improved diagnostic tests; (3) the rapid development, production, and distribution of definitive medical countermeasures (i.e., vaccines); (4) the targeted and effective use of antiviral medications and other potentially scarce medical resources to treat symptomatic individuals; (5) the judicious application of community infection control measures; (6) effective communication of risk reduction strategies to the private sector and to individuals; and (7) the full collaboration of the public and the private sector. A dynamic and resourceful public health and medical response has the potential to save lives by delaying the occurrence of outbreaks, decreasing the proportion of the population who develop influenza or become critically ill, and reducing the burden on critical health care facilities. For such a response to occur, Federal, State, local, and tribal officials must ensure that all stakeholders understand their responsibilities and are adequately prepared to play their part, they must prioritize the use of scarce resources, and they must ensure the continuity of essential government, emergency, and medical services.

Fortunately, we live in an era of great medical and scientific progress. Today we have a better understanding of the influenza virus and the illness that it causes than ever before. Vaccinology is making rapid strides and we are learning more about the use of adjuvants and other dose-sparing strategies. Two new and effective antiviral medications (oseltamivir and zanamivir) have received Food and Drug Administration (FDA) approval in the last 7 years. We understand much more about the transmission dynamics and epidemiology of influenza than we did at the time of the last pandemic, in 1968. We have better international and domestic disease surveillance systems and we have developed a national network of diagnostic laboratories incorporating standardized reagents and protocols. Since September 11, 2001, we have made significant investments in all aspects of public health emergency preparedness. We are, in short, better prepared than ever to meet the immense challenge posed by a pandemic.

But the challenge will be formidable. We do not understand why some influenza viruses are efficiently transmitted and some are not. In the event of a pandemic, we will have to overcome severe shortfalls in surge capacity in our health care facilities. Our current vaccine production capabilities cannot keep pace with an evolving pandemic. We lack adequate stockpiles of antiviral medications and plans to distribute the supplies we have. Most surveillance systems do not operate in real time. We cannot quantify the value of many infection control strategies and do not know the optimal timing for or sequencing of those that would affect entire communities. Finally, and perhaps most importantly, members of the public may not appreciate the importance of the care they will provide to ill family members, the degree to which they can modify their risk of becoming ill, nor the extent to which their collective actions will shape the course of a pandemic.

Key Considerations

The overarching strategic goals of the *Strategy* are to: (1) stop, slow, or limit the spread of disease; (2) mitigate disease, suffering, and death; and (3) sustain infrastructure and mitigate impact to the economy and the functioning of society. These goals are not sequential but mutually supportive. The objective of the *Strategy* is to accomplish all three goals, to whatever extent possible, at all times during a pandemic.

Epidemiology

The transmission of a communicable agent between individuals is a chance event, the probability of which varies according to the nature and intimacy of their interactions. Epidemics occur when, on average, an infected individual transmits infection to more than one other person (R_0, or reproductive rate, >1). Conversely, and critically, outbreaks of infectious disease will diminish and ultimately terminate when, on average, an infected individual transmits infection to less than one other person (reproductive rate less than one). *The key to stopping an epidemic is to bring the reproductive rate below 1 and keep it there through whatever means, or combination of means, feasible.* These means can include the administration of effective vaccines or antiviral prophylaxis, the identification and isolation of infected individuals and quarantine of their contacts, and the implementation of appropriate infection control and social distancing measures.

The velocity of an epidemic — the speed with which an epidemic spreads through a community — is a function of the basic reproductive rate for the disease in question and how long it takes for infected individuals to infect others (generation time, or T_g). Influenza is moderately infectious but has a very short generation time. Recent estimates have suggested that while the reproductive rate for most strains of influenza is less than 2, the generation time may be as little as 2.6 days. These parameters predict that in the absence of disease containment measures the number of cases of epidemic influenza will double about every 3 days. It is important to note that the magnitude of the reproductive rate determines the intensity of measures required to halt transmission, while the components of the generation time — that is, the duration of the latent and infectious periods — determine how and when these measures must be applied.

Patients with influenza typically become infectious after about 1 to 1.5 days and prior to becoming symptomatic. At about 2 days, most infected persons will develop symptoms of illness, the spectrum and severity of which may vary considerably. Understanding the natural history of influenza makes it possible to assess potential response measures and determine the factors critical for their success. Given that 2 days will elapse between infection and illness in most cases, for example, a significant percentage of infected persons who travel internationally to the United States and are asymptomatic when boarding a flight will still be well upon arrival and will not be detected by screening at the border.

Pivotal Importance of Initial Conditions

While we cannot predict the severity of a pandemic before it begins, the initial analysis of the characteristics of the virus and its epidemiology will tell us much about the way in which the pandemic will unfold. The cardinal determinants of the public health response to a pandemic will be its severity, as defined by the ability of the pandemic virus to cause severe morbidity and mortality, especially in otherwise low-risk populations, and the availability and effectiveness of vaccine and antiviral medications.[15] Decisions about the prioritization and distribution of medical countermeasures; the content of risk communication campaigns; the application of community infection control measures; and whether and when to make adjustments in the delivery of care commensurate with available resources are interrelated and all fundamentally determined by these factors, which will be known from the beginning of an outbreak. These are the critical triggers that will dictate the actions of public health authorities.

Severe pandemics, for example, pose the greatest threat to critical infrastructure and national security. Groups receiving priority access to medical countermeasures during a severe pandemic will reflect the need to maintain infrastructure and security functions. When vaccine and antiviral drug supplies are very limited, targeting necessarily will be narrower and the importance of community infection control measures will be greater. An inadequate supply of countermeasures in the setting of a severe pandemic would also be an indication to authorities to expand surge capacity and prepare to alter standards of care by expanding staff, extending the defined roles of providers, and establishing infirmaries. Public messaging to health care professionals, other stakeholders, and the general public would seek to prepare them for a severe pandemic and the shortage of medical countermeasures. It would not be necessary to wait for numbers of cases to rise exponentially.

Greater vaccine and antiviral drug supply, on the other hand, would permit more flexibility in the strategies and objectives for the use of medical countermeasures. Preservation of critical infrastructure and security functions would still be crucial, but consideration might also be given to efforts to decrease transmission of infection in communities through the early immunization of children or by providing post-exposure prophylaxis to household contacts of ill persons. Anticipating a pandemic caused by a highly pathogenic virus, authorities would still move to expand surge capacity and prepare to change the way care is delivered by expanding staff, extending the defined roles of providers, and establishing infirmaries. Public messaging would be tailored accordingly.

In a less severe pandemic, where infrastructure and security concerns are not as significant, efforts could be focused on protecting those at high risk for severe disease and death from the beginning, especially if supplies of medical countermeasures are inadequate. Public health authorities might recommend home care, with or without isolation, for the great majority of patients and the costs and benefits of community infection control measures would be calculated differently.

---

[15] It is important to emphasize that the severity of a pandemic is a function not of the attack rate or transmissibility of the virus, both of which appear to be relatively constant between pandemics, but of its ability to produce severe illness or death. The severity of illness caused by a strain of influenza with pandemic potential will be quickly apparent, although continued monitoring and analysis will be necessary to refine initial assessments.

The value of a decision framework based on pandemic severity and the supply of vaccines and antiviral medications is that such a framework facilitates decisive and concrete pre-pandemic planning and allows the construction, in advance, of response algorithms and decision trees. It is important to caveat these observations by noting that since antiviral resistance can develop over time and the virulence of circulating strains may change as the virus adapts to its human hosts, ongoing monitoring for antiviral resistance and geographically circumscribed or more global changes in vaccine effectiveness or viral pathogenicity during a pandemic will be essential. Strategies for use of vaccine and antiviral medications that are in short supply may shift in response to such observations or as the supply of countermeasures changes over time.

Maintaining Situational Awareness

Surveillance

The goal of influenza surveillance is to track novel influenza subtypes and detect clusters of severe human infection heralding the emergence of strains with pandemic potential, so as to facilitate early and aggressive attempts at containment. International surveillance programs and goals are described in Chapter 4 - International Efforts. Domestic surveillance goals include detection of initial U.S. cases if the pandemic begins abroad, defining its spread, elucidating health impacts and high-risk groups, and monitoring characteristics of the virus, including antigenic and genetic changes, and changes in antiviral resistance patterns.

The Federal Government collects outpatient, hospital, and mortality surveillance data through a variety of systems and networks, and in recent years has improved its capability to aggregate and analyze data in real time. Unfortunately, current systems do not provide sufficient depth and coverage to guide all elements of the national response, and a great deal of analysis and time is required to assess the consequences of seasonal influenza outbreaks and the effectiveness of the annual vaccine. To remedy this shortcoming, and to enhance their own situational awareness, State and local public health departments should make it a priority to establish or enhance influenza surveillance systems within their jurisdictions. To improve national surveillance capabilities, the National Biosurveillance Integration System (NBIS) has been established to provide an all-source biosurveillance common operating picture to improve early-warning capabilities and facilitate national response activities through better situational awareness.

In the event of a pandemic, States should be prepared to increase diagnostic testing for influenza as well as the frequency of reporting to the Centers for Disease Control and Prevention (CDC). Early detection of pandemic virus at a local level requires the collection and testing of appropriate specimens as recommended. The most intense testing will be necessary during the early stages of a pandemic, when detecting the introduction of the virus into a State or community is the primary goal.

Response

Maintaining situational awareness during a pandemic will be extremely difficult. In addition to the surveillance and disease reporting activities described above, Federal, State, and local authorities will also be called upon to collect, analyze, integrate, and report information about the status of their hospitals and health care systems, critical infrastructure, and materiel requirements, and they will be called upon to supply such information at a time when their capabilities may be eroded by significant absenteeism.

Hospital and health care resource tracking can and should be performed in real time. The identification of stress points and focal insufficiencies in real time will permit the burden of patient care to be distributed across health care systems more equitably, preserving core functionalities despite significant and even extreme surges in demand. Additionally, the early recognition of increased systemic loads could serve as a trigger to public health officials to implement or promote more stringent disease containment measures and to make adjustments in the delivery of care commensurate with available resources.

Implementing disease containment and infection control measures is likely to impose significant costs on affected communities. Determining the optimal timing and thresholds for interventions with significant associated costs will be difficult in the absence of quantitative data about their effectiveness and the benefits they will confer. Insights into the biology and patterns of transmission of pandemic influenza, as well as the efficacy of various disease containment strategies, will evolve in real time and should be tractable to analysis and modeling.

Role of Rapid and Reliable Diagnostic Tests

During periods of heightened surveillance for the emergence of novel influenza strains and early in a pandemic, when disease is localized in one or several countries, both clinical and epidemiological (e.g., exposure) characteristics are important for surveillance and case detection. As the pandemic begins to spread, rapid diagnostic tests may be widely used to distinguish influenza A from other respiratory illnesses. Once pandemic disease is widespread, cases will be identified primarily by clinical presentation. Historically, most patients with pandemic influenza have presented with signs and symptoms similar to those of seasonal influenza, although in some the presentation is more fulminant and progresses very rapidly.

Rapid diagnostic tests for influenza are screening tests for influenza virus infection that provide results within 60 minutes and can be used for individuals or groups. Diagnostic tests will be most critical in the early phases of a pandemic, when identification of the first cases in a locality is important, and they may also be useful as the epidemic declines and pandemic disease becomes less prevalent. Depending on their sensitivity and specificity, such tests might also facilitate screening of travelers at ports of entry or prior to boarding inbound flights. At present, widely available rapid diagnostic tests and testing protocols do not distinguish between specific subtypes and strains of influenza and, because of their suboptimal sensitivity and specificity, cannot even definitively distinguish between influenza and other causes of similar illness. Because the available diagnostic tests have differing sensitivities, specificities, and technical requirements, they may find use in different settings and for different purposes during a pandemic.

New technologies and new approaches are driving down costs and improving the specificity and sensitivity of rapid diagnostic tests to the point that subtype- and strain-specific tests may be available for large-scale screening within the next couple of years. If these tests can be packaged in a way that facilitates their use in non-clinical settings, their potential to facilitate disease containment efforts will be even greater, by allowing more effective screening of travelers (and thus the more targeted application of movement restrictions) or even by identifying patients before they become symptomatic or infectious. The Federal Government will continue to support research in this area, in an effort to promote such advances.

In the interim, existing diagnostic technologies must be used to greatest effect to rapidly screen individuals infected with pandemic influenza. To this end, the Department of Health and Human Services (HHS), the Department of Agriculture (USDA), the Department of Energy (DOE), the Environmental Protection Agency (EPA), the Department of Defense (DOD), the Federal Bureau of Investigation (FBI), and the Department of Homeland Security (DHS) participate, with State and local public health laboratories, in the Laboratory Response Network (LRN), the member laboratories of which have adopted uniform diagnostic standards, protocols, and reagents, and can perform subtype- and strain-specific confirmation testing for influenza. HHS and the private sector have also developed high-throughput rapid diagnostic kits that will undergo field testing by U.S. and Southeast Asian scientists and public health officials to ascertain the utility and robustness of these products.

Countermeasure Production, Prioritization, Distribution, and Security

The optimal way to control the spread of a pandemic and reduce its associated morbidity and mortality is through the use of vaccines. Broadly speaking, vaccines may be divided into those that are developed against strains of animal influenza viruses that have caused isolated infections in humans, which may be regarded as "pre-pandemic" vaccines, and those that are developed against strains that have evolved the capacity for sustained and efficient human-to-human transmission ("pandemic" vaccines). Because emergence in human populations necessarily reflects genetic changes within the pandemic virus, pre-pandemic vaccines may be a good or poor match for — and offer greater or lesser protection against — the pandemic strain that ultimately emerges.

Current FDA-licensed inactivated influenza vaccines are based on technologies developed more than 30 years ago. Scientists first select the three virus strains that they expect to circulate in the United States during the following season. These strains are then adapted to grow in fertilized chicken eggs and manufacturers inject each adapted virus strain separately into millions of eggs, which are subsequently incubated to produce influenza virus. Large batches of these eggs are harvested and the viral particles that are obtained are inactivated, chemically disrupted, and blended into a single vaccine product that includes all three influenza virus strains. A single dose of the trivalent vaccine contains 15 ug of hemagglutinin for each of the three antigenic components. The total dose (45 ug) is approximately the amount of purified virus obtained from the allantoic fluid of one egg. Current manufacturing processes thus require manufacturers to procure one fertilized chicken egg for every dose of vaccine produced and are dependent on the timely availability of vaccine seed strains.

Antiviral medications can be used for treatment or prophylaxis of people exposed to influenza. Currently only two classes of medication — the neuraminidase inhibitors and the adamantanes — demonstrate efficacy against circulating influenza viruses. Both classes of medication are most effective if administered in the earliest stages of infection. Adamantane resistance emerges fairly quickly (adamantane-resistant H5N1 influenza already circulates, for example) and does not appear to affect viral fitness, in terms of the transmissibility of the virus or its ability to produce illness. Resistance to oseltamivir, the oral neuraminidase inhibitor, emerges more slowly but has been associated with treatment failure in patients with H5N1 influenza. Resistance to zanamivir, the inhaled neuraminidase inhibitor, has not been documented in immunocompetent hosts, but its efficacy in treating patients with H5N1 or other subtypes and strains with pandemic potential requires further assessment.

Production

The Federal Government has established two primary vaccine goals: (1) establishment and maintenance of stockpiles of pre-pandemic vaccine adequate to immunize 20 million persons against influenza strains that present a pandemic threat; and (2) expansion of domestic influenza vaccine manufacturing surge capacity for the production of pandemic vaccines for the entire domestic population within 6 months of a pandemic declaration.

While progress can be made toward the first goal with current egg-based manufacturing methods, the existing domestic influenza vaccine manufacturing base lacks sufficient surge capacity to meet the second. Moreover, since populations have no baseline immunity to strains of influenza with pandemic potential, it is highly probable that more vaccine antigen will be required per person to induce protective immunity. The amount of vaccine antigen that is currently manufactured is matched to the usual requirements for seasonal influenza vaccine, and not the requirements for a pandemic vaccine, which may require significantly more hemagglutinin per person than a seasonal vaccine to induce an effective immune response. Furthermore, in the event of a pandemic it is likely that bulk influenza vaccine manufactured outside the United States (and accounting for about 40 percent of annual domestic supply) will be unavailable. Thus, the measures taken by the Federal Government over the past several years to ensure a secure egg supply and support the expansion and diversification of influenza vaccine manufacturing capacity will require significant enhancement and acceleration.

The Federal Government has adopted a three-pronged strategy to secure the required surge capacity for pre-pandemic and pandemic vaccines. Current initiatives fall broadly under the categories of advanced vaccine development, establishment, and expansion of new U.S. vaccine manufacturing facilities, and vaccine acquisition. In keeping with our goal of developing a rapid response vaccine manufacturing capability, we will support the advanced development of cell-based influenza vaccine candidates. The Federal Government will also support the renovation of existing U.S. manufacturing facilities that produce other FDA-licensed cell-based vaccines or biologics as well as the establishment of new domestic cell-based influenza vaccine manufacturing facilities. To accommodate pre-pandemic vaccine needs without disturbing seasonal influenza vaccine manufacturing campaigns, the Federal Government will continue through 2008 to procure H5N1 vaccine from manufacturers of U.S.-licensed influenza vaccines. With these and other initiatives, the pandemic vaccine capacity goal for the United States may be within reach by the end of 2010.

Improvements in vaccine technology may alleviate some vaccine capacity concerns. Dose-sparing strategies for influenza vaccines that are currently under evaluation may reduce the requirement for vaccine antigen per dose and/or allow for effective immunization with a single shot. In the future, broad-spectrum influenza vaccines may supplement seasonal and pandemic influenza vaccines to provide broader virus specificity and longer persistence of enhanced immunity, especially in the populations most vulnerable to influenza — children, the elderly, and the chronically ill.

The Federal Government has established two primary goals for stockpiling existing antiviral medications: (1) establishment and maintenance of stockpiles adequate to treat 75 million persons, divided between Federal and State stockpiles; and (2) establishment and maintenance of a Federal stockpile of 6 million treatment courses reserved for containment efforts. In an effort to expand the medical armamentarium, the Federal Government is also supporting research projects to optimize dosing strategies for existing antiviral medications, identify novel drug targets, and develop compounds that inhibit viral entry, replication, and maturation.

---

[16] Cell-based manufacturing methods use mammalian cells to grow the influenza viruses used in the vaccine and offer a number of advantages. Vaccine manufacturers can bypass the step needed to adapt the virus strains to grow in eggs. Cells may be frozen in advance and large volumes grown quickly. U.S. licensure and manufacture of influenza vaccines produced in cell culture also will provide security against risks associated with egg-based production, such as shortages and the potential for egg supplies to be contaminated by various poultry-based diseases. Finally, the new cell-based influenza vaccines will provide an option for people who are allergic to eggs and therefore unable to receive the currently licensed vaccines. It should be noted that certain issues must be addressed by extensive testing and characterization prior to the banking and use of mammalian cells for vaccine production. For example, such cells may be at risk of contamination with various disease-causing organisms affecting the animals from which the cells or cell-growth media components were derived, and there may be tumorigenicity concerns with cells that may be useful for high-yield manufacturing.

Prioritization

The Federal Government is developing guidelines to assist State and local governments and the private sector in defining groups that should receive priority access to scarce medical countermeasures. Priority recommendations will reflect the pandemic response goals of limiting mortality and severe morbidity; maintaining critical infrastructure and societal function; diminishing economic impacts; and maintaining national security. Limiting transmission also may be an objective. Antiviral prophylaxis of household contacts of infected individuals and vaccination of children may decrease disease spread in affected communities but would require large quantities of drug and vaccine. If supplies and public health resources were sufficient, these strategies might be pursued in certain settings.

Priorities for vaccine and antiviral drug use will vary based on pandemic severity as well as the vaccine and drug supply. In settings of very limited vaccine and drug supply, narrow targeting and efficient use are required. Vaccine may be reserved for critical personnel, while antiviral medications are reserved for symptomatic individuals who are at high risk of serious complications or death. With greater availability, it may be feasible to expand priority groups and implement strategies to limit disease transmission. Recognizing that no single priority list is appropriate for all scenarios, Federal guidance will be developed for multiple contingencies.

The use of pre-pandemic vaccine will be targeted to maintain critical societal functions through the protection of critical infrastructure personnel and to protect those who are at greater risk of early exposure and infection during a pandemic, such as health care providers or first responders. Pre-pandemic vaccination objectives may include primary immunization if the match between the pre-pandemic vaccine and the circulating virus is close, or priming the immune system to respond more rapidly and robustly to an initial dose of pandemic vaccine, when it becomes available, if the match is suboptimal.

Recommendations put forward by the Advisory Committee on Immunization Practices and the National Vaccine Advisory Committee are included in the *HHS Pandemic Influenza Plan* and provide initial guidance to Federal, State, local, and tribal partners regarding many of the potential target groups being considered.

Distribution

When sustained and efficient human-to-human transmission of a potential pandemic influenza strain is documented anywhere in the world, the Federal Government will develop and distribute recommendations on target groups for vaccine and antiviral drugs. These recommendations will reflect data from the pandemic and available supplies of medical countermeasures in light of the considerations outlined above. These recommendations will be provided to Federal health care providers and State, local, and tribal authorities.

A treatment course of oseltamivir for adults and adolescents ages 13 and above is 1 capsule taken twice daily for 5 days, or 10 capsules. A typical prophylaxis course for adults and adolescents is one capsule taken once daily for at least 10 days, although oseltamivir has been shown to be safe and effective when taken for up to 6 weeks. Because prophylaxis requires significantly more medication, results in the administration of a scarce medical resource to people who might not have become sick in any case, and only reduces risk during the period when the medication is being taken, current plans propose using antiviral medication stockpiles only for treatment once a pandemic is underway. Prophylactic use of antiviral medications will be reserved for initial containment efforts and other highly select circumstances.

Given the highly distributed nature of a pandemic, the need to deliver antiviral prophylaxis within 2 days of exposure or to provide therapy to infected patients within 2 days of the onset of symptoms presents significant unresolved logistical challenges. It will be necessary to develop and exercise pandemic influenza countermeasure distribution plans in each of the States and territories and public-private partnerships supporting the seamless, efficient, and timely distribution of these countermeasures may also be required.

Security

It is conceivable that criminal elements may try to take advantage of medical countermeasure scarcity and citizens' fears regarding a pandemic by producing and distributing counterfeit vaccines and antiviral medications. The Federal Government will aggressively monitor efforts to produce and distribute counterfeit drugs, both domestically and internationally, and ensure that existing laws are vigorously enforced in order to deter such conduct, protect the integrity of our drug supply, and maintain public confidence.

Reducing Disease Transmission and Rates of Illness

While preventing a pandemic after person-to-person transmission becomes well established may be impossible, the systematic application of disease containment measures can significantly reduce disease transmission rates with concomitant reductions in the intensity and velocity of any pandemics that do occur. The goals of disease containment after a pandemic is underway are to delay the spread of disease and the occurrence of outbreaks in U.S. communities, to decrease the clinical attack rate in affected communities, and to distribute the number of cases that do occur over a longer interval, so as to minimize social and economic disruption and to minimize, so far as possible, hospitalization and death. Investigation of early local outbreaks of pandemic influenza will provide helpful clinical and epidemiological information and support real-time modeling of pandemic response measures.

The primary strategies for preventing pandemic influenza are the same as those for seasonal influenza: vaccination; early detection and treatment with antiviral medications; and the use of infection control measures to prevent transmission. However, when a pandemic begins, a vaccine might not be widely available, and the supply of antiviral drugs may be limited. The ability to limit transmission and delay the spread of the pandemic will therefore rely primarily on the appropriate and thorough application of infection control measures in health care facilities, the workplace, the community, and for individuals at home. CDC recommendations in this regard are described at length in Supplement 4 of the *HHS Pandemic Influenza Plan.*

In the initial stages of a domestic outbreak, it might be feasible to perform case tracking and contact tracing, with isolation of individuals with known pandemic influenza and voluntary quarantine of their close contacts. Antiviral post-exposure prophylaxis targeted at contacts of the first cases identified in the United States may slow the spread of the pandemic. Quarantine of case contacts has played an important role in the management of outbreaks of other diseases transmitted by large-particle droplets, but its role in containing influenza has not been fully defined.

Depending on the severity of a pandemic and its anticipated effects on health care systems and the functioning of critical infrastructure, communities may recommend or implement general measures to promote social distancing and the disaggregation of disease transmission networks. As a general rule, the value of such measures will be greatest if the interventions are implemented early in the course of a community outbreak and sustained until definitive countermeasures are available. In the case of a pandemic, where it may not be possible to delay the spread of disease indefinitely, the goal of such measures will be to decrease the clinical attack rate and to distribute the number of cases that do occur over a longer interval, so as to minimize social and economic disruption.

Some social distancing measures, such as the recommendation to maintain one-yard spatial separation between individuals or the recommendation to businesses to conduct meetings by teleconference, will be sustainable indefinitely at comparatively minimal cost, whereas others (e.g., implementation of "snow day" restrictions) are associated with substantial costs and can be sustained only for limited periods. Low-cost or sustainable social distancing measures should be introduced immediately after a community outbreak begins, while the more costly and non-sustainable measures should be reserved for situations in which the need for disease containment is critical. Decisions as to how and when to implement such social distancing measures will be made on a community-by-community basis, with the Federal Government providing technical support and guidance to local officials.

The clinical attack rates for seasonal and pandemic influenza are highest among children. Closure of schools and targeted vaccination of children have demonstrated efficacy in diminishing community influenza rates. Modeling supports school closure as an effective means of reducing overall attack rates within communities and suggests that the value of this intervention is maximized if school closure occurs early in the course of a community outbreak. Cancellation of non-essential public gatherings, restrictions on long-distance travel, and social distancing within the workplace could also potentially decrease rates of influenza transmission, but the real-world effectiveness of these interventions has not been quantified. Measures to be considered within schools and in the workplace are described in Chapter 9.

"Snow day" restrictions — the recommendation or mandate by authorities that individuals and families limit social contacts by remaining within their households — should reduce community transmission rates and would afford protection to households where infection has not yet occurred. How long and how effectively snow day restrictions can be maintained has not been determined and thus the value of such restrictions has not been quantified. For maximum effectiveness and to the extent possible, snow day restrictions should be maintained for at least two incubation periods, as defined by epidemiological analysis of the circulating pandemic strain. In the absence of definitive countermeasures (i.e., an effective vaccine), snow day restrictions will serve to disrupt but not stop community transmission of influenza. The uses of snow day restrictions during a pandemic will vary. They might be employed to decompress health care facilities by temporarily reducing the rate of new infections within an affected community. The optimal timing for the implementation of snow day restrictions has not been determined but should be tractable to modeling. The economic impacts of snow day restrictions could be quite large and should be weighed against the likely health benefits.

Geographic Quarantine *(Cordon Sanitaire)*

Geographic quarantine is the isolation, by force if necessary, of localities with documented disease transmission from localities still free of infection. It has been used intermittently throughout history in efforts to contain serious epidemics and must be differentiated from the quarantine of case contacts, where exposure to an infectious agent but not infection per se has been confirmed. Geographic quarantine results in the detention, within an epidemic zone, of persons who may or may not have been exposed to the pathogen in question. Some nations, notably Australia in the fall of 1918, have imposed reverse geographic quarantines, in an effort to keep epidemic disease out. The value of efforts to impose modified forms of reverse geographic quarantine is discussed at greater length in Chapter 5. In summary, even if such efforts prove unsuccessful, delaying the spread of the disease could provide the Federal Government with valuable time to activate the domestic response.

Once influenza transmission has occurred in multiple discrete locations, and it is clear that containment efforts have failed, the value of conventional geographic quarantine as a disease containment measure in any particular locality will be profoundly limited. Whether geographic quarantine should play a role in efforts to contain an outbreak of influenza with pandemic potential at its source will depend on the area and population affected, whether the implementation of a *cordon sanitaire* is feasible, the likelihood of success of other public health interventions, the ability of authorities to provide for the needs of the quarantined population, and in all likelihood geopolitical considerations that are beyond the scope of this chapter. The implementation of conventional geographic quarantine imposes significant opportunity costs and may result in the diversion of significant resources and assets that might be used to better effect supporting less draconian disease containment measures.

Quarantine at the level of families and individuals is a legitimate public health intervention that figured prominently in the public health response to severe acute respiratory syndrome (SARS). It is important to underscore that the value of individual quarantine as a public health intervention is determined by the biology of the agent against which it is directed. Because influenza infection can be transmitted by persons who are not ill, and because viral shedding occurs prior to the onset of clinical illness, isolation of ill persons or exclusion from work of those who are ill will reduce but not prevent transmission in public settings. Because of influenza's short generation period, isolation and quarantine must be implemented very quickly to have an impact and will not be as effective as for a disease like SARS or smallpox where the generation time is longer and asymptomatic shedding of virus does not appear to be significant. Nevertheless, the value of isolating patients with pandemic influenza and quarantining their contacts is clearly supported by recent modeling efforts.

Expanding Medical Surge Capacity

While a pandemic may strain hundreds of communities simultaneously, each community will experience the pandemic as a local event. In the best of circumstances, patients and health care resources are not easily redistributed; in a pandemic, conditions would make the sharing of resources and burdens even more difficult. The Federal Government will provide medical countermeasures, resources, and personnel, if available, in support of communities experiencing pandemic influenza, but communities should anticipate that in the event of multiple simultaneous outbreaks, the Federal Government may not possess sufficient medical resources or personnel to augment local capabilities. The development of medical and public health mutual aid arrangements through the Emergency Management Assistance Compact (EMAC) and other mechanisms is encouraged, but States and localities should anticipate that all sources of external aid may be compromised during a pandemic.

Personnel

During a pandemic, the number of persons seeking medical care is expected to increase significantly and overcrowding may lead hospital and other health care institutions to adjust clinical care algorithms in order to optimize the allocation of scarce resources. Since most health professionals are already geographically dispersed, local and State governments are in a position to take primary responsibility for identifying, registering, and coordinating volunteer medical and health care personnel within their jurisdictions to respond to any surge in demand for health care. HHS has partnered with States and localities through the Medical Reserve Corps and the Emergency System for the Advanced Registration of Volunteer Health Professionals (ESAR-VHP) Programs to develop locally sponsored emergency response teams and state-based volunteer registries to recruit, credential, and mobilize health care personnel in the event of a large scale medical emergency.

Medical Standards of Care

If a pandemic overwhelms the health and medical capacity of a community, it will be impossible to provide the level of medical care that would be expected under pre-pandemic circumstances. It may be necessary because of hospital overcrowding to establish pre-hospital facilities and alternate-care sites to provide supplemental capacity. In some circumstances, it may be necessary to apply triage principles in the hospital to regulate which patients gain access to intensive care units (ICUs) and ventilators, and it is likely that vaccine, pharmaceuticals, and other medical materiel will also be rationed. Non-clinical personnel and family members may be asked to assist with administrative and environmental tasks, while qualified clinicians may be asked to perform unfamiliar functions such as staffing temporary medical care facilities, visiting patients in their homes, or providing medical advice via on-line or hot-line connections.

The terms 'altered' and 'degraded' standards of care have often been applied to such situations in both government documents and the medical literature. The legal and ethical 'standard of care,' however, is what is reasonably expected of medical systems and providers and is determined by extant circumstances. Relevant conditions include the availability of hospital, ICU, or specialty care beds; medical equipment and materiel; and personnel who are trained and qualified to provide care. As in all situations involving the allocation of scarce medical resources, the standard of care will be met if resources are fairly distributed and are utilized to achieve the greatest benefit. In a pandemic, hospital and ICU beds, ventilators, and other medical services may be rationed. As in other situations of scarce medical resources, preference will be given to those whose medical condition suggests that they will obtain greatest benefit from them. Such rationing differs from approaches to care in which resources are provided on a first-come, first-served basis or to patients with the most severe illnesses or injuries.

Given the strain that a pandemic would place on a community's medical system, it will be necessary for hospitals, medical providers, and oversight agencies to maximize hospital bed surge capacity, and triage and treat patients in a manner that affords each the best chance of survival and recovery within the limits of available resources. In addition, the public must be informed regarding when, how, and where to obtain medical care. In all cases, the goal should be to provide care and allocate scarce equipment, supplies, and personnel in a way that saves the largest number of lives. Planning should therefore include thresholds for altering triage algorithms and otherwise optimizing the allocation of scarce resources. Where prospective and mature data are available, changes in clinical care algorithms should be evidence-based.

In planning for a prolonged mass casualty event, it must be recognized that persons with unrelated medical conditions will continue to require emergency, acute, and chronic care. It is important to keep the health care system functioning and to deliver the best care possible to preserve as many lives as possible. Planning a health and medical response to a mass casualty event must be comprehensive, community-based, and coordinated at the regional level. In making adjustments in the delivery of care because of constrained resources, individual autonomy, privacy, and dignity should be protected to the extent possible and reasonable under the circumstances. Finally, clear communication with the public is essential before, during, and after a mass casualty event such as a pandemic.

Availability of Medical Materiel

Health care facilities typically maintain limited inventories of supplies on-site and depend on just-in-time restocking programs. Replenishment of critical inventories is thus dependent upon an intact supply chain from manufacturing and distribution to transportation and receiving. During a pandemic there would be an increased demand for both consumable and durable resources. Examples of critical supplies are listed in Supplement 3 to the *HHS Pandemic Influenza Plan*. Competition for these resources at a time of increased demand could result in critical shortages.

Manufacturers and suppliers are likely to report inventory shortages because of the massive simultaneity of need and supply chains may also be disrupted by the effects of a pandemic on critical personnel. Medical facilities should make provision for these considerations in their planning efforts and consider stockpiling critical medical materiel individually or collaborating with other facilities to develop local or regional stockpiles maintained under vendor managed inventory systems.

Facilities

Health care facilities will face increased demand for isolation wards, intensive care unit beds, and ventilators. Historical comparisons and recent severe seasonal influenza epidemics suggest that U.S. health care facilities would be overwhelmed with influenza patients during a pandemic. Extrapolating from the 1918 pandemic, a severe pandemic could result at its peak in the need for significantly more hospital and intensive care unit beds than the U.S. health care system currently supports.

Because of the intense but transient demand for clinical care areas, and because cohorting of patients with pandemic influenza in common treatment areas is an acceptable response to hospital overcrowding, establishing infirmaries in armories or other facilities of opportunity to supplement existing health care facilities is a reasonable consideration for those not critically ill. Suitable spaces can be identified in the pre-pandemic phase, medical materiel and supplies can be stockpiled prospectively, and actions to stand up the infirmary commenced in the early stages of an outbreak. The Federal Government has assembled a limited number of Federal Medical Stations (FMSs), which are scalable, modular, 250-bed deployable caches that require 40,000 square feet of enclosed space and an enabling environment (i.e., loading docks, electrical power source systems, climate control, communications, information technology support) and are configured to provide basic but essential medical care.[17]

Psychosocial Concerns

During a pandemic, psychosocial issues may play significantly contribute to, or hinder, the effectiveness of the response. Public anxiety and subjective perception of risk during the initial phases will impact the degree of medical surge; overall compliance with quarantine, snow days, and other control procedures; and participation of the workforce, including health care workers, in response efforts. In later stages of the epidemic, other psychosocial factors may also emerge. During the 1918-1919 "Spanish flu," for example, people experienced significant distress due to loss of family members and anxiety about work, food, transportation, and basic infrastructure, while the SARS outbreak in 2003 led to psychological distress for health care workers and the general public because of social isolation, stigmatization of groups perceived to be high risk, and general fears about safety and health. While most people are resilient and will need minimal psychological support to cope with catastrophic events such as an influenza pandemic, it is imperative that planning for behavioral health reactions be undertaken to support affected populations and possibly reduce the occurrence of long-term psychological distress. Such planning should involve efforts to recruit, credential, and mobilize mental health and substance abuse personnel (as part of personnel efforts discussed above), along with the development of materials on psychological self-care and related topics, including a plan for dissemination of such materials.

---

[17] Staffing for FMS units is not provided automatically but must be drawn from available Federal, State, or local medical personnel.

Emergency Medical Services

Emergency Medical Services (EMS) provide critical pre-hospital care and transportation and the individuals engaged in these services are among the high priority groups considered for vaccination. However, when a pandemic begins, a vaccine may not be widely available, and the supply of antiviral drugs may be limited. Illness and absenteeism may adversely affect these services and local governments and hospitals may need to explore alternative methods of transporting patients.

Pre-hospital EMS transportation capability will play a critical role in responding to requests for assistance, providing treatment, and in triaging patients. 9-1-1 call centers/public safety answering points (PSAPs) will experience a significant surge in calls and will determine how and when EMS units are dispatched. Coordination and communication between public health, PSAPs, EMS, and hospital officials will be necessary to ensure optimal patient care as hospital bed availability and pre-hospital resources are strained. Planners should consider modifying PSAP call-taker and dispatch protocols and developing pandemic-specific pre-hospital triage and treatment protocols. A robust statewide or regional system for monitoring PSAP medical calls, EMS responses and transports, and hospital bed availability will be critical for tracking and responding to a pandemic.

Persons with emergency medical licensure not engaged in transporting patients could potentially provide support to personnel working in hospitals and infirmaries and could, with additional education, training and legal authority, broaden their scopes of practice during the emergency and, for instance, administer vaccinations to the public or other emergency support personnel.

Home-based Care

Given that most persons with pandemic influenza will experience typical influenza symptoms, most persons who seek care can be managed appropriately by outpatient providers using a home-based approach. Appropriate management of outpatient pandemic influenza cases may reduce the risk of progression to severe disease and thereby reduce demand for inpatient care. A system of effective home-based care would decrease the burden on health care providers and hospitals and lessen exposure of uninfected persons to persons with influenza. Telephone call centers should be established or augmented within affected communities to provide advice on whether to stay home or to seek care. Home health care providers and organizations can provide follow-up for those managed at home, decreasing potential exposure of the public to persons who are ill and may transmit infection.

Fatality Management

Given the anticipated increase in the number of deaths associated with an influenza pandemic, hospitals and health care facilities working with State, local, or tribal health officials and medical examiners should assess current capacity for refrigeration of deceased persons, discuss mass fatality plans and identify temporary morgue sites, and determine the scope and volume of supplies needed to handle an increased number of deceased persons.

Risk Communication

Government and public health officials must communicate clearly and continuously with the public prior to and throughout a pandemic. To maintain public confidence and to enlist the support of individuals and families in disease containment efforts, public officials must provide unambiguous and consistent guidance on what individuals can do to protect themselves, how to care for family members at home, when and where to seek medical care, and how to protect others and minimize the risks of disease transmission.

Individuals will, in general, respond to a pandemic and to public health interventions in ways that they perceive to be congruent with their interests and their instinct for self-preservation, and public health authorities should tailor their risk communication campaigns and interventions accordingly. The public will respond favorably to messages that acknowledge its concerns, allay anxiety and uncertainty, and provide clear incentives for desirable behavior. The information provided by public health officials should therefore be useful, addressing immediate needs, but it should also help private citizens recognize and understand the degree to which their collective actions will shape the course of a pandemic.

Providing regular messages through a single spokesperson with professional credibility is highly desirable. Conveying clinical information requires particular care to ensure that a lay audience can understand it. Distinguishing between political and professional messages is essential. Provisions should be made for communication in languages other than English and for those with disabilities.

Other important objectives for communication campaigns include providing information to the public about the status of the response; providing anticipatory guidance and dispelling unrealistic expectations regarding the delivery of health and medical care; providing guidance on how to obtain information about the status of missing persons; and providing information related to influenza complications, including where to seek help if people are having significant difficulties in coping with personal losses or fears about the pandemic.

Regulatory / Financial / Legal Matters

More than one in four Americans receive health care coverage through Medicare, Medicaid, the State Children's Health Insurance Program (SCHIP), the Veterans Health Administration, TRICARE, or other Federal programs. Ensuring access to, and timely payment for, covered services during a pandemic will be critical to maintaining a functional health care infrastructure. It may also be necessary to extend certain waivers or develop incident-specific initiatives or coverage to facilitate access to care. Pandemic influenza response activities may exceed the budgetary resources of responding Federal and State government agencies, requiring compensatory legislative action.

Depending on the severity of a pandemic, certain requirements may be waived or revised to facilitate efficient delivery of health care services. For example, certain Emergency Medical Treatment and Active Labor Act (EMTALA), Medicare, Medicaid, SCHIP, and Health Insurance Portability and Accountability Act (HIPAA) requirements may be waived following a declaration of a public health emergency by the Secretary of HHS and a Presidential declaration of a major disaster or emergency. The authority to waive or amend legal requirements during a pandemic corresponds with the level of government that issues the requirements, whether Federal, State, or local. Statutes and rules may provide flexibility without waiver or revision. For example, HIPAA regulations allow covered entities to disclose patient information in circumstances that could arise during a pandemic, including disclosures: to provide treatment; to public health authorities for disease prevention and control and public health surveillance, investigations, and interventions; to lessen an imminent threat to health and safety; and to contact family members, guardians, or caretakers. In all cases, it will be important to make providers and institutions aware of the established legal framework, so that it is clear which authorities and regulations do or do not apply in a given situation.

Prior to the declaration of a public health emergency, State and local planners should examine existing State public health and medical licensing laws, interstate emergency management compacts and mutual aid agreements, and other legal and regulatory arrangements to determine the extent to which they meet potential new threats. Waivers granted at any level are likely to be targeted to an affected area for a temporary and specified period of time. In the case of an evolving pandemic, it will therefore be important to have the flexibility to extend or expand such waivers as needed.

Roles and Responsibilities

The responsibility for preparing for, detecting, and responding to influenza outbreaks is shared by everyone. This includes private citizens, health care providers, the private sector, State, local, and tribal public health authorities, and the Federal Government. State, local, and tribal governments, the private sector, and the Federal Government all have important and interdependent roles in preparing for, responding to, and recovering from a pandemic. Effective management of the Nation's medical and public health response systems during a pandemic will require coordinated action by all segments of government and society.

State, local, and tribal governments are primarily responsible for detecting and responding to disease outbreaks and implementing measures to minimize the consequences of an outbreak. The Federal Government supports detection and response in many ways, including providing response personnel and expertise, response materiel, diagnostic reference services and testing support, and funding for certain response activities. It is anticipated that the potentially catastrophic nature of a pandemic may overwhelm local, State, and tribal capabilities. Federal agencies will be called upon to provide additional support, but even those resources may be overwhelmed at the peak of a pandemic.

The Federal Government

The Federal Government will use all capabilities within its authority to support the private sector and State, local, and tribal public health authorities in preparedness and response activities. It will increase readiness to sustain essential Federal public health and medical functions during a pandemic and provide public health and medical support services under the *National Response Plan* (NRP). It will be prepared to advise State, local, and tribal governments and the medical and public health communities at large on how to deploy scarce medical resources, use and sequence community infection control measures, and address the medical challenges posed by pandemic influenza. It will perform surveillance for and monitor the progress of a pandemic on a national and international scale, support the development and production of medical countermeasures, and sponsor research on influenza viruses with pandemic potential. It will provide financial support and technical assistance to State, local, and tribal governments as they develop pandemic preparedness plans.

Department of Health and Human Services: HHS's primary responsibilities are those actions required to protect the health of all Americans, including communication of information related to pandemic influenza, leading international and domestic efforts in surveillance and detection of influenza outbreaks, ensuring the provision of essential human services, implementing measures to limit spread, and providing recommendations related to the use, distribution, and allocation of countermeasures and to the provision of care in mass casualty settings. HHS will support rapid containment of localized outbreaks domestically and provide guidance to State, local, and tribal public health authorities on the use, timing, and sequencing of community infection control measures. HHS also supports biomedical research and development of new vaccines and medical countermeasures.

Department of Homeland Security: Pursuant to Homeland Security Presidential Directive 7 (HSPD-7), DHS coordinates overall domestic incident management and Federal response procedures under the NRP and National Incident Management System (NIMS). Under the NRP, DHS is responsible for coordinating the protection of the Nation's critical infrastructure, and within the framework of Emergency Support Function #8 - Public Health and Medical Services (ESF #8) for the deployment of available NDMS medical, mortuary, and veterinary response assets.

Department of Defense: The primary responsibility of DOD is to preserve national security by protecting American forces, maintaining operational readiness, and sustaining critical military missions. DOD's first priority with respect to protecting human health will be to ensure sufficient capability to provide medical care to DOD forces and beneficiaries. DOD can provide medical, public health, transportation, logistical, communications, and other support consistent with existing legal authorities and to the extent that DOD's National Security preparedness is not compromised. Ideally, the human and technical resources of the National Guard should be balanced between support to the Governors of the individual States and the overall needs of national security.

Department of Veterans Affairs: VA provides health care, monetary benefits, and burial benefits to our Nation's veterans. VA's priority with respect to protecting human health is to deliver health care to enrolled veterans and beneficiaries. VA also has a mission to provide medical surge capacity for treatment of casualties arising from DOD operations and can provide other support to the extent that VA's mission to serve veterans is not compromised.

Department of Labor: DOL's primary responsibilities are those actions required to protect the health and safety of workers, including communication of information related to pandemic influenza to workers and employers, and other relevant activities.

State, Local, and Tribal Entities

State, local, and tribal entities should have credible pandemic preparedness plans that address key response issues and outline strategies to mitigate the human, social, and economic consequences of a pandemic. They will initiate the request for the delivery and be primarily responsible for the distribution of medical countermeasures released from national stockpiles. States should be prepared to face challenges in the availability of essential commodities, demands for health care services that exceed existing capacity, and public pressure to enforce infection control measures in ways that may hinder the delivery of emergency services and supplies and exacerbate the economic repercussions of the pandemic. States, localities, and tribal entities should work to improve communication between public health departments and both private sector partners, such as health care facilities, community- and faith-based organizations, and clinical laboratories that are likely to be involved in the response to a pandemic. State, local, and tribal public health departments should coordinate their planning efforts with local Federal health care facilities.

The Private Sector and Critical Infrastructure Entities

The private sector will play an integral role in preparedness before a pandemic begins and should be part of the national response. Businesses and corporations, especially those within sectors constituting the Nation's critical infrastructure, should develop continuity of operations plans that provide for workforce health protection and ensure that essential functions and vital services can be performed in the setting of significant absenteeism. Businesses and corporations should be prepared for public health interventions and recommendations that may increase absenteeism. Elements of the private sector concerned with health care should be prepared to support local, State, national, and international efforts to contain or mitigate a pandemic.

Individuals and Families

Private citizens must recognize and understand the degree to which their personal actions will govern the course of a pandemic. The success or failure of infection control measures is ultimately dependent upon the acts of individuals, and the collective response of 300 million Americans will significantly influence the shape of the pandemic and its medical, social, and economic outcomes (see *Individual, Family, and Community Response to Pandemic Influenza* between Chapters 5 and 6). Individuals will, in general, respond to a pandemic and to public health interventions in ways that they perceive to be congruent with their interests and their instinct for self-preservation, and public health authorities should tailor their risk communication campaigns and interventions accordingly. Institutions in danger of becoming over-whelmed will rely on the voluntarism and sense of civic and humanitarian duty of ordinary Americans. The talents and skills of individuals will prove crucial in our Nation's response to a pandemic.

Actions and Expectations

6.1. Pillar One: Preparedness and Communication

Preparedness and transparency are critical elements of the Strategy and the foundation of efforts to detect, contain, limit, delay, and mitigate a pandemic. Activities that should be undertaken before a pandemic to ensure preparedness and to communicate expectations and responsibilities to all levels of government and society are described below.

a. Planning for a Pandemic

6.1.1. Continue to work with States, localities, and tribal entities to establish and exercise pandemic response plans.

6.1.1.1. The Federal Government shall, and State, local, and tribal governments should, define and test actions and priorities required to prepare for and respond to a pandemic, within 6 months. Measure of performance: completion and communication of national, departmental, State, local, and tribal pandemic influenza response plans; actions and priorities defined and tested.

6.1.1.2. HHS, in coordination with DHS, shall review and approve State Pandemic Influenza plans to supplement and support DHS State Homeland Security Strategies to ensure that Federal homeland security grants, training, exercises, technical, and other forms of assistance are applied to a common set of priorities, capabilities, and performance benchmarks, in conformance with the National Preparedness Goal, within 12 months. Measure of performance: definition of priorities, capabilities, and performance benchmarks; percentage of States with plans that address priorities, identify capabilities, and meet benchmarks.

6.1.1.3. DHS, in coordination with HHS, DOJ, DOT, and DOD, shall be prepared to provide emergency response element training (e.g., incident management, triage, security, and communications) and exercise assistance upon request of State, local, and tribal communities and public health entities within 6 months. Measure of performance: percentage of requests for training and assistance fulfilled.

6.1.2. **Build upon existing domestic mechanisms to develop medical and veterinary surge capacity within or across jurisdictions to match medical requirements with capabilities.**

6.1.2.1. All health care facilities should develop and test infectious disease surge capacity plans that address challenges including: increased demand for services, staff shortages, infectious disease isolation protocols, supply shortages, and security.

6.1.2.2. HHS, in coordination with DHS, DOD, and VA, shall develop a joint strategy defining the objectives, conditions, and mechanisms for deployment under which NDMS assets, U.S. Public Health Service (PHS) Commissioned Corps, Epidemic Intelligence Service (EIS) officers, and DOD/VA health care personnel and public health officers would be deployed during a pandemic, within 9 months. Measure of performance: interagency strategy completed and tested for the deployment of Federal medical personnel during a pandemic.

6.1.2.3. HHS, in coordination with DHS, DOT, DOD, and VA, shall work with State, local, and tribal governments and leverage Emergency Management Assistance Compact agreements to develop protocols for distribution of critical medical materiel (e.g., ventilators) in times of medical emergency within 6 months. Measure of performance: critical medical material distribution protocols completed and tested.

6.1.2.4. HHS, in coordination with DOD and VA, in collaboration with medical professional and specialty societies, within their domains of expertise, shall develop guidance for allocating scarce health and medical resources during a pandemic, within 6 months. Measure of performance: guidance developed and disseminated.

6.1.2.5. HHS shall package and offer to the States and Territories the core operating components of an ESAR-VHP system within 6 months and encourage all States and tribal entities to implement the ESAR-VHP program by providing technical assistance and orientations at State and territory request to implement and operate Federal guideline (ESAR-VHP) compliant systems within 12 months. Measure of performance: guidance and technical assistance, as requested, provided to States to implement ESAR-VHP capability, compliant with Federal guidelines, in all States and U.S. territories.

6.1.2.6. HHS, in coordination with the USA Freedom Corps and Citizen Corps programs, shall continue to work with States and local communities to expand the Medical Reserve Corps program by 20 percent within 12 months. Measure of performance: increase number of Medical Reserve Corps units by 20 percent, from 350 to 420 units.

6.1.2.7.   HHS, in coordination with DHS, DOD, VA and the USA Freedom Corps and Citizen Corps programs, shall prepare guidance for local Medical Reserve Corps coordinators describing the role of the Medical Reserve Corps during a pandemic, within 3 months. Measure of performance: guidance materials developed and published on Medical Reserve Corps website (www.medicalreservecorps.gov).

6.1.2.8.   DHS, in coordination with the USA Freedom Corps, shall direct other Citizen Corps programs to prepare guidance detailing appropriate pandemic preparedness activities for each program, within 3 months. Measure of performance: guidance materials developed and published on Citizen Corps website and component program websites.

b. Communicating Expectations and Responsibilities

6.1.3.   Work to ensure clear, effective, and coordinated risk communication, domestically and internationally, before and during a pandemic. This includes identifying credible spokespersons at all levels of government to effectively coordinate and communicate helpful, informative messages in a timely manner.

6.1.3.1.   HHS, in coordination with DHS, DOS, DOD, VA, and other Federal partners, shall develop, test, and implement a Federal Government public health emergency communications plan (describing the government's strategy for responding to a pandemic, outlining U.S. international commitments and intentions, and reviewing containment measures that the government believes will be effective as well as those it regards as likely to be ineffective, excessively costly, or harmful) within 6 months. Measure of performance: containment strategy and emergency response materials completed and published on www.pandemicflu.gov; communications plan implemented.

6.1.3.2.   HHS, in coordination with DHS, shall develop, test, update and implement (if necessary) a multilingual and multimedia public engagement and risk communications strategy within 6 months. Measure of performance: risk communication material completed and published on **www.pandemicflu.gov** and other venues; State summit meetings held.

6.1.3.3.   HHS, in coordination with DHS, DOD, and the VA, and in collaboration with State, local, and tribal health agencies and the academic community, shall select and retain opinion leaders and medical experts to serve as credible spokespersons to coordinate and effectively communicate important and informative messages to the public, within 6 months. Measure of performance: national spokespersons engaged in communications campaign.

6.1.4.   Provide guidance to the private sector and critical infrastructure entities on their role in the pandemic response, and considerations necessary to maintain essential services and operations despite significant and sustained worker absenteeism.

6.1.4.1.   State, local, and tribal public health and health care authorities, in collaboration with DHS, HHS, and the Department of Labor (DOL), should coordinate emergency communication protocols with print and broadcast media, private industry, academic, and nonprofit partners within 6 months. Measure of performance: coordinated messages from communities identified above.

6.1.4.2.   DOT, in cooperation with HHS, DHS, and DOC, shall develop model protocols for 9-1-1 call centers and public safety answering points that address the provision of information to the public, facilitate caller screening, and assist with priority dispatch of limited emergency medical services, within 12 months. Measure of performance: model protocols developed and disseminated to 9-1-1 call centers and public safety answering points.

c. Producing and Stockpiling Vaccines, Antiviral Medications, and Medical Material

6.1.5.   Encourage and subsidize the development of State-based antiviral stockpiles to support response activities.

6.1.5.1.   HHS shall encourage and subsidize the development of State, territorial, and tribal antiviral stockpiles to support response activities within 18 months. Measure of performance: State, territorial, and tribal stockpiles established and antiviral medication purchases made toward goal of aggregate 31 million treatment courses.

6.1.6.   Ensure that our national stockpile and stockpiles based in States and communities are properly configured to respond to the diversity of medical requirements presented by a pandemic, including personal protective equipment, antibiotics, and general supplies.

6.1.6.1.   HHS, in coordination with DOD, VA, and State, local, and tribal partners, shall define the mix of antiviral medications to include in the Strategic National Stockpile (SNS) and State stockpiles and develop recommendations for how the different agents are to be used, within 6 months. Measure of performance: development of policy concerning the selection, relative proportions, and use of antiviral medications in SNS and State stockpiles.

6.1.6.2.   HHS, in coordination with DOD, VA, and State, local, and tribal partners, shall define critical medical material requirements for stockpiling by the SNS and States to respond to the diversity of needs presented by a pandemic, within 9 months. Measure of performance: requirements defined and guidance provided on stockpiling.

6.1.6.3.   DOD, as part of its departmental implementation plan, shall conduct a medical materiel requirements gap analysis and procure necessary materiel to enhance Military Health System surge capacity, within 18 months. Measure of performance: gap analysis completed and necessary materiel procured.

6.1.6.4.   HHS, DOD, VA and the States shall maintain antiviral and vaccine stockpiles in a manner consistent with the requirements of FDA's Shelf Life Extension Program (SLEP) and explore the possibility of broadening SLEP to include equivalently maintained State stockpiles, within 6 months. Measure of performance:

compliance with SLEP requirements documented; decision made on broadening SLEP to State stockpiles.

6.1.7.   Establish domestic production capacity and stockpiles of countermeasures to ensure sufficient antiviral medications and vaccine for front-line personnel and at-risk populations, including military personnel.

6.1.7.1.   HHS, in coordination with DHS, DOJ, VA, and in collaboration with State, local, and tribal partners, shall determine the national medical countermeasure requirements to ensure the sustained functioning of medical, emergency response, and other front-line organizations, within 12 months. Measure of performance: more specific definition of sectors and personnel for priority access to medical countermeasures and quantities needed to protect those groups; guidance provided to State, local, and tribal governments and to infrastructure sectors for various scenarios of pandemic severity and medical countermeasure supply.

6.1.7.2.   HHS shall establish and maintain stockpiles of pre-pandemic vaccines adequate to immunize 20 million persons against influenza strains that present a pandemic threat, as soon as possible within the constraints of industrial capacity. Measure of performance: procurement of 20 million courses of pre-pandemic vaccine against influenza strains presenting a pandemic threat.

6.1.7.3.   HHS in collaboration with State/local partners shall procure and allocate sufficient stockpiles of countermeasures to ensure continuity of critical medical and emergency response operations, within 18 months, within the constraints of industrial capacity. Measure of performance: sufficient quantities of antiviral medications and other countermeasures procured and distributed between SNS and State stockpiles.

6.1.7.4.   DOD shall establish stockpiles of vaccine against H5N1 and other influenza subtypes determined to represent a pandemic threat adequate to immunize approximately 1.35 million persons for military use within 18 months of availability. Measure of performance: sufficient vaccine against each influenza virus determined to represent a pandemic threat in DOD stockpile to vaccinate 1.35 million persons.

6.1.8.   Establish domestic production capacity and stockpiles of countermeasures to ensure sufficient vaccine to vaccinate the entire U.S. population within 6 months of the emergence of a virus with pandemic potential.

6.1.8.1.   HHS shall work with the pharmaceutical industry toward the goal of developing, within 60 months, domestic vaccine production capacity sufficient to provide vaccine for the entire U.S. population within 6 months after the development of a vaccine reference strain. Measure of performance: domestic vaccine manufacturing capacity in place to produce 300 million courses of vaccine within 6 months of development of a vaccine reference strain during a pandemic.

6.1.9. **Establish domestic production capacity and stockpiles of countermeasures to ensure antiviral treatment for those who contract a pandemic strain of influenza.**

6.1.9.1. HHS shall, to the extent feasible, work with antiviral drug manufacturers and large distributors to develop agreements supporting the Federal procurement of available stocks of antiviral drugs both during the pre-pandemic and pandemic periods, within 12 months. Measure of performance: new antiviral medications procured by SNS, within the constraints of industrial capacity; Federal contracts in place with antiviral drug manufacturers and distributors.

6.1.9.2. HHS, in collaboration with the States, shall purchase sufficient quantities of antiviral drugs to treat 25 percent of the U.S. population, with reserve of 6 million treatment courses for outbreak containment within 18 months, within the constraints of industrial capacity. Measure of performance: 50 million treatment courses of antiviral drugs procured by SNS; States and tribes make stockpile purchases toward aggregate 31 million treatment course goal.

6.1.9.3. DOD shall procure 2.4 million treatment courses of antiviral medications and position them at locations worldwide within 18 months. Measure of performance: aggregate 2.4 million treatment courses of antiviral medications in DOD stockpiles.

6.1.10. **Facilitate appropriate coordination of efforts across the vaccine manufacturing sector.**

6.1.10.1. HHS, in coordination with the private sector, shall assess the ability of U.S.-based pharmaceutical manufacturing facilities to contribute surge capacity and to retrofit existing facilities for pandemic vaccine production. This assessment will be completed within 6 months and should inform efforts to expand vaccine capacity. Measure of performance: completed assessment.

6.1.10.2. HHS, in coordination with DHS, DOD, VA, DOC, DOJ, and Treasury, shall assess within whether use of the Defense Production Act or other authorities would provide sustained advantages in procuring medical countermeasures, within 6 months. Measure of performance: analytical report completed on the advantages/disadvantages of invoking the Defense Production Act to facilitate medical countermeasure production and procurement.

6.1.11. **Address regulatory and other legal issues to the expansion of our domestic vaccine production capacity.**

6.1.11.1. HHS shall assess its existing authorities and develop a plan of action to address any regulatory or other legal issues related to the expansion of domestic vaccine production capacity within 12 months. Measure of performance: regulatory and legal issues identified in assessment.

6.1.11.2. HHS shall develop a protocol and decision tools to implement liability protections and compensation, as authorized by the Public Readiness and Emergency Preparedness Act (Pub. L. 109-148), within 6 months. Measure of performance: publication of protocol and decision tools.

6.1.12.   Expand the public health recommendations for domestic seasonal influenza vaccination and encourage the same practice internationally.

6.1.12.1.   HHS shall collaborate with health care providers, industry partners, and State, local, and tribal public health authorities to develop public information campaigns and other mechanisms to stimulate increased seasonal influenza vaccination, within 12 months. Measure of performance: domestic vaccine use increased relative to historical norms.

d. Establishing Distribution Plans for Medical Countermeasures, Including Vaccines and Antiviral Medications

6.1.13.   Develop credible countermeasure distribution mechanisms for vaccine and antiviral agents prior to and during a pandemic.

6.1.13.1.   HHS, in coordination with DHS, DOD, VA, and DOJ, and in collaboration with State, local, and tribal partners and the private sector, shall ensure that States, localities, and tribal entities have developed and exercised pandemic influenza countermeasure distribution plans, and can enact security protocols if necessary, according to pre-determined priorities (see below) within 12 months. Measures of performance: ability to activate, deploy, and begin distributing contents of medical stockpiles in localities as needed established and validated through exercises.

6.1.13.2.   HHS, in coordination with DOD, VA, States, and other public sector entities with antiviral drug stockpiles, shall coordinate use of assets maintained by different organizations, within 12 months. Measure of performance: plans developed for coordinated use of antiviral stockpiles.

6.1.13.3.   HHS, in collaboration with State, territorial, tribal, and local health care delivery partners, shall develop and execute strategies to effectively implement target group recommendations described below, within 12 months. Measure of performance: guidance on strategies to implement target group recommendations developed and disseminated to State, local, and tribal authorities for inclusion in pandemic response plans.

6.1.13.4.   HHS, in coordination with DOD, VA, and in collaboration with State, local, and tribal governments and private sector partners, shall assist in the development of distribution plans for medical countermeasure stockpiles to ensure that delivery and distribution algorithms have been planned for each locality for antiviral distribution. Goal is to be able to distribute antiviral medications to infected patients within 48 hours of the onset of symptoms within 12 months. Measure of performance: distribution plans developed.

6.1.13.5.   HHS, in coordination with DHS, DOS, DOD, DOL, VA, and in collaboration with State, local, and tribal governments and private sector partners, shall develop plans for the allocation, distribution, and administration of pre-pandemic vaccine, within 9 months. Measure of performance: department plans developed and guidance disseminated to State, local, and tribal authorities to facilitate development of pandemic response plans.

6.1.13.6. DOT, in coordination with HHS, DHS, State, local, and tribal officials and other EMS stakeholders, shall develop suggested EMS pandemic influenza guidelines for statewide adoption that address: clinical standards, education, treatment protocols, decontamination procedures, medical direction, scope of practice, legal parameters, and other issues, within 12 months. Measure of performance: EMS pandemic influenza guidelines completed.

6.1.13.7. HHS, in coordination with DHS, DOT, DOD, and VA, shall work with State, local, and tribal governments and private sector partners to develop and test plans to allocate and distribute critical medical materiel (e.g., ventilators with accessories, resuscitator bags, gloves, face masks, gowns) in a health emergency, within 6 months. Measure of performance: plans developed, tested, and incorporated into department plan, and disseminated to States and tribes for incorporation into their pandemic response plans.

6.1.13.8. DOD shall supply military units and posts, installations, bases, and stations with vaccine and antiviral medications according to the schedule of priorities listed in the DOD pandemic influenza policy and planning guidance, within 18 months. Measure of performance: vaccine and antiviral medications procured; DOD policy guidance developed on use and release of vaccine and antiviral medications; and worldwide distribution drill completed.

6.1.13.9. HHS, in coordination with DOD, VA, and in collaboration with State, territorial, tribal, and local partners, shall develop/refine mechanisms to: (1) track adverse events following vaccine and antiviral administration; (2) ensure that individuals obtain additional doses of vaccine, if necessary; and (3) define protocols for conducting vaccine- and antiviral-effectiveness studies during a pandemic, within 18 months. Measure of performance: mechanism(s) to track vaccine and antiviral medication coverage and adverse events developed; vaccine- and antiviral-effectiveness study protocols developed.

6.1.13.10. DOJ, in coordination with HHS, DHS, DOS, and DOC, shall lead the development of a joint strategic plan to ensure international shipments of counterfeit vaccine and antiviral medications are detected at our borders and that domestic counterfeit drug production and distribution is thwarted through aggressive enforcement efforts. Measure of performance: joint strategic plan developed; international and domestic counterfeit drug shipments prevented or interdicted.

6.1.14. Prioritize countermeasure allocation before an outbreak, and update this prioritization immediately after the outbreak begins based on the at-risk populations, available supplies, and the characteristics of the virus.

6.1.14.1. HHS, in coordination with DHS and Sector-Specific Agencies, DOS, DOD, DOJ, DOL, VA, Treasury, and State/local governments, shall develop objectives for the use of, and strategy for allocating, vaccine and antiviral drug stockpiles during pre-pandemic and pandemic periods under varying conditions of countermeasure supply and pandemic severity within 3 months. Measure of performance:

clearly articulated statement of objectives for use of medical countermeasures under varying conditions of supply and pandemic severity.

6.1.14.2.   HHS, in coordination with DHS and Sector-Specific Agencies, DOS, DOD, DOL, VA, Treasury, and State/local governments, shall identify lists of personnel and high-risk groups who should be considered for priority access to medical countermeasures, under various pandemic scenarios, according to strategy developed in compliance with 6.1.14.1, within 9 months. Measure of performance: provisional recommendations of groups who should receive priority access to vaccine and antiviral drugs established for various scenarios of pandemic severity and medical countermeasure supply.

6.1.14.3.   HHS, in coordination with DHS and Sector-Specific Agencies, DOS, DOD, DOL, and VA, shall establish a strategy for shifting priorities based on at-risk populations, supplies and efficacy of countermeasures against the circulating pandemic strain, and characteristics of the virus within 9 months. Measure of performance: clearly articulated process in place for evaluating and adjusting pre-pandemic recommendations of groups receiving priority access to medical countermeasures.

6.1.14.4.   HHS, in coordination with DHS and Sector-Specific Agencies, DOS, DOD, DOL, VA, and Treasury, shall present recommendations on target groups for vaccine and antiviral drugs when sustained and efficient human-to-human transmission of a potential pandemic influenza strain is documented anywhere in the world. These recommendations will reflect data from the pandemic and available supplies of medical countermeasures. Measure of performance: provisional identification of priority groups for various pandemic scenarios through interagency process within 2-3 weeks of outbreak.

e. Advancing Scientific Knowledge and Accelerating Development

6.1.15.   Ensure that there is maximal sharing of scientific information about influenza viruses between governments, scientific entities, and the private sector.

6.1.15.1.   HHS shall develop capability, protocols, and procedures to ensure that viral isolates obtained during investigation of human outbreaks of influenza with pandemic potential are sequenced and that sequences are published on GenBank within 1 week of confirmation of diagnosis in index case, within 6 months. Measure of performance: viral isolate sequences from outbreaks published on GenBank within 1 week of confirmation of diagnosis.

6.1.15.2.   HHS shall increase and accelerate genomic sequencing of known human and avian influenza viruses and shall rapidly make this sequence information publicly available, within 6 months. Measure of performance: increased throughput of genomes sequenced (versus FY 2005 baseline) and decreased time interval between completion of sequencing and publication on GenBank.

6.1.15.3.   HHS shall develop protocols and procedures to ensure timely reporting to Federal agencies and submission for publication of data from HHS-supported influenza vaccine, antiviral medication, and diagnostic evaluation studies, within 6 months. Measure of performance: study data shared with Federal agencies within 1 month of analysis and publication of clinical trial data following completion of studies.

6.1.16. Accelerate the development of cell culture technology for influenza vaccine production and establish a domestic production base to support vaccination demands.

6.1.16.1. HHS shall continue to support the advanced development of cell-culture based influenza vaccine candidates. Measure of performance: research grants and/or contracts awarded to develop cell-culture based influenza vaccines against currently circulating influenza strains with pandemic potential within 6 months.

6.1.16.2. HHS shall support the renovation of existing U.S. manufacturing facilities that produce other FDA-licensed cell-based vaccines or biologics and the establishment of new domestic cell-based influenza vaccine manufacturing facilities, within 36 months. Measure of performance: contracts awarded for renovation or establishment of domestic cell-based influenza vaccine manufacturing capacity.

6.1.17. Use novel investment strategies to advance the development of next-generation influenza diagnostics and countermeasures, including new antiviral medications, vaccines, adjuvant technologies, and countermeasures that provide protection across multiple strains and seasons of the influenza virus.

6.1.17.1. HHS shall continue to support the development and clinical evaluation of novel vaccines and vaccination strategies (e.g., adjuvants, alternative delivery systems, common epitope vaccines). Measure of performance: research grants and/or contracts awarded to support the development of influenza vaccines (including polyvalent influenza vaccines), adjuvants and dose-sparing strategies, and more efficient delivery systems within 12 months, leading to initiation of phase I and II clinical trials to evaluate influenza vaccines and vaccination strategies.

6.1.17.2. HHS shall collaborate with the pharmaceutical, medical device, and diagnostics industries to accelerate development, evaluation (including the evaluation of dose-sparing strategies), licensure, and U.S.-based production of new antiviral drugs and diagnostics. Development activities should include design of preclinical and clinical studies to collect safety and efficacy information across multiple strains and seasons of circulating influenza illness, and advance design of protocols to obtain additional updated information to support revisions in product usage during circulation of novel strains and evolution of pandemic spread. Such collaborations should involve early and frequent discussions with the FDA to explore the use of accelerated regulatory pathways towards product approval or licensure. Collaborations concerning diagnostic tests should include CDC to facilitate access to pandemic virus samples for validation testing and ensure that the test is one that can be used to promote and protect the public health during an influenza pandemic. Measure of performance: initiation of clinical trials of new influenza antiviral drugs and diagnostics.

6.1.17.3.   HHS, in coordination with DHS, shall develop and test new point-of-care and laboratory-based rapid influenza diagnostics for screening and surveillance, within 18 months. Measure of performance: new grants and contracts awarded to researchers to develop and evaluate new diagnostics.

6.1.17.4.   HHS shall increase access to standardized influenza reagents for use in influenza tests and research, within 6 months. Measure of performance: standardized influenza reagents distributed to domestic and international partners within 3 business days of a request.

6.2. Pillar Two: Surveillance and Detection

The ability to contain or delay the spread of pandemic influenza depends critically upon the early detection of outbreaks. Within the United States, we will work to establish surveillance systems and reporting mechanisms that provide continuous, real-time "situational awareness" to public health authorities at all levels of government. We will also work to enhance laboratory capacity, develop new and improved rapid diagnostic tests, and consolidate real-time analytical and modeling capabilities to support response activities.

a. Ensuring Rapid Reporting of Outbreaks

6.2.1.   Support the development and sustainment of sufficient U.S. and host nation laboratory capacity and diagnostic reagents in affected regions and domestically, to provide rapid confirmation of cases in animals or humans.

6.2.1.1.   HHS shall provide guidance to public health and clinical laboratories on the different types of diagnostic tests and the case definitions to use for influenza at the time of each pandemic phase. Guidelines for the current pandemic alert phase will be disseminated within 3 months. Measure of performance: dissemination on www.pandemicflu.gov and through other channels of guidance on the use of diagnostic tests for H5N1 and other potential pandemic influenza subtypes.

6.2.1.2.   HHS shall ensure that testing by reverse transcriptase-polymerase chain reaction (RT-PCR) for H5N1 and other influenza viruses with pandemic potential is available at LRN laboratories and CDC within 3 months. Measure of performance: RT-PCR for H5N1 and other potential pandemic influenza subtypes and strains in use at CDC and LRN laboratories.

6.2.1.3.   HHS, in coordination with DOD, VA, USDA, DHS, EPA, and other partners, in collaboration with its LRN Reference Laboratories, shall be prepared within 6 months to conduct laboratory analyses to detect pandemic subtypes and strains in referred specimens and conduct confirmatory testing, as requested. Measure of performance: initial testing and identification of suspect pandemic influenza specimens completed at LRN Reference and National Laboratories within 24 hours.

6.2.1.4.   All Federal, State, local, tribal, and private sector medical facilities should ensure that protocols for transporting influenza specimens to appropriate reference laboratories are in place within 3 months. Measure of performance: transportation protocols for laboratory specimens detailed in HHS, DOD, VA, State, territorial, tribal, and local pandemic response plans.

6.2.1.5.   State, local, and tribal entities should be prepared, in the event of a pandemic, to increase diagnostic testing for influenza and increase the frequency of reporting to CDC.

6.2.2.   Advance mechanisms for "real-time" clinical surveillance in domestic acute care settings such as emergency departments, intensive care units, and laboratories to provide tribal, local, State, and Federal public health officials with continuous awareness of the profile of illness in communities, and leverage all Federal medical capabilities, both domestic and international, in support of this objective.

6.2.2.1.   HHS shall be prepared to provide ongoing information from the national influenza surveillance system on the pandemic's impact on health and the health care system, within 6 months. Measure of performance: surveillance data aggregated and disseminated every 7 days, or as often as the situation warrants, to DHS, Sector-Specific Agencies, and State, territorial, tribal, and local partners.

6.2.2.2.   HHS, in coordination with Federal, State, local, tribal, and private sector partners, shall develop real-time (same-day) tracking capabilities of pneumonia or influenza hospitalizations and influenza deaths to enhance its surveillance capabilities at the onset of and during a pandemic, within 12 months. Measure of performance: real-time (same-day) nationwide hospital census and mortality tracking system is operational for use during a pandemic.

6.2.2.3.   HHS, in coordination with DOD and VA, shall expand the number of hospitals and cities participating in the BioSenseRT program to improve the Nation's capabilities for disease detection, monitoring, and situational awareness within 12 months. Measure of performance: number of hospitals (including DOD and VA facilities) participating in the BioSenseRT program increased to 350 hospitals in 42 cities.

6.2.2.4.   HHS shall reduce the time between reporting of virologic laboratory data from State, local, tribal, and private sector partners and collation, analysis, and reporting to key stakeholders, within 6 months. Measure of performance: time delay between receipt of data and collation, analysis, and reporting of results of 7 days or less.

6.2.2.5.   HHS shall increase the frequency of reporting and the number and geographic location of reporting health care providers from which outpatient surveillance data are collected through the Sentinel Provider Network (SPN), the Emerging Infections Program (EIP) influenza project, and the New Vaccine Surveillance Network (NVSN), within 6 months. Measure of performance: number of reporting healthcare providers increased to one or more per 250,000 population.

6.2.2.6.   HHS shall improve the speed at which it performs mortality surveillance through the 122 Cities Mortality Reporting System within 3 months. Measure of performance: mortality data collected at CDC within 1 week of decedent's demise increased by 25 percent compared with 2005.

6.2.2.7. DHS, in collaboration with HHS, DOD, VA, USDA, and other Federal departments and agencies with biosurveillance capabilities and real-time data sources, shall enhance NBIS capabilities to ensure the availability of a comprehensive and all-source biosurveillance common operating picture throughout the Interagency, within 12 months. Measure of performance: NBIS provides integrated surveillance data to DHS, HHS, USDA, DOD, VA, and other interested interagency customers.

6.2.2.8. HHS, in coordination with DHS, DOD, and VA, and in collaboration with State, local, and tribal authorities, shall be prepared to collect, analyze, integrate, and report information about the status of hospitals and health care systems, health care critical infrastructure, and medical materiel requirements, within 12 months. Measure of performance: guidance provided to States and tribal entities on the use and modification of the components of the National Hospital Available Beds for Emergencies and Disasters (HAvBED) system for implementation at the local level.

6.2.2.9. DOD shall enhance influenza surveillance efforts within 6 months by: (1) ensuring that medical treatment facilities (MTFs) monitor the Electronic Surveillance System for Early Notification of Community-based Epidemics (ESSENCE) and provide additional information on suspected or confirmed cases of pandemic influenza through their Service surveillance activities; (2) ensuring that Public Health Emergency Officers (PHEOs) report all suspected or actual cases through appropriate DOD reporting channels, as well as to CDC, State public health authorities, and host nations; and (3) posting results of aggregated surveillance on the DOD Pandemic Influenza Watchboard; all within 18 months. Measure of performance: number of MTFs performing ESSENCE surveillance greater than 80 percent; DOD reporting policy for public health emergencies, including pandemic influenza completed.

6.2.2.10. State, local, and tribal public health departments should develop relationships with hospitals and health care systems within their jurisdictions to facilitate collection of real-time or near real-time clinical surveillance data from domestic acute care settings such as emergency departments, intensive care units, and laboratories.

6.2.2.11. State, local, and tribal public health departments should provide weekly reports on the overall level of influenza activity in their States or localities, with assistance from CDC epidemiologists and field officers posted within each State health department in collecting and reporting these data.

6.2.3. Develop and deploy rapid diagnostics with greater sensitivity and reproducibility to allow onsite diagnosis of pandemic strains of influenza at home and abroad, in animals and humans, to facilitate early warning, outbreak control, and targeting of antiviral therapy.

6.2.3.1.   HHS, in coordination with DHS and DOD, shall work with pharmaceutical and medical device company partners to develop and evaluate rapid diagnostic tests for novel influenza subtypes including H5N1 within 18 months. Measure of performance: new investment in research to develop influenza diagnostics; new rapid diagnostic tests, if found to be useful, are available for influenza testing, including for novel influenza subtypes.

6.2.3.2.   HHS, in coordination with DHS, DOD, and VA, shall compile an inventory of all research and product development work on rapid diagnostic testing for influenza and shall reach consensus on sets of requirements meeting national needs and a common test methodology to drive further private-sector investment and product development, within 6 months. Measure of performance: inventory developed and requirements paper disseminated.

6.2.3.3.   HHS, in coordination with DOD, VA, and DHS, shall encourage and expedite private-sector development of rapid subtype- and strain-specific influenza point-of-care tests within 12 months of the publication of requirements. Measure of performance: rapid point-of-care test available in the marketplace within 18 months.

6.2.3.4.   HHS-, DOD-, and VA-funded hospitals and health facilities shall have access to improved rapid diagnostic tests for influenza A, including influenza with pandemic potential, within 6 months of when tests become available.

6.2.3.5.   State, local, and tribal public health departments should acquire and deploy rapid diagnostic tests that are specific and sensitive for pandemic influenza strains, as soon as those tests are available. Measure of performance: diagnostic tests, if found to be useful, are accessible to federally funded health facilities.

b. Using Surveillance to Limit Spread

6.2.4.   Develop and exercise mechanisms to provide active and passive surveillance during an outbreak, both within and beyond our borders.

6.2.4.1.   HHS, in coordination with DHS, DOD, VA, USDA, and DOS, shall be prepared, within 12 months, to continuously evaluate surveillance and disease reporting data to determine whether ongoing disease containment and medical countermeasure distribution and allocation strategies need to be altered as a pandemic evolves. Measure of performance: analyses of surveillance data performed at least weekly during an outbreak with timely adjustment of strategic and tactical goals, as required.

6.2.4.2.   DHS, in coordination with Sector-Specific Agencies, HHS, DOD, DOJ, and VA, and in collaboration with the private sector, shall be prepared to track integrity of critical infrastructure function, including the health care sector, to determine whether ongoing strategies of ensuring workplace safety and operational continuity need to be altered as a pandemic evolves, within 6 months. Measure of performance: tracking system in place to monitor integrity of critical infrastructure function and operational continuity in near real time.

6.2.4.3.   DOD and VA shall be prepared to track and provide personnel and beneficiary health statistics and develop enhanced methods to aggregate and analyze data documenting influenza-like illness from its surveillance systems within 12 months. Measure of performance: influenza tracking systems in place and capturing beneficiary clinical encounters.

6.2.5.   Develop rapid-response modeling capability to improve decision making during a pandemic.

6.2.5.1.   HHS, in coordination with DOD and DHS, shall develop and maintain a real-time epidemic analysis and modeling hub that will explore and characterize response options as a support to policy and decision makers within 6 months. Measure of performance: modeling center with real-time epidemic analysis capabilities established.

6.3. Pillar Three: Response and Containment

In approaching the problem of pandemic influenza, the U.S. Government endorses a layered strategy of response and containment. As outlined in the other chapters of this document, the United States is working with other nations and relevant international organizations to detect and contain outbreaks of animal influenza with pandemic potential with the aim of preventing its spread to humans. In the event of sustained and efficient human-to-human transmission of an influenza virus with pandemic potential, all reasonable actions to contain the epidemic at its source and to delay its introduction to the United States should be attempted. If such efforts fail, all instruments of national power will be directed to limiting or otherwise delaying the spread of disease; minimizing suffering and death; sustaining critical infrastructure and a Constitutional form of government; and reducing the economic and social effects of the pandemic.

a. Containing Outbreaks

6.3.1.   Encourage all levels of government, domestically and globally, to take appropriate and lawful action to contain an outbreak within the borders of their community, province, State, or nation.

6.3.1.1.   State, local, and tribal pandemic preparedness plans should address the implementation and enforcement of isolation and quarantine, the conduct of mass immunization programs, and provisions for release or exception.

6.3.2.   Provide guidance, including decision criteria and tools, to all levels of government on the range of options for infection control and containment, including those circumstances where social distancing measures, limitations on gatherings, or quarantine authority may be an appropriate public health intervention.

6.3.2.1.   HHS, in coordination with DHS, DOT, Education, DOC, DOD, and Treasury, shall provide State, local, and tribal entities with guidance on the combination, timing, evaluation, and sequencing of community containment strategies (including travel restrictions, school closings, snow days, self-shielding, and quarantine during a pandemic) based on currently available data, within 6 months, and update this guidance as additional data becomes available. Measure of performance: guidance provided on community influenza containment measures.

6.3.2.2.   HHS shall provide guidance on the role and evaluation of the efficacy of geographic quarantine in efforts to contain an outbreak of influenza with pandemic potential at its source, within 3 months. Measure of performance: guidance available within 72 hours of initial outbreak.

6.3.2.3.   HHS, in coordination with DHS and DOD and in collaboration with mathematical modelers, shall complete research identifying optimal strategies for using voluntary home quarantine, school closure, snow day restrictions, and other community infection control measures, within 12 months. Measure of performance: guidance developed and disseminated on the use of community control.

6.3.2.4.   As appropriate, DOD, in consultation with its Combatant Commanders (COCOM), shall implement movement restrictions and individual protection and social distancing strategies (including unit shielding, ship sortie, cancellation of public gatherings, drill, training, etc.) within their posts, installations, bases, and stations. DOD personnel and beneficiaries living off-base should comply with local community containment guidance with respect to activities not directly related to the installation. DOD shall be prepared to initiate within 18 months. Measure of performance: the policies/procedures are in place for at-risk DOD posts, installations, bases, stations, and for units to conduct an annual training evaluation that includes restriction of movement, shielding, personnel protection measures, health unit isolation, and other measures necessary to prevent influenza transmission.

6.3.2.5.   All HHS-, DOD-, and VA-funded hospitals and health facilities shall develop, test, and be prepared to implement infection control campaigns for pandemic influenza, within 3 months. Measure of performance: guidance materials on infection control developed and disseminated on www.pandemicflu.gov and through other channels.

6.3.2.6.   All health care facilities should develop, test, and be prepared to implement infection control campaigns for pandemic influenza, within 6 months.

6.3.2.7.   HHS, in coordination with DHS, DOC, DOL, and Sector-Specific Agencies, and in collaboration with medical professional and specialty societies, shall develop and disseminate infection control guidance for the private sector, within 12 months. Measure of performance: validated, focus group-tested guidance developed, and published on **www.pandemicflu.gov** and in other forums.

6.3.3.   Emphasize the roles and responsibilities of the individual in preventing the spread of an outbreak, and the risk to others if infection control practices are not followed.

6.3.3.1.   HHS, in coordination with DHS, VA, and DOD, shall develop and disseminate guidance that explains steps individuals can take to decrease their risk of acquiring or transmitting influenza infection during a pandemic, within 3

months. Measure of performance: guidance disseminated on
www.pandemicflu.gov and through VA and DOD channels.

6.3.3.2.   HHS, in coordination with DHS, DOD, VA, and DOT and in collaboration with State, local, and tribal partners, shall develop and disseminate lists of social distancing behaviors that individuals may adopt within 6 months and update guidance as additional data becomes available. Measure of performance: guidance disseminated on **www.pandemicflu.gov** and through other channels.

b. Leveraging National Medical and Public Health Surge Capacity

6.3.4.   Implement State, local, and tribal public health and medical surge plans, and leverage all Federal medical facilities, personnel, and response capabilities to support the national surge requirement.

6.3.4.1.   Major medical societies and organizations, in collaboration with HHS, DHS, DOD, and VA, should develop and disseminate protocols for changing clinical care algorithms in settings of severe medical surge. Measure of performance: evidence-based protocols developed to optimize care that can be provided in conditions of severe medical surge.

6.3.4.2.   HHS, in coordination with DHS, DOD, and VA, and in collaboration with States, localities, tribal entities, and private sector health care facilities, shall develop strategies and protocols for expanding hospital and home health care delivery capacity in order to provide care as effectively and equitably as possible, within 6 months. Measure of performance: guidance and protocols developed and disseminated.

6.3.4.3.   HHS shall work with State Medicaid and SCHIP programs to ensure that Federal standards and requirements for reimbursement or enrollment are applied with the flexibilities appropriate to a pandemic, consistent with applicable law. Preliminary strategies shall be developed within 6 months. Measure of performance: draft policies and guidance developed concerning emergency enrollment in and reimbursement through State Medicaid and SCHIP programs during a pandemic.

6.3.4.4.   DHS assets, including NDMS medical materiel and mobile medical units, and HHS assets, such as the USPHS Commissioned Corps and FMSs, shall be deployed in a manner consistent with pre-defined strategic considerations. Measure of performance: development, within 6 months, of strategic principles for deployment of Federal medical assets in a pandemic; consistency of deployments during a pandemic with these principles.

6.3.4.5.   DHS shall activate NDMS teams, if available, to augment efforts of State, local, and tribal governments as part of the Federal response. Measure of performance: number of NDMS teams activated and deployed during a pandemic.

6.3.4.6.   HHS shall deploy the USPHS Commissioned Corps and FMSs, if available and in combination or separately as circumstances warrant, to augment efforts of

State/local governments as part of the Federal response. Measure of performance: USPHS Commissioned Corps personnel trained on FMSs within 9 months; Commissioned Corps personnel and FMSs deployed within 72 hours of order to mobilize during a pandemic.

6.3.4.7.   DOD shall enhance its public health response capabilities by: (1) continuing to assign epidemiologists and preventive medicine physicians within key operational settings; (2) expanding ongoing DOD participation in CDC's EIS Program; and (3) within 18 months, fielding specific training programs for PHEOs that address their roles and responsibilities during a public health emergency. Measure of performance: all military PHEOs fully trained within 18 months; increase military trainees in CDC's EIS program by 100 percent within 5 years.

6.3.4.8.   All hospitals should be prepared to treat patients with pandemic influenza (i.e., equipped and ready to care for: (1) a limited number of patients infected with a pandemic influenza virus, or other novel strain of influenza, as part of normal operations; and (2) a large number of patients in the event of escalating transmission of pandemic influenza).

6.3.4.9.   All hospitals and health care systems should develop, test, and be ready to employ business continuity plans and identify the critical links in their supply chains as well as sources of emergency.

6.3.4.10.   All health care systems, individually or collaborating with other facilities to develop local or regional stockpiles maintained under vendor managed inventory systems, should consider stockpiling consumable critical medical materiel (including but not limited to food, fuel, water, N95 respirators, surgical and /or procedural masks, gowns, and ethyl-alcohol based gels) sufficient for the peak period of a pandemic wave (2-3 weeks).

6.3.5.   Activate plans to distribute medical countermeasures, including non-medical equipment and other material, from the Strategic National Stockpile and other distribution centers to Federal, State, local, and tribal authorities.

6.3.5.1.   HHS, in coordination with DHS, DOL, Education, VA, and DOD, shall develop and disseminate guidance and educational tools that explain steps individuals can take to decrease their risk of acquiring or transmitting influenza infection during a pandemic, within 6 months. Measure of performance: interim guidance disseminated on **www.pandemicflu.gov** and through VA, DOD, and other channels within 3 months; complementary educational tools on social distancing, personal hygiene, mask use, and other infection control precautions developed within 6 months.

6.3.5.2.   HHS, in collaboration with State, local, and tribal governments, shall develop and disseminate recommendations for the use, if any, of antiviral stockpiles for targeted post-exposure prophylaxis in civilian populations, within 3 months. Measure of performance: States, localities, and tribal entities have received recommendations for incorporation into response plans.

6.3.5.3.   HHS, in coordination with DHS, shall allocate and assure the effective and secure distribution of public stocks of antiviral drugs and vaccines when they become available. HHS and DHS are currently prepared to distribute stockpile as soon as countermeasures become available. Measure of performance: number of doses of vaccine and treatment courses of antiviral medications distributed.

6.3.6.   Address barriers to the flow of public health, medical, and veterinary personnel across State and local jurisdictions to meet local shortfalls in public health, medical, and veterinary capacity.

6.3.6.1.   Prior to the declaration of a public health emergency, State, local, and tribal public health authorities should examine existing Federal laws, regulations, and requirements, State public health and medical licensing laws, the provisions of interstate emergency management compacts and mutual aid agreements, and other legal and regulatory arrangements to determine the extent to which they address barriers to the flow of qualified public health and medical personnel across jurisdictional lines or between health care facilities.

c. Sustaining Infrastructure, Essential Services, and the Economy

6.3.7.   Determine the spectrum of infrastructure-sustainment activities that the U.S. military and other government entities may be able to support during a pandemic, contingent upon primary mission requirements, and develop mechanisms to activate them.

6.3.7.1.   HHS, in coordination with DHS, DOD, VA, and DOT, and as the lead for ESF #8, shall identify public health and medical capabilities required to support a pandemic response and work with other supporting agencies to identify and deploy or otherwise deliver the required capability or asset, if available. Measure of performance: inventory of public health and medical capabilities within 6 months; available public health or medical capabilities or assets deployed or delivered during a pandemic.

6.3.7.2.   DOD and VA assets and capabilities shall be postured to provide care for military personnel and eligible civilians, contractors, dependants, other beneficiaries, and veterans and shall be prepared to augment the medical response of State, territorial, tribal, or local governments and other Federal agencies consistent with their ESF #8 support roles, within 3 months. Measure of performance: DOD and VA pandemic preparedness plans developed; in a pandemic, adequate health response provided to military and associated personnel.

6.3.7.3.   VA shall develop draft emergency policies and directives allowing VA personnel and resources to be used for the treatment of non-veteran patients with pandemic influenza within 3 months. Measure of performance: emergency policies and directives drafted.

6.3.7.4.   VA shall develop, test, and implement protocols and policies allowing VA personnel and resources to be used for the treatment of non-veteran patients during health emergencies, within 3 months. Measure of performance: protocols and policies developed and implemented.

6.3.7.5. DOD shall develop and implement guidelines defining conditions under which Reserve Component medical personnel providing health care in non-military health care facilities should be mobilized and deployed, within 18 months. Measure of performance: guidelines developed and implemented.

d. Ensuring Effective Risk Communication

6.3.8. Ensure that timely, clear, coordinated messages are delivered to the American public from authoritative sources at all levels of government and assist the governments of affected nations to do the same.

6.3.8.1. HHS, in coordination with DHS, DOD, and VA, shall develop and disseminate a risk communication strategy within 6 months, updating it as required. Measure of performance: implementation of risk communication strategy on **www.pandemicflu.gov** and elsewhere.

6.3.8.2. DOD and VA, in coordination with HHS, shall develop and disseminate educational materials, coordinated with and complementary to messages developed by HHS but tailored for their respective departments, within 6 months. Measure of performance: up-to-date risk communication material published on DOD and VA pandemic influenza websites, HHS website **www.pandemicflu.gov,** and in other venues.

CHAPTER 7 — PROTECTING ANIMAL HEALTH

Introduction

Influenza viruses that cause severe disease outbreaks in animals, especially birds, are believed to be a likely source for the emergence of a human pandemic influenza virus. The avian influenza type A "H5N1" virus currently found in parts of Asia, Europe, and Africa is one of particular concern due to its demonstrated ability to infect both birds and mammals, including humans. Whether or not this H5N1 virus develops the ability to transmit efficiently between humans and cause a human pandemic, there will inevitably be other influenza viruses in animals that will pose such a threat in the future.

Most influenza viruses found in birds and other animals do not pose any threat to humans, but a few may have the potential to become a human pandemic strain and must be eradicated or otherwise controlled when they occur. Although there is no definitive way to identify all influenza viruses in animals that may have human pandemic potential, such potential could be evidenced by the ability of a virus that infects birds or other animals to also cause illness in humans or to cause illness in both birds and other animals.

Influenza viruses that cause severe illness and death in birds or other animals are known as "highly pathogenic" for the species in which that illness occurs. Some avian influenza viruses, such as the H5N1 in Asia, Europe, and Africa, cause high mortality in chickens and are referred to as highly pathogenic avian influenza (HPAI) viruses. Such avian viruses are generally of the H5 or H7 type, although not all H5 and H7 viruses are highly pathogenic for chickens. However, all H5 and H7 types have the potential to mutate into a highly pathogenic strain. In order to protect poultry and other birds in the United States, and also minimize or eliminate the possibility that a human pandemic strain might emerge from such viruses, all HPAI viruses or other H5 or H7 avian influenza viruses that infect domestic poultry in the United States will be eradicated or otherwise controlled. Because H5 and H7 types are not the only influenza A viruses that may have the potential to emerge as a human pandemic strain, other type A influenza viruses in animals that show evidence of human pandemic potential will also be eradicated or otherwise controlled.

Until a human pandemic influenza virus emerges, there is no way to know whether that virus will be able to infect and be transmitted by birds or other animals, or if it will "only" be transmissible from human-to-human. While it is possible that a human pandemic strain of influenza virus could infect and be transmitted by birds or other animals, it is probably unlikely.[18] In any case, if a human pandemic strain emerges, it will be very important to confirm through experimental and epidemiologic studies whether or not the virus can also infect, and be transmitted by, birds or other animals, so that any measures needed to mitigate the threat to humans and the impacts on poultry or other animals can be implemented.

A human pandemic influenza virus could emerge outside the United States or within our borders. Because of the potential for the HPAI H5N1 virus to become a pandemic strain, many international animal health initiatives are currently underway through the U.S. Agency for International Development

---

[18] It cannot be known what specific characteristics a human pandemic influenza virus will possess, but the virus will have to be able to efficiently bind to the receptors of, and replicate in, human respiratory cells, in order to be transmitted efficiently from human-to-human. Such a virus would not likely also be able to efficiently bind to cell receptors and replicate efficiently in avian hosts, due to differences in receptor specificity and other species-specific factors. A slightly greater, but still low, likelihood may exist for a virus adapted to humans to also replicate in swine.

and the International Partnership on Avian and Pandemic Influenza to assist affected countries with control of the current outbreak. Many more international activities are planned (see Chapter 4 - International Efforts). The more that can be done through these efforts to address fundamental issues related to the detection and control of viruses with pandemic potential in birds or other animals, the lower the risk will be for the emergence of a human pandemic strain.

Regardless of where the risk for emergence exists, we must be prepared to respond appropriately. If an influenza virus with human pandemic potential is introduced into domestic birds or other animals in the United States, despite all international efforts to prevent it, we must detect and eradicate the virus as quickly as possible. If it is found in wild birds, efforts will be directed at preventing introduction into domestic birds or other susceptible animals, rather than eradication.

Key Considerations

The Department of Agriculture (USDA) has a history of success in working with Federal partners, State, local, and tribal entities, and the poultry industry to eradicate avian influenza viruses, including HPAI and H5 or H7 viruses with the potential to become HPAI, that have been introduced into U.S. poultry. Significant outbreaks of HPAI or potential HPAI in poultry were eradicated in 1984 and 2002, as was a smaller outbreak in 2004.

Although such eradication efforts may help to protect human health, they can result in significant costs due to poultry production losses from bird depopulation activities and from quarantine or other movement restrictions placed on birds. But eradication of these viruses also protects the production of U.S. poultry, worth almost $29 billion in 2004, including broiler production worth more than $20 billion. The United States is the second largest exporter of poultry meat in the world and our trading partners are not only concerned about HPAI, but also increasingly wary of importing poultry or poultry products from any country that may have avian influenza viruses with the potential to become highly pathogenic.

The economic consequences of an HPAI outbreak in the United States would depend on its size, location, and type, and on the amount of time necessary to eradicate the outbreak. Production losses would depend on the proximity of the outbreak to major poultry areas, but with limited backyard flocks and strong biosecurity in large facilities, any outbreak would likely be contained with only modest production losses. The most economically significant recent outbreak of avian influenza in the United States occurred in 1983 and 1984, primarily in Pennsylvania and Virginia. That outbreak affected mainly layer flocks and resulted in the depopulation of 17 million birds and destruction of 14 million eggs. While the amount of birds and eggs destroyed was small relative to total annual U.S. production, the loss of breeder and laying flocks had a greater impact than implied by the destruction of the birds and eggs since they represent future production. Losses were estimated at $65 million.

Unlike domestic birds, wild bird species are highly dispersed, highly mobile, and occupy a wide range of native habitats. These characteristics render any effort to eradicate avian influenza in wild bird populations impractical. The Department of the Interior (DOI), which is responsible for managing wild migratory birds under Federal law and international treaty, works closely with State wildlife agencies, other Federal agencies, and partners to conserve wild migratory bird populations through the management of habitats, regulation of sport hunting, and other management actions. The DOI maintains an intensive research and data management capability that allows it to track the movement of birds during the migration season, identify migratory stopover sites, and inform its partners of migratory bird arrivals.

USDA and DOI share the responsibility for managing the consequences of wildlife disease. USDA has the lead role in preventing the introduction of disease from wildlife to domestic birds and conducts a broad range of disease research, surveillance, and management activities associated with this role. DOI has the lead role in managing healthy wildlife populations for the benefit of the American public and conducts comprehensive field and laboratory wildlife disease investigations and disease research with emphasis on the ecology of disease and its impact on wild populations, surveillance, and management. The USDA and DOI programs complement one another such that the full range of management needs resulting from wildlife disease is addressed. Should H5N1 or any other HPAI virus be detected in wild birds, the departments will work together on a unified response, to include conducting additional surveillance of wild birds and recommending biosecurity measures to prevent interactions between domestic and wild birds.

Response Planning

To respond effectively to an introduction of influenza in birds or other animals in the United States, Federal and State/tribal-level response plans and resources must be in place. Once in place, plans should regularly be updated at the Federal, State, tribal, and animal industry sector levels, and exercised among those levels. Emergency management roles must be clearly defined and understood at all levels. The *National Response Plan* (NRP) and the National Incident Management System (NIMS) provide a response structure, but response plans for disease outbreaks in animals must be exercised between all levels so that roles and functions are clearly understood prior to a response.

Communicating and Mitigating Risks

There will be a need for timely and clear communication about the risks associated with the introduction of influenza and how to mitigate them, especially at the level of the individual producer or animal owner. Significant misconceptions may exist about risks, and accurate and open communication will be crucial in correcting any misconceptions. Owners and producers of birds or other animals at risk for influenza must understand their critical role in protecting those animals from infection and in reporting any illness that may indicate the presence of a pathogenic influenza virus. Similarly, State and tribal wildlife management authorities must understand their roles in identifying and reporting illness in wild animals that may presage the emergence of highly pathogenic influenza.

USDA currently conducts a multilevel outreach and education campaign called "Biosecurity for the Birds" to provide disease and biosecurity information to poultry producers, especially those with "backyard" production. The information provides guidance to bird owners and producers on preventing introduction of disease and mitigating spread of disease should it be introduced. The campaign also encourages producers to report sick birds, thereby increasing surveillance opportunities for avian influenza.

Animal industry groups should develop industry-specific standards for biosecurity and plans for outbreak response. Standards and plans should be as specific as required to deal with a highly contagious disease like influenza, but in particular need to address issues related to the zoonotic potential of an influenza outbreak. Response plans also need to help ensure successful eradication of the disease, yet preserve as much continuity of normal animal production activities as possible before, during, and after the outbreak. This kind of planning will require collaboration with Federal, State, local, and tribal entities to address issues that might otherwise negatively impact animal production during a disease response.

DOI conducts outreach to Federal, State, and tribal wildlife authorities, and the public through a multi-faceted program of technical products related to wildlife disease. Through a series of bulletins, websites, and other means, the DOI alerts and advises those who may come into contact with infected wildlife. Using this advice, State and tribal wildlife agencies should develop specific standards for biosecurity and plans for outbreak response. These plans need to address conditions specific to wildlife populations.

Animal outbreaks caused by influenza viruses with human pandemic potential, including those known to cause human illness, present challenges for preparedness and response due to the zoonotic potential of such viruses and the resulting risk for infection and illness in persons exposed to infected animals, carcasses, or animal waste. Mitigation of these risks requires specific planning, including working with public health and occupational health and safety professionals to determine requirements for personal protective equipment (PPE), seasonal influenza vaccination, and/or antiviral prophylaxis for personnel performing response functions with potential exposure to virus. Plans also need to address the logistical requirements for providing the necessary worker protection and the safe disposal of animal carcasses and animal waste.

Resources for a Response

Potentially large quantities of response materiel will need to be distributed expeditiously and accurately. As prescribed in Homeland Security Presidential Directive 9, USDA has established a National Veterinary Stockpile (NVS) that can be rapidly distributed in the event of an animal disease outbreak. The NVS has a variety of materiel that would be necessary for a response to an influenza outbreak, including PPE, disinfectant, diagnostic reagents, and antiviral medication (for responders). In addition to the NVS materiel, there are currently 40 million doses of avian influenza vaccine available for use in poultry, should an outbreak occur. Half these doses are for an H5 virus and half are for an H7 virus. However, in the event of a large scale outbreak of avian influenza, additional stockpiles of avian influenza vaccine may be needed. In addition to vaccines, there will be a need for diagnostic reagents, equipment, and other materiel to be available for rapid deployment to the site(s) of an influenza outbreak in animals, especially in poultry or other birds.

Research and Development

Perhaps even more important than having the planning, communication, and response resources in place, is ensuring that we have the scientific knowledge and tools necessary to detect and respond to an influenza outbreak in animals. Research and development will play a vital role in our preparedness to protect animals against influenza infection, detect infections when they occur, and respond effectively to influenza outbreaks caused by viruses with human pandemic potential. Enhancement of our knowledge of the ecology of influenza viruses, viral evolution, novel influenza strains that emerge in animals, and the determinants of virulence of influenza viruses in animal populations is essential. Better tools are needed for detection of influenza viruses in the environment, for providing immunity to avian populations, and for validating disease response strategies. All of this will require an appropriate infrastructure for animal health research and development. Most critically, there must be an adequate amount of laboratory research space that meets biosafety requirements appropriate for conducting animal studies using an influenza virus with pandemic potential. Deficiencies in research facility capacity will limit development of science-based solutions for the prevention, management, and control or eradication of influenza in animal populations.

Rapid Detection

Although a human influenza pandemic may emerge outside the United States, early detection of influenza viruses with pandemic potential in animals within the United States is critical to minimizing the chances of a human pandemic strain emerging here. A robust surveillance system in domestic animals and wildlife is required to ensure detection. Such surveillance of animals needs to integrate with human influenza surveillance activities at a national level. It is important for results of animal surveillance to serve as an input that may help target human surveillance efforts, relative to temporal, geographic, or other risk factors, especially if an influenza virus with human pandemic potential is detected in birds or other animals in the United States.

An extensive amount of influenza surveillance is currently conducted in poultry and wild birds in the United States. Commercial poultry operations are monitored for avian influenza through the National Poultry Improvement Plan (NPIP), and birds moving through the U.S. live bird marketing system (LBMS) are also tested for avian influenza. Wild birds are examined for avian influenza viruses through efforts involving the DOI, USDA, State wildlife authorities, and universities. Surveys of waterfowl and shore birds have been conducted in Alaska since 1998 looking for the presence of avian influenza viruses. Diagnostic testing of samples from these domestic and wild birds is carried out by many Federal, State, university, and private laboratories, including DOI's National Wildlife Health Center (NWHC) and USDA's National Veterinary Services Laboratories (NVSL) and Southeast Poultry Research Laboratory.

In addition to surveillance performed specifically to detect avian influenza in domestic and wild birds, the USDA employs specially trained wildlife disease biologists to survey for wildlife diseases and respond to disease outbreaks through its National Wildlife Disease Surveillance and Emergency Response System. This system ensures support to existing programs with appropriate sample collection, information exchange, and additional laboratory infrastructure. The USDA and State animal health authorities also employ specially trained veterinarians, called foreign animal disease diagnosticians, to investigate suspected cases of exotic disease in poultry and other influenza-susceptible species that are reported from USDA-accredited veterinary practitioners and from animal owners. Veterinary practitioners also submit specimens from sick birds and other influenza-susceptible species to State and university veterinary diagnostic laboratories, almost 40 of which have the capability to perform a rapid screening test for HPAI viruses as part of the National Animal Health Laboratory Network (NAHLN), a cooperative effort between USDA and the American Association of Veterinary Laboratory Diagnosticians.

Although substantial surveillance activities are already in place in the United States to detect avian influenza viruses with human pandemic potential in domestic poultry, enhancing surveillance in domestic animals (including at slaughter and processing) and wildlife will help ensure that reporting of these events will occur as early as possible. Animal populations that are most critical for additional surveillance activities are poultry and wild birds, not only in terms of increased numbers tested but also in the geographic distribution of testing to increase the probability of detection. In particular, domestic birds moving through the LBMS, farmed waterfowl and game birds, and migratory waterfowl and shore birds are important targets for increased avian influenza testing. Concomitant with increased targeting for animal sampling is the need for an increased capability to perform the necessary diagnostic testing to detect influenza viruses in those samples. Specifically, there is a need to enhance the capabilities of diagnostic laboratories participating in avian influenza surveillance of wild birds, and of commercial birds in the LBMS and in the NPIP, to be equivalent to those of laboratories in the NAHLN.

To fully utilize data collected as part of the national surveillance for influenza viruses with pandemic potential in animal populations, capabilities for capturing, analyzing, and sharing data must be in place. A database is needed to provide a means for evaluating the types of surveillance that should be conducted in the future, where the surveillance is needed, and the numbers of samples that must be collected. Such a database will also facilitate sharing of critical information with other animal health and public health partners working to detect influenza viruses, especially those viruses that may have human pandemic potential.

Coordinated Response

Detection of an outbreak of avian or other influenza virus with human pandemic potential in an animal population in the United States will demand a rapid and coordinated response by Federal, State, and tribal entities, industry partners, and other stakeholders. Initially there will be a State, local, and/or tribal response supported by USDA (for domestic animals) or both USDA and DOI (for wildlife). If the scope of the outbreak is beyond the immediate resource capabilities of USDA/DOI and the animal health officials in an affected State or tribal entity, USDA can implement an integrated Federal, State, tribal, and local response utilizing all necessary Federal resources under the NRP and Emergency Support Function #11 - Agriculture and Natural Resources (ESF #11). USDA is the coordinator of ESF #11 for an animal disease response, with DOI serving as the primary agency responsible for issues related to the protection of natural and cultural resources, including wildlife, endangered species, and migratory birds. Because of the general zoonotic potential of influenza outbreaks in birds or other animals, USDA will work closely with the Department of Health and Human Services (HHS), the coordinator of Emergency Support Function #8 - Public Health and Medical Services (ESF #8). Outbreaks known to have both human and animal infections will be investigated jointly by public health authorities, including HHS, and animal health authorities, including USDA, that will then work together to implement appropriate response strategies.

The response will be organized using the Incident Command System as prescribed by the NIMS. Depending on the circumstances of the outbreak and the animal population involved, the Secretary of Agriculture may declare an "extraordinary emergency" to enhance the response authorities of the USDA. If necessary, USDA would make a request to the Department of Homeland Security (DHS) for declaration of an Incident of National Significance that would invoke the full support of NRP coordination mechanisms. If the outbreak becomes extremely large, there will be a need to utilize all potential sources of support. To meet the demand for skilled responders, it may be necessary to have licensed veterinary practitioners cross jurisdictional boundaries, either State or national, to assist in the response. These boundaries can present barriers to veterinarians wishing to work as responders in any jurisdiction where they are not already licensed to practice.

Goals

Overall, the goals for protecting animals against influenza viruses with human pandemic potential (or against a human pandemic virus, should it be able to infect animals) include: developing new capabilities in influenza preparedness, prevention, detection, and response; planning and preparedness for response to an outbreak; detecting influenza infections in animals, especially poultry and wild birds; and eradicating or controlling influenza outbreaks in animals that present a risk to human or animal health.

Roles and Responsibilities

The responsibility for preparing for, detecting, and responding to influenza infections in birds or other animals, domestic or wild, is shared by everyone associated with the animals at risk. This includes animal owners, animal industry groups, State, local, and tribal wildlife management and animal health authorities, and the Federal Government. All these individuals and entities have important and interdependent roles in animal health-related activities.

The Federal Government

The Federal Government will use all capabilities within its authority to support the private sector and State, local, and tribal animal health authorities in preparedness, surveillance, and response activities related to animal disease outbreaks. It will increase readiness to sustain essential Federal animal health functions during a human pandemic and provide animal health support services under the NRP.

Department of Agriculture: USDA is responsible for protecting American livestock, including poultry, from exotic or foreign animal diseases, such as HPAI. It advises individuals, the private sector, and State, local, and tribal entities, on appropriate biosecurity measures both before and after a disease is introduced, and helps to develop, support, and carry out surveillance for disease agents of concern. USDA provides diagnostic reference services and primary testing support, both prior to an outbreak and during an outbreak response. USDA stockpiles vaccines for possible use in a response to an outbreak of influenza with human pandemic potential in animals, and sponsors research on influenza viruses with pandemic potential and on vaccines that might be effective in controlling them. It provides assistance to the private sector and State, local, and tribal entities, in the development of influenza preparedness and response plans. Under the NRP, DHS has overall incident management coordination responsibilities and USDA will be the coordinator for ESF #11 for the response to a highly contagious disease like influenza, implementing an integrated national-level response with industry, State, local, and tribal responders. It provides response personnel, materiel, technical expertise, and funding for certain disease control and eradication activities. USDA is also responsible for providing Federal leadership to Federal, State, and tribal entities in managing problems caused by nuisance wildlife, including native wildlife, invasive species, and exotic animals. USDA partners with the DOI and others to coordinate the Federal Government's surveillance strategy for the early detection of HPAI in wild migratory birds and other wildlife when appropriate. USDA administers a National Wildlife Disease Surveillance and Emergency Response Program that is responsible for conducting daily surveillance on wildlife diseases, such as HPAI, and responding to a variety of emergencies including natural disasters and disease outbreaks. USDA also inspects and monitors meat, poultry, and egg products sold in interstate and foreign commerce to ensure products for public consumption are inspected for signs of disease.

Department of the Interior: DOI is responsible for managing and protecting certain wildlife, including migratory birds, under various laws and treaties and for protecting public health on more than 500 million acres of Federal land across the country. DOI coordinates the Federal Government's surveillance of wild migratory birds for the presence of HPAI virus, coordinates Federal surveillance with related surveillance activities of State, fish, and wildlife agencies, and provides leadership and support in the area of wildlife disease research and diagnostics to Federal and State natural resource agencies. DOI's NWHC works with department bureaus, as well as State, tribal, and other Federal entities, on wildlife disease investigations, providing the best available science and technical support for issues related to wildlife health and disease. This biosafety level 3 laboratory is actively involved in targeted surveillance of migratory birds and shorebirds, as well as wildlife morbidity and mortality event investigations to identify causative agents of wildlife disease. In the event of an HPAI outbreak in wild migratory birds, DOI will work with Federal and State natural resource, agricultural health, and public health agencies to support timely and effective response.

Department of Health and Human Services: HHS's primary responsibilities are those actions required to protect the health of all Americans, including communication of information related to pandemic influenza, leading international and domestic efforts in surveillance and detection of influenza outbreaks, ensuring the provision of essential human services, implementing measures to limit spread, and providing recommendations related to the use, distribution, and allocation of countermeasures and to the provision of care in mass casualty settings. HHS supports research, education, and prevention projects addressing the Nation's pressing agricultural health and safety problems, evaluating agricultural injury and disease prevention, and developing and evaluating control technologies to prevent illness and injuries among agricultural workers and their families. Through its Centers for Agricultural Disease and Injury Research, Education, and Prevention program, HHS supports consultation and/or training to researchers, health and safety professionals, graduate/professional students, and agricultural extension agents and others in a position to improve the health and safety of agricultural workers.

Department of Homeland Security: While DHS has overall incident management coordination responsibilities, it is also a support agency to USDA under ESF #11 - Agriculture and National Resources. Under this annex, DHS may provide additional support in interdicting adulterated products in transport and at ports of entry; subject-matter expertise and technical assistance (e.g., Customs and Border Protection Agricultural Specialists); and air and transport services (e.g., U.S. Coast Guard), as needed, for personnel and laboratory samples. DHS's Homeland Security Operations Center will also receive updates from USDA. In the event of a zoonotic disease outbreak, DHS will coordinate with USDA and HHS to release public information.

Department of Defense: In the event that an animal health emergency exceeds the capability of civil authorities, the Department of Defense (DOD) may provide defense support of civil authorities in accordance with the NRP and appropriate DOD Directives, as well as other procedures and authorities that exist for requesting assistance from DOD. If authorized by the Secretary of Defense, DOD can provide personnel, equipment, facilities, materials, and pharmaceuticals to the extent that national security readiness is not compromised. USDA may request and receive support from DOD in the event that the presence of animal/plant diseases and/or pests, endemic or exotic, constitutes an actual or potential emergency. For the purposes of this plan, an emergency is defined as any sudden negative economic impact, either perceived or real, such as a "foreign animal disease" event or a natural disaster that threatens the viability of U.S. animal agriculture and thereby the food supply of the United States.

State, Local, and Tribal Entities

State, local, and tribal entities are primarily responsible for detecting and responding to disease outbreaks and implementing measures to minimize the consequences of an outbreak. State, local, and tribal entities should have preparedness plans that address key issues in dealing with a disease outbreak in animals. They will be the first line of defense in limiting the spread of disease. Appropriate movement controls for susceptible birds or other animals and their products, and the ability to implement those controls, will be essential. For that purpose, there may be a need to integrate State, local, and tribal law enforcement entities into an animal disease response plan. Reporting mechanisms for use in early identification of suspect cases of influenza in animal populations should be established, as should mechanisms for communicating with the local animal agriculture community about influenza and response activities.

The Private Sector and Critical Infrastructure Entities

The private sector plays an integral role in preparedness for, and successful response to, an animal disease outbreak. Animal industry groups should develop standards for biosecurity and plans for outbreak response that help ensure successful eradication of the disease yet preserve as much continuity of normal animal production activities as possible during the outbreak.

Individuals and Families

Animal owners should practice appropriate biosecurity to prevent or minimize the risk of disease introduction prior to an outbreak, and must comply with quarantines or other movement restrictions to prevent or minimize the spread of disease during an outbreak.

Actions and Expectations

7.1. Pillar One: Preparedness and Communication

To help ensure that response plans can be successfully implemented, a capability must exist to rapidly provide personnel for response activities and surge capacity for veterinary diagnostic laboratories. If an influenza outbreak occurs in animals, owners and producers of susceptible animals, as well as natural resource managers, must understand their role, and the role of Federal, State, and tribal entities, in responding to an influenza outbreak in domestic animals or wildlife and limiting spread of the disease. Stockpiled materiel and vaccines need to be increased, and additional research and development is essential, including simulation modeling to refine disease mitigation strategies.

a. Planning for a Pandemic

7.1.1. Support the development and exercising of avian and pandemic response plans.

7.1.1.1.   USDA, in coordination with DHS, HHS, DOD, and DOI, and in partnership with State and tribal entities, animal industry groups, and (as appropriate) the animal health authorities of Canada and Mexico, shall establish and exercise animal influenza response plans within 6 months. Measure of performance: plans in place at specified Federal agencies and exercised in collaboration with States believed to be at highest risk for an introduction into animals of an influenza virus with human pandemic potential.

7.1.2. Continue to work with States, localities, and tribal entities to develop medical and veterinary surge capacity plans.

7.1.2.1.   USDA shall partner with State and tribal entities to establish, organize, train, and exercise incident management teams and a veterinary reserve corps within 12 months. Measure of performance: a veterinary reserve corps and incident management teams trained for each of the States believed to be at highest risk for an introduction into an animal population of an influenza virus with human pandemic potential.

7.1.2.2.   USDA, in coordination with DOD, HHS, DHS, and DOI, shall partner with States and tribal entities to ensure sufficient veterinary diagnostic laboratory surge capacity for response to an outbreak of avian or other influenza virus with human pandemic potential, within 6 months. Measure of performance: plans and necessary agreements to meet laboratory capacity needs for a worst case scenario influenza outbreak in animals validated by utilization in exercises.

b. Communicating Expectations and Responsibilities

7.1.3. **Provide guidance and support to poultry, swine, and related industries on their role in responding to an outbreak of avian influenza, including ensuring the protection of animal workers and initiating or strengthening public education campaigns to minimize the risks of infection from animal products.**

7.1.3.1.   USDA, in coordination with DHS, shall develop, disseminate, and encourage adoption of best practices and recommendations for maintaining the biosecurity of animals, especially poultry and swine, against infection and spread of influenza viruses and for reporting suspected cases of influenza with human pandemic potential in animals to State or Federal authorities, within 4 months. Measure of performance: incorporation of best practices by industry.

7.1.3.2.   USDA, in coordination with DHS, shall partner with State and tribal entities, and industry groups representing poultry and swine producers and processors, and other stakeholders, to define and exercise response roles and capabilities within 9 months. Measure of performance: exercises involving State or tribal entities, at least one poultry industry group, and one swine industry group, conducted and after action reports produced.

7.1.3.3.   HHS, in coordination with USDA, DHS, and the Department of Labor (DOL), shall work with the poultry and swine industries to provide information regarding strategies to prevent avian and swine influenza infection among animal workers and producers, within 6 months. Measure of performance: guidelines developed and disseminated to poultry and swine industries.

7.1.3.4.   USDA, in coordination with DOI, shall collaborate with DHS and other Federal partners, with State, local, and tribal partners, including State wildlife authorities, and with industry groups and other stakeholders, to develop guidelines to reduce the risk of transmission between domestic animals and wildlife during an animal influenza outbreak, within 6 months. Measure of performance: guidelines for various outbreak scenarios produced, disseminated, and incorporated by partners.

7.1.3.5.   DOI, in coordination with USDA, shall work with other Federal, State, and tribal partners to develop appropriate response strategies for use in the event of an outbreak in wild birds, within 4 months. Measure of performance: coordinated response strategies in place that can rapidly be tailored to a specific outbreak scenario.

c. Producing and Stockpiling Vaccines, Antiviral Medications, and Medical Material

7.1.4. **Expand the domestic supply of avian influenza vaccine to control a domestic outbreak of avian influenza in bird populations.**

7.1.4.1.   USDA shall augment the current stockpile of 40 million doses of avian influenza vaccine with an additional 70 million doses within 9 months. Measure of performance: avian influenza vaccine stockpiles increased to 110 million doses.

7.1.4.2.   USDA shall stockpile diagnostic reagents, PPE, antiviral medication for protection of response personnel, and other response materiel within 9 months. Measure of performance: materiel pre-positioned for rapid delivery to areas where poultry or other animals are believed to be at highest risk for an introduction of an influenza virus with human pandemic potential.

d. Advancing Scientific Knowledge and Accelerating Development

7.1.5.   Ensure that there is maximal sharing of scientific information about influenza viruses between governments, scientific entities, and the private sector.

7.1.5.1.   USDA and DOI shall perform research to understand better how avian influenza viruses circulate and are transmitted in nature, in order to improve information on biosecurity distributed to local animal owners, producers, processors, markets, auctions, wholesalers, distributors, retailers, and dealers, as well as wildlife management agencies, rehabilitators, and zoos, within 18 months. Measure of performance: completed research studies provide new information, or validate current information, on the most useful biosecurity measures to be taken to effectively prevent introduction, and limit or prevent spread, of avian influenza viruses in domestic and captive animal populations.

7.1.5.2.   USDA and DOI shall perform research to develop and validate tools that will facilitate environmental surveillance for avian influenza viruses, especially in wild birds, through the evaluation of feathers, feces, water, or nesting material, within 24 months. Measure of performance: new environmental surveillance tools researched and made available for use by Federal, State, tribal, university, and other entities performing avian influenza surveillance.

7.1.5.3.   USDA shall sequence genomes of all available avian influenza viruses to provide diagnostic sequences, identify possible vaccine antigens, and provide potential information on viral evolution, relationships, and determinants of virulence within 12 months. Measure of performance: genomes of avian influenza viruses sequenced and submitted to GenBank, and information reported on potential diagnostic sequences and viral relationships.

7.1.5.4.   USDA shall perform research to improve vaccines and mass immunization techniques for use against influenza in domestic birds within 36 months. Measure of performance: an effective avian influenza vaccine that can be delivered simultaneously to multiple birds ready for commercial development.

7.1.5.5.   USDA, in coordination with DHS, shall identify any deficiencies relative to needs for Federal animal research facility capacity, including appropriate biosafety levels, for performing studies of avian, swine, and other animal influenza viruses with pandemic potential, and establish a plan of action to ensure that needed facilities will be available to carry out those studies, within 6 months. Measure of performance: deficiencies in capacity of Federal animal research facilities identified and plans developed for addressing those needs.

7.1.5.6.   USDA, in coordination with DHS, DOI, and DOD, shall partner with State and tribal authorities to refine disease mitigation strategies for avian influenza in poultry or other animals through outbreak simulation modeling, within 6 months. Measure of performance: simulation models produced and reports issued on the results of influenza outbreak scenario modeling.

7.2. Pillar Two: Surveillance and Detection

Even with the large amount of surveillance and significant diagnostic capabilities currently targeted at detecting avian influenza, additional actions need to be taken to help ensure rapid detection of influenza in birds or other animals, bolster our diagnostic capabilities, and improve our ability to analyze and share surveillance data.

a. Ensuring Rapid Reporting of Outbreaks

7.2.1.   Expand our domestic livestock and wildlife surveillance activities to ensure early warning of the spread of an outbreak to our shores.

7.2.1.1.   DOI and USDA shall collaborate with State wildlife agencies, universities, and others to increase surveillance of wild birds, particularly migratory water birds and shore birds, in Alaska and other appropriate locations elsewhere in the United States and its territories, to detect influenza viruses with pandemic potential, including HPAI H5N1, and establish baseline data for wild birds, within 12 months. Measure of performance: reports detailing geographically appropriate wild bird samples collected and influenza virus testing results.

7.2.1.2.   USDA and DOI shall collaborate to develop and distribute information to State and tribal entities on the detection, identification, and reporting of influenza viruses in wild bird populations, within 6 months. Measure of performance: information distributed and a report available describing the type, amount, and audiences for the information.

7.2.1.3.   USDA shall work with State and tribal entities, and industry groups, to perform surveys of game birds and waterfowl raised in captivity, and implement surveillance of birds at auctions, swap meets, flea markets, and public exhibitions, within 12 months. Measure of performance: samples collected at 50 percent of the largest auctions, swap meets, flea markets, and public exhibitions held in at least five States or tribal entities believed to be at highest risk for an avian influenza introduction.

7.2.1.4.   USDA shall work with State and tribal entities to provide additional personnel in additional locations to increase the number of facilities inspected and number of samples collected for avian influenza virus testing within the LBMS, within 12 months. Measure of performance: number of facilities inspected and sampled increased by 50 percent compared to previous year.

7.2.2. Support the development and sustainment of sufficient U.S. and host nation laboratory capacity and diagnostic reagents in affected regions and domestically, to provide rapid confirmation of cases in animals or humans.

7.2.2.1.   USDA shall increase the capacity of the NVSL and the NAHLN to process influenza surveillance samples from commercial and LBMS sources, as well as wild birds, and develop and contract for the production of test reagents for distribution at no cost to collaborating State and industry laboratories within 12 months. Measure of performance: national capacity for laboratory testing increased by 100 percent compared to previous year and contracts for production of required avian influenza test reagents in place.

7.2.2.2.   USDA shall partner with State and tribal entities to provide additional support for laboratory activities associated with NPIP surveillance for avian influenza within 12 months. Measure of performance: cooperative support agreements with States and tribal entities developed and implemented.

7.2.2.3.   DOI and USDA shall increase the wild bird testing capacity of the NWHC and the National Wildlife Research Center, respectively, to process avian influenza samples from wild birds, within 12 months. Measure of performance: national wild bird testing capacity for avian influenza virus increased by 50 percent compared to previous year.

b. Using Surveillance to Limit Spread

7.2.3. Expand and enhance mechanisms for screening and monitoring animals that may harbor viruses with pandemic potential.

7.2.3.1.   USDA shall develop an integrated database, or enhance existing databases, to support the national initiative for comprehensive surveillance for influenza viruses with pandemic potential in domestic animals using data collected from multiple sources, within 12 months. Measure of performance: functioning animal influenza surveillance database producing reports for a variety of queries and supporting multiple analyses of data.

7.2.3.2.   DOI, in coordination with USDA, shall work with State and tribal entities, universities, and others to implement the Avian Influenza Data Clearinghouse developed by the NWHC to support the integrated surveillance program for influenza in wild birds within 12 months. Measure of performance: a functional wild bird influenza data clearinghouse utilized by multiple stakeholders.

7.3. Pillar Three: Response and Containment

If an outbreak of influenza occurs in birds or other animals in the United States it will be necessary to respond rapidly and in a coordinated manner with Federal, State, and tribal officials, industry partners, natural resource managers, and other stakeholders. The capability to utilize all possible Federal sources of wildlife management and veterinary response surge capacities will need to be in place. In order to prevent the outbreak from spreading, the movements of susceptible species of domestic animals and their products must be controlled or halted in the outbreak "control area." During an outbreak it will be essential to implement an effective communication strategy to keep stakeholders and the public informed of response activities and to clearly elucidate and put into perspective the risks and hazards that may exist and how to mitigate them.

a. Containing Outbreaks

7.3.1.   Provide guidance for States, localities, and industry on best practices to prevent the spread of avian influenza in commercial, domestic, and wild birds, and other animals.

7.3.1.1.   USDA, in coordination with DHS, HHS, DOI, and the Environmental Protection Agency, shall partner with State and tribal entities, animal industries, individual animal owners, and other affected stakeholders to eradicate any influenza outbreak in commercial or other domestic birds or domestic animals caused by a virus that has the potential to become a human pandemic strain, and to safely dispose of animal carcasses. Measure of performance: at least one incident management team from USDA on site within 24 hours of detection of such an outbreak.

7.3.1.2.   USDA shall coordinate with DHS and other Federal, State, local, and tribal officials, animal industry, and other affected stakeholders during an outbreak in commercial or other domestic birds and animals to apply and enforce appropriate movement controls on animals and animal products to limit or prevent spread of influenza virus. Measure of performance: initial movement controls in place within 24 hours of detection of an outbreak.

7.3.1.3.   USDA shall be prepared to provide near real-time technical information and policy guidance for State and tribal entities, animal industries, and individuals, on best practices to prevent the spread of avian influenza in commercial and other domestic birds and animals during an outbreak, within 4 months. Measure of performance: information and guidance distributed within 72 hours of confirmed outbreak and report available describing type and amount of information, and audiences to whom delivered.

7.3.1.4.   DOI shall coordinate with Federal, State, local, and tribal officials to identify and apply appropriate measures to limit the spread of influenza virus should an outbreak occur in free-ranging wildlife populations. Measure of performance: initial control measures implemented within 24 hours of detection of an outbreak in free-ranging wildlife.

b. Leveraging National Medical and Public Health Surge Capacity

7.3.2.   Activate plans to distribute medical countermeasures, including non-medical equipment and other material, from the Strategic National Stockpile and other distribution centers to Federal, State, and local authorities.

7.3.2.1.   USDA shall activate plans to distribute veterinary medical countermeasures and materiel from the NVS to Federal, State, local, and tribal influenza outbreak responders within 24 hours of confirmation of an outbreak in animals of influenza with human pandemic potential, within 9 months. Measure of performance: NVS materiel distributed within 24 hours of confirmation of an outbreak.

7.3.3.   Address barriers to flow of public health, medical, and veterinary personnel across State and local jurisdictions to meet local shortfalls in public health, medical, and veterinary capacity.

7.3.3.1.   USDA, in coordination with DOS, shall partner with appropriate international, Federal, State, and tribal authorities, and with veterinary medical associations, including the American Veterinary Medical Association, to reduce barriers that inhibit veterinary personnel from crossing State or national boundaries to work in an animal influenza outbreak response, within 9 months. Measure of performance: agreements or other arrangements in place to facilitate movement of veterinary practitioners across jurisdictional boundaries.

7.3.4.   Determine the spectrum of public health, medical, and veterinary surge capacity activities that the U.S. military and other government entities may be able to support during a pandemic, contingent upon primary mission requirements, and develop mechanisms to activate them.

7.3.4.1.   USDA shall assess the outbreak response surge capacity activities that other Federal partners, including the DOD, may be able to support during an outbreak of influenza in animals and ensure that mechanisms are in place to request such support, within 6 months. Measure of performance: written assessment completed and all necessary activation mechanisms in place.

c. Ensuring Effective Risk Communication

7.3.5.   Work with State and local governments to develop guidelines to assure the public of the safety of the food supply and mitigate the risk of exposure from wildlife.

7.3.5.1.   USDA, in coordination with DHS, DOI, and HHS, shall work with State, local, and tribal partners, industry groups, and other stakeholders to develop, clear and coordinated pre-scripted public messages that can later be tailored to the specifics of a given outbreak and delivered by trained spokespersons, within 3 months. Measure of performance: appropriate informational and risk mitigation messages developed prior to an outbreak, then shared with the public within 24 hours of an outbreak.

7.3.5.2.   USDA and HHS, in coordination with DHS, State, local, and tribal partners, industry groups, and other stakeholders, shall develop guidelines to assure the public of the safety of the food supply during an outbreak of influenza in animals, within 6 months. Measure of performance: guidelines for various outbreak scenarios produced and shared with partners; within first 24 hours of an outbreak, appropriately updated guidelines on food safety shared with the public.

7.3.5.3.   USDA, in coordination with DOI, shall collaborate in working with Federal partners, with State, local, and tribal partners, including State wildlife authorities, and with industry groups and other stakeholders, to update and distribute guidelines to reduce the risk of transmission between domestic animals and wildlife and reduce the risk of spread to other wildlife species during an animal influenza outbreak. Measure of performance: guidelines updated and shared with the public within first 24 hours of an outbreak.

CHAPTER 8 — LAW ENFORCEMENT, PUBLIC SAFETY, AND SECURITY

Introduction

If a pandemic influenza outbreak occurs in the United States, it is essential that governmental entities at all levels continue to provide essential public safety services and maintain public order. It is critical that all stakeholders in State and local law enforcement and public safety agencies, whose primary responsibility this is, be fully prepared to support public health efforts and to address the additional challenges they may face during such an outbreak. Federal law enforcement and military officials should be prepared to assist in a lawful and appropriate manner, and all involved should be familiar with the established protocols for seeking such assistance and have validated plans to provide that assistance.

Key Considerations

State, local, tribal, and private sector entities have primary responsibility for the public safety and security of persons and non-Federal property within their jurisdictions, and are typically the first line of response and support in these functional areas. However, the unique challenges that might confront State, local, tribal, and private sector entities could require them to request additional assistance, either of a logistical or operational nature, from within their States, from other States pursuant to a mutual aid compact, or from the Federal Government. Civil disturbances and breakdowns in public order might occur in several different situations: as health care facilities are overwhelmed with those seeking care and treatment for themselves or family members; as persons vie for limited doses of vaccines and antiviral medications; as supply-chain disruptions cause shortages in basic necessities; as individuals attempt to leave areas where outbreaks have occurred or where containment measures are in place, and, potentially, in border communities if neighboring countries are impacted. 9-1-1 emergency call centers and public safety answering points may be overwhelmed with calls for assistance, including requests to transport influenza patients.

In addition to facing these challenges and dealing with the day-to-day situations they normally face, State, local, and tribal law enforcement agencies may be called upon to enforce movement restrictions or quarantines, thereby diverting resources from traditional law enforcement duties. To add to these challenges, law enforcement and public safety agencies can also expect to have their uniform and support ranks reduced significantly as a result of the pandemic, especially if they are not vaccinated.

It also essential to protect the health and safety of law enforcement and public safety and security workers to ensure these critical personnel can safely and effectively perform their assigned roles given these additional challenges.

Response Planning

It is essential that as part of State, local, and tribal overall pandemic response planning, their respective law enforcement and public safety agencies formulate comprehensive response plans based on in-depth understanding of the salient facts regarding a potential influenza outbreak and the related issues. The plans should establish close coordination and communications protocols between law enforcement and public safety agencies and public health and medical officials. Responsible elected officials, emergency management officials, public health officials, and members of the law enforcement and emergency response communities should then undergo training related to the execution of their plans and participate in exercises and other activities to ensure their ability to execute their plan if necessary. Such exercises will raise their awareness of the pertinent issues and initiate dialogue concerning issues such as interagency cooperation, incident command, and agency-specific roles and responsibilities during a pandemic influenza outbreak.

As part of the planning process, outreach and coordination should also be conducted with respect to private sector entities responsible for safeguarding and sustaining critical infrastructure during an outbreak. It is essential that the services provided by these entities continue without interruption and that those private sector personnel responsible for providing security develop plans to continue to provide security despite the effects pandemic influenza will have on their respective workforces and the understanding that the availability of local law enforcement resources to respond or otherwise assist may be limited.

While this chapter outlines the types of Federal assistance that can be provided when States, territories, and localities need assistance, especially direct law enforcement assistance, planning officials should note that the Federal Government's ability to provide such assistance across the United States will be limited due to the relatively small numbers of Federal law enforcement personnel available to assist as well as the effects the outbreak will have on the Federal Government workforce. The ability of military personnel will likewise depend on many factors including whether such support is feasible in light of other national defense functions being provided at the time, and the impact of the pandemic on military personnel.

Understanding the Legal Framework

Because emergency management in public health emergencies will depend heavily on the effective use of relevant legal authorities, public health, law enforcement, and emergency management officials, and fire and EMS first responders will benefit from joint training on the legal authorities essential to effective response in public health emergencies *before* the emergency occurs. While significant progress has been made since the terrorist attacks on September 11, 2001, in establishing joint investigative protocols and linkages among the key components of public health, emergency management, law enforcement, and emergency response communities, an influenza pandemic will present new challenges, and it is important that all concerned understand their roles and the governing legal authorities so that they can coordinate their efforts under a complex set of Federal, State, tribal, and local laws. Federal, State, local, and tribal governments should review their legal authorities to respond to an influenza pandemic, identify needed changes in the law, and pursue legislative action as appropriate.

Sharing Ideas and Experiences

To facilitate coordination and planning at all levels and to identify issues, key Federal, State, local, and tribal law enforcement and public safety officials should be brought together with subject matter experts, including those in the public health and medical community, to discuss the influenza preparedness and response issues they may face, including maintaining civil order and how to effectively implement and enforce a quarantine or other restrictive measures. The unique needs and challenges faced by departments and agencies of all sizes should be considered. Those with relevant experience dealing with actual incidents such as the Toronto SARS experience should also be consulted. Their findings should result in the publication of best practices and model protocols, which should then be disseminated to their colleagues and counterparts throughout the Nation.

Protecting Law Enforcement and Public Safety Personnel

Ensuring the health and safety of law enforcement officers and others who may be called upon to respond in a pandemic influenza outbreak or any other public health emergency is critical. The law enforcement and public safety community should take appropriate protective measures to minimize their risk of infection, and selected personnel should be provided training to ensure they are knowledgeable about these measures. Law enforcement personnel should obtain immunizations or other prophylaxis in accordance with the priorities established for the circumstance in the event quantities are limited.

Continuity of Operations

Agencies should have continuity plans to ensure essential services are provided if significant numbers of their employees become ill during the outbreak as well as if disruptions in other sectors they depend on occur. Ideally such plans should address issues such as the reassignment of personnel to perform critical functions, encouraging personnel to have plans to take care of their families while they are assigned to critical functions, and determining at what point it would be necessary to seek additional assistance.

Outside Assistance

To prepare for the possibility that assistance from partners such as the National Guard may be required to supplement State or local law enforcement and public safety response agencies that are undermanned or overwhelmed, State and local officials should prepare in advance the processes and procedures for assessing the need for such forces and how they will be utilized in the event they are needed. Critical to this contingency is a clear understanding within the law enforcement and public safety community as to the processes that will be required to request such augmentation. Additionally, appropriate joint training should be provided as necessary to Guard forces and the potential supported agencies to ensure they are prepared for their possible missions. Once training has been completed, joint exercises between Guard units and law enforcement and other emergency responders would allow them to work through command and control and interoperability issues.

Conducting Training and Preparedness Exercises

Once all law enforcement and public safety stakeholders have formulated their plans, they should engage in joint discussions, training, and exercises to ensure that plans at the Federal, State, tribal, and local levels are effectively integrated. These discussions should identify issues such as how the Incident Command System (ICS) will function during a pandemic influenza outbreak if there are requirements for a quarantine or other similar restrictive efforts to deal with an extraordinary situation. While most incidents are managed at the local level by a member of the fire or law enforcement community, it may well be that local officials choose to designate a public health official to coordinate their response. Regardless of who is in the lead, however, public health and medical officials should participate in training on ICS policies and procedures, since they will undoubtedly be key players in these incidents and it is likely that many of them will not have had prior experience or training in this area. All Hazard Incident Management Team training would also be beneficial as it would bring together law enforcement, fire and rescue, public health, public works, and other key personnel so that each discipline learns how to work together with other disciplines.

Implementing Control Measures

While a detailed discussion of quarantine and related containment measures that may be implemented in the event of a pandemic influenza outbreak are set forth in Chapter 6 of this Implementation Plan (Plan), a brief outline of those measures is warranted here. The main goal of these containment measures is to delay the spread of disease and resulting adverse effects. Once cases are observed in the United States, early cases may be isolated from others (in a hospital or elsewhere) and their contacts (who may have been exposed) could be asked to remain out of contact with others for a period of time (voluntary quarantine). Other social distancing measures may be recommended or mandated by communities. These measures could involve recommendations on limiting personal contact, work-at-home options, limits on public gatherings, and school closures.

Geographic quarantine (*cordon sanitaire*) is the isolation of localities with documented disease transmission from localities still free of infection. It has been used occasionally throughout history in efforts to contain serious epidemics. It is important to distinguish this from the quarantine of case contacts described above, where exposure to an infectious agent, but not infection per se, has been confirmed. Although it is very unlikely that public health professionals would recommend a geographic quarantine once influenza transmission is observed in different locations, State, local, and tribal entities should still consider plans to assist with the implementation of such a measure. Whether geographic quarantine would be implemented by public health officials to contain an outbreak of influenza with pandemic potential at its source will depend on a number of factors including both the feasibility of implementing the quarantine and the ability of authorities to provide for the needs of the quarantined population.

Planning for the enforcement of quarantine or other control measures at the local level will likewise require extensive advance planning among stakeholders. Procedures for requesting mutual aid from other State and local jurisdictions should be examined and updated as necessary. Difficult issues such as rules on the use of force to enforce quarantine if necessary and what to do with those who refuse to be quarantined should be settled as much as possible in advance of any quarantine implementation. Jurisdictions with international borders or international airports should coordinate in advance with Federal officials who may be required to quarantine persons arriving in the United States. States, local, and tribal entities may also seek Federal assistance in enforcing their own quarantines, so planning should also address the mechanism for doing so. Although it is quite unlikely to be used, quarantine of a geographic area will present especially unique challenges, as it will likely require close coordination between agencies from overlapping or adjacent jurisdictions.

Readiness through Situational Awareness

While law enforcement and public safety officials are not generally expected to play an active role in surveillance and detection, they should maintain close communication with public health, EMS, and fire rescue officials who will likely be more engaged in disease surveillance efforts. This will enable them to plan and prepare as needed. As the possibility of an outbreak grows they should continue to test response plans, policies, and procedures and update them as required to ensure a continuous state of preparedness. The Federal Bureau of Investigation (FBI) will closely monitor events through coordination with the Centers for Disease Control and Prevention (CDC) and take appropriate action in the event that it is suspected that there was deliberate human intervention in the spread of the pandemic.

Law Enforcement Response During an Outbreak

During the course of a pandemic influenza outbreak, State, local, and tribal law enforcement and public safety agencies will be conducting operations in accordance with their established plans and protocols. It is possible that the *National Response Plan* (NRP) will be activated and it is likely that State, local, and tribal operations will be coordinated through emergency operations centers. In the event that State and local authorities and tribal entities need additional law enforcement assistance, established procedures, as set forth below, must be followed to obtain such assistance.

State, Local, and Tribal Law Enforcement

In the event of a civil disturbance, including rioting or looting, State and local law enforcement will normally provide the first response pursuant to State and local law. Consistent with State law, the Governor may deploy National Guard as needed to prevent or respond to civil disturbances. Mutual aid agreements, such as Emergency Management Assistance Compacts, may also be used to obtain assistance from both within States and from neighboring States.

Federal Law Enforcement

Federal agencies with law enforcement capabilities may investigate and respond to Federal crimes and conduct security measures as a result of a domestic emergency.

Emergency Federal Law Enforcement Assistance

The Federal Government may assist a State in maintaining order at the request of a Governor when State and local resources are overwhelmed and not capable of an effective response. There are two primary ways the Federal Government can provide such assistance: (1) providing Federal law enforcement personnel; and (2) pursuant to exceptions to the Posse Comitatus Act, 18 U.S.C. § 1385, when civilian law enforcement resources are inadequate, by the President directing the Armed Forces to assist with civilian law enforcement functions.

When Federal departments and agencies are requested to provide public safety and security support, the assistance is provided through the mechanism of Emergency Support Function #13 – Public Safety and Security (ESF #13) of the NRP. ESF #13 provides Federal public safety and security assistance to support prevention, preparedness, response, and recovery priorities in circumstances where locally available resources are overwhelmed or are inadequate, or where a unique Federal capability is required.

Civilian Federal Law Enforcement Assistance

Under the Emergency Federal Law Enforcement Assistance Act, 42 U.S.C. § 10501 et seq., the Attorney General may provide law enforcement assistance, including Federal personnel, in response to a Governor's written request, when he determines that such assistance is necessary to provide an adequate response to a law enforcement emergency. The provisions define a law enforcement emergency as an uncommon situation requiring law enforcement resources that threatens to become of serious or epidemic proportions, and for which State and local resources are inadequate to protect lives or property, or to enforce criminal laws. To the extent Federal personnel would be used to enforce State or local law, they should be deputized or otherwise authorized under State or local law to exercise the key law enforcement powers (arrest, search, seizure) involved in enforcing those laws.

Use of the Military for Law Enforcement Duties

Although the primary mission of the Department of Defense (DOD) is the defense of the United States, the Department may, with approval of the Secretary of Defense, provide logistical support for law enforcement operations that does not involve the use of law enforcement powers such as arrest authority. In addition, in certain situations DOD personnel may be directed by the President -- traditionally only as a last resort and in support of civilian authorities -- to perform actual law enforcement responsibilities.

The Law Enforcement Role in Containment

Although as set forth above there are less-intrusive strategies for stopping the spread of disease, response to an influenza pandemic could require more restrictive measures such as isolation or quarantine and offer social distancing measures such as movement restrictions. Most States have broad quarantine authorities enacted pursuant to their police powers. The Federal Government also has statutory authority to order a quarantine to prevent the introduction, transmission, or spread of communicable diseases from foreign countries into the United States or from one State or possession into any other State or possession. "Influenza caused by novel or re-emergent influenza viruses that are causing, or have the potential to cause, a pandemic" is on the list of specified communicable diseases for which Federal quarantine is available.

State Quarantine

If necessary, State and local law enforcement agencies, with assistance from their State's National Guard as needed, will normally enforce quarantines or other containment measures ordered by State or local authorities. Customs and Coast Guard officers may assist in enforcing State quarantines at the direction of the Secretary of Health and Human Services. At the request of State and local authorities, if author-ized under the Emergency Law Enforcement Assistance Act, and with appropriate deputations under Federal, State, and local law, Federal law enforcement officers can assist in State and local quarantine enforcement. If directed by the President pursuant to the Insurrection Act, the military may suppress domestic unrest associated with resistance to a State quarantine.

Federal Quarantine and Other Movement Restrictions

Borders: The President has the authority to bar entry into the United States of aliens who have pandemic influenza if he determines that entry is detrimental to the interests of the United States. The Secretary of Health and Human Services may prohibit the entry of persons or property from foreign countries where the entry of such persons or property would present a serious danger of the introduc-tion of a communicable disease. The Department of Homeland Security (DHS) has broad general authority pursuant to the customs and immigration laws to examine merchandise, cargo, conveyances, and persons upon their entry to the United States to ensure that imports comply with U.S. law, and to seize and forfeit vessels, animals, or other things used in the unlawful importation or transportation of articles contrary to U.S. law. Customs and Coast Guard officers are required to aid in the enforcement of Federal quarantine rules and regulations. Furthermore, Customs and Coast Guard officers and "military officers commanding in any fort or station upon the seacoast" are required to aid in the enforcement of State quarantines.

Air and other Transportation modes: The Federal Aviation Administration (FAA) can order United States flag air carriers not to enter designated airspace of a foreign country (e.g., to keep airspace clear for rescue operations). If FAA determines that an emergency exists related to safety in air commerce that requires immediate action, FAA may prescribe regulations and issue orders immediately to meet that emergency. Likewise, the Transportation Security Administration (TSA) Assistant Secretary may issue regulations or security directives immediately to protect transportation security in all modes of transport.

Rail: Any movement in the United States by rail carrier (including commuter rail but excluding urban rapid transit not connected to the general system of rail transportation) may be stopped, redirected, or limited by the authority of the Surface Transportation Board (STB) or the Federal Railroad Administration (FRA), or both, irrespective of the commodity involved. FRA may issue an emergency order imposing any restrictions or prohibitions necessary to abate what FRA determines is an emergency situation involving a hazard of death or personal injury caused by unsafe conditions or practices.

Persons Arriving From Foreign Countries and Traveling Between States

Pursuant to regulation, the CDC may quarantine individuals arriving from foreign countries or possessions who are reasonably believed to be infected with or exposed to any of the communicable diseases specified by the President in an Executive Order. In addition, CDC may quarantine individuals reasonably believed to be infected with or exposed to such diseases and traveling from one State or possession into another.

Roles and Responsibilities

The Federal Government

Federal law enforcement officials are responsible for contingency planning relating to public safety and security missions in support of the Federal response to a pandemic. In particular, certain agencies are assigned specific security and other responsibilities in the NRP's ESF #13 and Emergency Support Function #8 - Public Health and Medical Services (ESF #8).

Department of Justice: The Attorney General, as the chief law enforcement officer of the United States, with appropriate coordination with other Federal officials, is responsible by law (42 U.S.C. § 10521), for determining whether to authorize Federal law enforcement assistance, upon the written request of a Governor, in the case of a law enforcement emergency for which State and local resources are inadequate to protect lives or property, or to enforce criminal laws. This is separate and distinct from the role the Attorney General has, in coordination with the Secretary of the Department of Homeland Security, under ESF #13, which provides a mechanism for coordinating and providing Federal-to-Federal support or Federal support to State and local authorities to include non-investigative/non-criminal law enforcement, public safety, and security capabilities and resources.

Designated Department of Justice (DOJ) officials, including those in the United States Marshals Service (USMS), may deputize Federal law enforcement personnel from other agencies as Special Deputy United States Marshals to broaden their law enforcement authorities.

The USMS serves as the lead Federal law enforcement security component for the Strategic National Stockpile (SNS). A Memorandum of Agreement between the Department of Health and Human Services (HHS) and DOJ details previously agreed-upon responsibilities that are to be fulfilled by the USMS during the movement and transition of SNS assets. The USMS also works with HHS in coordinating with State and local law enforcement officials concerning SNS future planning, exercises, and operations.

The FBI is responsible for monitoring the outbreak situation as it develops for any indications that it may not be the result of natural causes and upon learning of such information, taking the appropriate investigative action as well as notifying the DHS Homeland Security Operations Center and the National Counterterrorism Center as set forth in the Biological Incident Annex of the NRP.

Department of Homeland Security: Pursuant to the NRP, the Secretary of DHS will coordinate all Federal operations within the United States to prepare for, respond to, and recover from terrorist attacks, natural disasters, and other emergencies. The Secretary of DHS is designated by Homeland Security Presidential Directive 5 as the "principal Federal official" for domestic incident management. Additionally, DHS agencies with law enforcement components have authority and responsibility to take actions related to the Federal response to an influenza pandemic, and may exercise authority over certain modes of transportation.

DHS, in conjunction with DOJ, is the co-coordinator for ESF #13 of the NRP. As such, they coordinate preparedness activities with ESF #13 supporting agencies and ensure that all activities performed under the purview of ESF #13 are related to the safety and security of the public. Many of DHS's operational elements also possess law enforcement capabilities that could be leveraged during a pandemic. For example, United States Secret Service, Customs and Border Protection, Immigration and Customs Enforcement, and TSA agents can assist State and local authorities with additional public safety and security requirements not only at ports of entry, but also in other locations, as required.

Department of Defense: DOD is responsible, at the direction of the President, for supplementing law enforcement resources with military personnel performing law enforcement functions. Such assistance ordinarily would be rendered only if civilian law enforcement agencies were overwhelmed and only if such assistance could be rendered without adversely affecting DOD's ability to perform its primary mission of defending the United States. The assistance may be provided if the President invokes the Insurrection Act at the request of a State or on his own, suppressing domestic violence or enforcing Federal law. DOD is a support agency to ESF #13 and may also provide public safety and security assistance of a logistical or support nature under the concept of Defense Support of Civil Authorities, when approved and directed by the Secretary of Defense.

States, Local, and Tribal Entities

State, local, and tribal law enforcement and public safety agencies have primary responsibility for providing public safety and security during a pandemic outbreak. These agencies are responsible for learning about the challenges they will face in a potential pandemic influenza outbreak and collaborating with the appropriate stakeholders in their respective jurisdictions. These stakeholders should include public health, judicial, fire service, corrections, and emergency management personnel. It is critical that these stakeholders develop comprehensive and mutually supporting plans that will enable them to continue their operations and respond to the challenges they will face in an outbreak.

The Adjutant General of each State, with guidance from DOD (including the National Guard Bureau) and assistance as appropriate for situations when State National Guard forces are either federalized or operating under a Title 32 status, are responsible for contingency planning and training to prepare Guard units within their State for public safety and security missions they may be assigned in a pandemic influenza outbreak.

Actions and Expectations

8.1. Pillar One: Preparedness and Communication

a. Planning for a Pandemic

8.1.1.   Develop Federal implementation plans on law enforcement and public safety, to include all components of the Federal Government and to address the full range of consequences of a pandemic, including human and animal health, security, transportation, economic, trade, and infrastructure considerations. Ensure appropriate coordination with State, local, and tribal governments.

  8.1.1.1.   States should ensure that pandemic response plans adequately address law enforcement and public safety preparedness across the range of response actions that may be implemented, and that these plans are integrated with authorities that may be exercised by Federal agencies and other State, local, and tribal governments.

  8.1.1.2.   DHS, in coordination with DOJ, HHS, DOL, and DOD, shall develop a pandemic influenza tabletop exercise for State, local, and tribal law enforcement/public safety officials that they can conduct in concert with public health and medical partners, and ensure it is distributed nationwide within 4 months. Measure of performance: percent of State, local, and tribal law enforcement/public safety agencies that have received the pandemic influenza tabletop exercise.

  8.1.1.3.   State, local, and tribal governments should review their legal authorities that may be needed to respond to an influenza pandemic, identify needed changes in the law, and pursue legislative action as appropriate.

  8.1.1.4.   DOJ shall ensure that appropriate Federal and State Court personnel are provided the information necessary to enable them to plan for the continuity of critical judicial functions during a pandemic. Measure of performance: this plan made available to all appropriate Federal and State court personnel.

  8.1.1.5.   States should ensure pandemic response plans address EMS, fire, public works, emergency management, and other emergency response and public safety preparedness.

8.1.2.   Continue to work with States, localities, and tribal entities to establish and exercise pandemic response plans.

  8.1.2.1.   DOJ, in coordination with HHS, DOL, and DHS, shall convene a forum for selected Federal, State, local, and tribal law enforcement/public safety personnel to discuss the issues they will face in a pandemic influenza outbreak and then publish the results in the form of best practices and model protocols within 4 months. Measure of performance: best practices and model protocols published and distributed.

8.1.2.2.   DOJ shall advise State Governors of the processes for obtaining emergency Federal law enforcement assistance, within 3 months. Measure of performance: all State Governors advised.

8.1.2.3.   DOJ shall advise State Governors of the processes for requesting Federal military assistance under the Insurrection Act, within 3 months. DOD, after coordination with DOJ, shall publish updated policy guidance on Military Assistance during Civil Disturbances, within 6 months. Measure of performance: all State Governors advised and guidance published.

8.1.2.4.   HHS and DOJ shall ensure consistency of the CDC Public Health Emergency Law Course with the *National Strategy for Pandemic Influenza (Strategy)*, this Plan and other Federal pandemic documents and then disseminate the CDC Public Health Emergency Law Course across the United States within 6 months. Measure of performance: distribution of presentations of reviewed public health emergency law course to all States.

8.1.2.5.   DOD, in consultation with DOJ and the National Guard Bureau, and in coordination with the States as such training applies to support of State law enforcement, shall assess the training needs for National Guard forces in providing operational assistance to State law enforcement under either Federal (Title 10) or State (Title 32 or State Active Duty) in a pandemic influenza outbreak and provide appropriate training guidance to the States and Territories for units and personnel who will be tasked to provide this support, within 18 months. Measure of performance: guidance provided to all States.

8.1.2.6.   DOD, in consultation with DOJ, shall advise State Governors of the procedures for requesting military equipment and facilities, training and maintenance support as authorized by 10 U.S.C. §§ 372-74, within 6 months. Measure of performance: all State Governors advised.

8.1.2.7.   DHS, in coordination with DOJ, DOD, DOT, HHS, and other appropriate Federal Sector-Specific Agencies, shall convene a forum for selected Federal, State, local, and tribal personnel to discuss EMS, fire, emergency management, public works, and other emergency response issues they will face in a pandemic influenza outbreak and then publish the results in the form of best practices and model protocols within 4 months. Measure of performance: best practices and model protocols published and distributed.

b. Communicating Expectations and Responsibilities

8.1.3.   Provide guidance to individuals on infection control behaviors they should adopt pre-pandemic, and the specific actions they will need to take during a severe influenza season or pandemic, such as self-isolation and protection of others if they themselves contract influenza.

8.1.3.1.   HHS, in coordination with DOL, shall provide clear guidance to law enforcement and other emergency responders on recommended preventive measures, including pre-pandemic vaccination, to be taken by law enforcement and emergency responders to minimize risk of infection from pandemic influenza, within 6 months. Measure of performance: development and dissemination of guidance for law enforcement and other emergency responders.

c. Establishing Distribution Plans for Vaccines and Antiviral Medications

8.1.4.   Develop credible countermeasure distribution mechanisms for vaccine and antiviral agents prior to and during a pandemic.

8.1.4.1.   State, local, and tribal law enforcement agencies should coordinate with appropriate medical facilities and countermeasure distribution centers in their jurisdictions (as recognized in Chapter 6, security at these facilities will be critical in the event of an outbreak) to coordinate security matters within 6 months.

8.3. Pillar Three: Response and Containment

a. Containing Outbreaks

8.3.1.   Encourage all levels of government, domestically and globally, to take appropriate and lawful action to contain an outbreak within the borders of their community, province, State, or nation.

8.3.1.1.   HHS, in coordination with DOJ, DOS, and DHS, shall determine when and how it will assist States in enforcing their quarantines and how it will enforce a Federal quarantine, within 9 months. Measure of performance: guidelines on quarantine enforcement available to all States.

b. Sustaining Infrastructure, Essential Services, and the Economy

8.3.2.   Determine the spectrum of infrastructure-sustainment activities that the U.S. military and other government entities may be able to support during a pandemic, contingent upon primary mission requirements, and develop mechanisms to activate them.

8.3.2.1.   DOJ, DHS, and DOD shall engage in contingency planning and related exercises to ensure they are prepared to maintain essential operations and conduct missions, as permitted by law, in support of quarantine enforcement and/or assist State, local, and tribal entities in law enforcement emergencies that may arise in the course of an outbreak, within 6 months. Measure of performance: completed plans (validated by exercise(s)) for supporting quarantine enforcement and/or law enforcement emergencies.

8.3.2.2.   DHS, in coordination with DOJ, DOD, DOT, HHS, and other appropriate Federal Sector-Specific Agencies, shall engage in contingency planning and related exercises to ensure they are prepared to sustain EMS, fire, emergency management, public works, and other emergency response functions during a pandemic, within 6 months. Measure of performance: completed plans (validated by exercise(s)) for supporting EMS, fire, emergency management, public works, and other emergency response functions.

CHAPTER 9 — INSTITUTIONS: PROTECTING PERSONNEL AND ENSURING CONTINUITY OF OPERATIONS

Introduction

It is the policy of the United States to have in place a comprehensive and effective program to ensure survival of our constitutional form of government, the uninterrupted continuation of national-level essential functions under all circumstances, and the resumption of all government functions and activities quickly following any disruption. This policy is in effect for all hazards but will require specialized planning in the event of an influenza pandemic.

Continuity of operations (COOP) is defined as the activities of individual Federal departments and agencies and their sub-components to ensure that the capability exists to continue essential agency functions across a wide range of potential emergencies. The Federal Executive Branch provides guidance on effective continuity planning in *Federal Preparedness Circular — 65, Federal Executive Branch Continuity of Operations* (FPC-65) and for State and local continuity planners in *Interim Guidance on Continuity of Operations Planning for State and Local Governments*. COOP planning at the State and local government level mirrors Federal guidance to ensure the continuation of services to each level of government's communities and constituents. Similarly, most businesses engage in business continuity planning, which outlines a set of procedures that define how a business will sustain or recover its critical functions in the event of an unplanned disruption to normal business operations. Such planning for an influenza pandemic must recognize that the next pandemic may come in waves, each lasting weeks or months, and pass through communities of all sizes across the United States and around the world.

Unlike many other catastrophic events, an influenza pandemic will not directly affect the physical infrastructure of an organization. While a pandemic will not damage power lines, banks, or computer networks, it will ultimately threaten all critical infrastructure by its impact on an organization's human resources by removing essential personnel from the workplace for weeks or months. Employers should include considerations for protecting the health and safety of employees during a pandemic in their business continuity planning.

The Federal Government recommends that government entities and the private sector plan with the assumption that up to 40 percent of their staff may be absent for periods of about 2 weeks at the height of a pandemic wave with lower levels of staff absent for a few weeks on either side of the peak. These absences may be due to employees who: care for the ill; are under voluntary home quarantine due to an ill household member; care for children dismissed from school; feel safer at home; or are ill or incapacitated by the virus. Because the movement of essential personnel, goods and services, and the maintenance of critical infrastructure are necessary during an event that spans weeks to months in any given community, effective continuity planning including protection of personnel during an influenza pandemic is a "good business practice" that must become part of the fundamental mission of all Federal, State, local, and tribal governmental departments and agencies, private sector businesses and institutions, and schools and universities.

The private sector will play an integral role in a community response to pandemic influenza by protecting employees' and customers' health and safety, and mitigating impact to the economy and the functioning of society. Because the private sector also owns and maintains approximately 85 percent of the U.S. critical infrastructure, it is imperative that business continuity plans include procedures to mitigate the potential disruptions caused by an influenza pandemic.

Numerous activities can be conducted now to plan for the potential of a pandemic, while other activities will require a plan for action when more information is available. This chapter provides guidance for organizations engaged in developing and improving plans to prepare for and respond to an influenza pandemic. All governmental departments and agencies at the Federal, State, local, and tribal levels, private sector businesses, and academic institutions must ensure that the capability exists to continue essential functions in the event of a disruption to normal operations. A checklist of key planning activities to supplement existing all-hazards business continuity plans for public and private organizations and businesses, schools and universities, and faith-based and community organizations is provided in Appendix A. Further guidance and references for these activities can be found at **www.pandemicflu.gov.**

Key Considerations

Planning Requirements for Pandemic Influenza Continuity of Operations

FPC-65 provides guidance on elements recognized across the Executive Branch as supportive of effective continuity planning. While the guidance in FPC-65 applies solely to the Federal Executive Branch, the planning elements that FPC-65 describes apply across all levels of government as well as the private sector and can be used to develop pandemic specific planning resources. Highlighted below are the 11 COOP program elements relevant to pandemic influenza planning.

1. Plans and Procedures

The foundation of a viable COOP program is the development and documentation of a COOP plan that, when implemented, will provide for the continued performance of an organization's essential functions under all circumstances. In order to reduce the pandemic threat, a portion of the COOP plan's objective should be to minimize the health, social, and economic impact of a pandemic on the United States.

2. Essential Functions

Essential functions are those functions that enable organizations to provide vital services, exercise civil authority, maintain the safety and well being of the general populace, and sustain the industrial/economic base in an emergency. During a pandemic, or any other emergency, these essential functions must be continued in order to facilitate emergency management and overall national recovery. Within the private sector, essential functions can be regarded as those core functions, services, and capabilities required to sustain business operations.

3. Delegations of Authority

Clearly pre-established delegations of authority are vital to ensuring that all organizational personnel know who has the authority to make key decisions in a COOP situation. Because absenteeism may reach a peak of 40 percent at the height of a pandemic wave, delegations of authority are critical.

4. Orders of Succession

An order of succession is essential to an organization's COOP plan to ensure personnel know who has authority and responsibility if the leadership is incapacitated or unavailable in a COOP situation. Since an influenza pandemic may affect regions of the United States differently in terms of timing, severity, and duration, businesses with geographically dispersed assets and personnel should consider dispersing their order of succession.

5. Alternate Operating Facilities

The identification and preparation of alternate operating facilities and the preparation of personnel for the possibility of an unannounced relocation of essential functions and COOP personnel to these facilities is part of COOP planning. Because a pandemic presents essentially simultaneous risk everywhere, the use of alternative operating facilities must be considered in a non-traditional way. COOP planning for pandemic influenza will involve alternatives to staff relocation/co-location such as social distancing in the workplace through telecommuting, or other means. In addition, relocation and redistribution of staff among alternative facilities may reduce the chance of infection impacting centralized critical operations staff simultaneously.

6. Interoperable and Effective Communications

The success of a viable COOP capability is dependent upon the identification, availability, and redundancy of critical communication systems to support connectivity of internal organizations, external partners, critical customers, and the public. Systems that facilitate communication in the absence of person-to-person contact can be used to minimize workplace risk for essential employees and can potentially be used to restrict workplace entry of people with influenza symptoms.

7. Critical Business Records and Databases

Businesses should identify, protect, and ensure the ready availability of electronic and hardcopy documents, references, records, and information systems needed to support essential functions. Pandemic influenza COOP planning must also identify and ensure the integrity of vital systems that require periodic maintenance or other direct physical intervention by employees.

8. Human Capital

Each organization must develop, update, exercise, and be able to implement comprehensive plans to protect its workforce. Although an influenza pandemic will not directly affect the physical infrastructure of an organization, a pandemic will ultimately threaten all operations by its impact on an organization's human resources. The health threat to personnel is the primary threat to continuity of operations during a pandemic.

9. Testing, Training and Exercises

Testing, training, and exercising of COOP capabilities are essential to assessing, demonstrating, and improving the ability of organizations to execute their COOP plans and programs during an emergency. Pandemic influenza COOP plans should test, train, and exercise sustainable social distancing techniques that reduce person-to-person interactions within the workplace.

10. Devolution of Control and Direction

Devolution is the capability to transfer authority and responsibility for essential functions from an organization's primary operating staff and facilities, to other employees and facilities, and to sustain operational capability under devolved authority for an extended period. Because local outbreaks will occur at different times, have variable durations, and may vary in their severity, devolution planning may need to consider rotating operations between regional/field offices as a pandemic wave moves throughout the United States.

11. Reconstitution

Reconstitution is the process by which an organization resumes normal operations. The objective during recovery and reconstitution after a pandemic is to expedite the return of normal services and operations as quickly as possible. Since a pandemic will not harm the physical infrastructure or facilities of an organization, and because long-term contamination of facilities is not a concern, the primary challenge for organizations after a pandemic will be the return to normal and bringing their systems back to full capacity. The mortality rate of a pandemic will depend on characteristics of the causative virus that cannot be predicted in advance, but for planning purposes it may be helpful to consider historical examples. The mortality rate of the 1918 pandemic in the United States — the worst influenza pandemic of the 20th century — is estimated to have been about 2 percent of those infected (about 0.5 percent of the total population). Using this historical information and current models of disease transmission, it is projected that a modern pandemic of equivalent lethality could lead to the deaths of 2 million people in the United States alone.

Continuity and Critical Infrastructure Protection

Public and private sector entities depend on certain critical infrastructure for their continued operations. Homeland Security Presidential Directive 7 (HSPD-7) identifies 17 critical infrastructure and key resources vital to national functioning.[19] Recognizing that more that 85 percent of the critical infrastructure is owned and operated by the private sector, the development of public-private partnership is paramount to securing our Nation's assets.[20]

Critical infrastructure protection (CIP) entails all the activities directed at safeguarding indispensable people, systems (especially communications), and physical infrastructure associated with the operations of the 17 critical infrastructure sectors. However, sustaining the operations of critical infrastructure under conditions of pandemic influenza will depend largely on individual organizations' development and implementation of (1) plans for business continuity under conditions of staffing shortages; and (2) plans to protect the health of their workforces. This is also true for maintaining economic activity generally, above and beyond the question of critical infrastructure. General recommendations for both of

---

[19] HSPD-7 defines critical infrastructure to include the following sectors: agriculture and food; public health and health care; drinking water and water treatment systems; energy (including the production, refining, storage, and distribution of oil and gas, and electric power except for nuclear facilities); banking and finance; national monuments and icons; defense industrial base; information technology; telecommunications; chemical; transportation systems (including mass transit, aviation, maritime, ground/surface, and rail and pipeline systems); emergency services; and postal and shipping. HSPD-7 defines key resources to include: dams; government facilities; commercial facilities; and nuclear reactors, material, and waste.

[20] HSPD-7 and the Interim National Infrastructure Protection Plan define an architecture for the Federal Government to coordinate with representatives of these critical infrastructure and key resource sectors. The Federal Government will use this structure to develop sector-specific guidance and share information. Private sector-led Sector Coordinating Councils are being established to work with their appropriate Sector-Specific Agencies via Government Coordinating Councils, which represent the government agencies that have a role in protecting the respective sectors. Currently, the Department of Homeland Security's (DHS) Office of Infrastructure Protection is finalizing the National Infrastructure Protection Plan. This finalized document will refine the public-private partnership model and a process for protecting critical infrastructure.

these areas are provided in this chapter.

COOP is one of the basic goals of CIP. During a pandemic, all critical infrastructure sectors might not be affected to the same degree or at the same time. Although pandemic influenza would be expected to affect the workforce across all sectors, a pandemic's impact in terms of demand for services may disproportionately affect several sectors including transportation, health care, agriculture, and emergency services. Sector-specific guidance and recommendations regarding transportation systems, health care, animal health, and emergency services (including law enforcement) are provided in Chapters 5, 6, 7, and 8, respectively. Development of more refined sector-specific guidance in partnership with critical infrastructure owners and operators will require further action.

Business Continuity Under Conditions of Staffing Shortages

Because an influenza pandemic would not damage physical infrastructure, the workplace would remain viable and day-to-day operations could continue based on the number of available personnel. Most organizations would not completely halt business operations because employees are ill. The organization may still need to produce products or provide services, interact with customers, and meet deadlines. A pandemic may result in an increase or decrease in demand for a business' products and/or services (e.g., effect of travel restrictions, restrictions on mass gatherings, need for hygiene supplies). Organizations should consider the potential impact of a pandemic on different product lines and/or production sites. Since essential functions are important at all times, it may be more appropriate to focus on day-to-day workload management during a pandemic. Consequently, organizations may need to rearrange priorities, rather than terminating daily operations or focusing only on essential functions as defined for a COOP situation.

Unlike other potential COOP situations that occur without warning, organizations can plan for a pandemic. Under normal conditions, if employees are on annual or sick leave, alternates are normally designated to provide back-up in the staff member's absence. To supplement the current workforce for conditions of significant absenteeism associated with a pandemic, organizations may consider cross-training and preparing ancillary workforce members (e.g., contractors, employees in other job titles/descriptions, retirees) to maintain daily functionality in the presence of anticipated staffing shortages.

Essential vs. Non-critical/Non-essential Services

Services provided by personnel may be categorized as critical or essential in light of their importance to business continuity (i.e., from the perspective of a business or organization) or in light of their contribution to maintaining critical infrastructure (i.e., from a societal or national perspective). Managers must make determinations about which employees perform essential functions at the business or organization level.

Organizations should carefully assess how a company functions, both internally and externally, to determine which staff, materials, procedures and equipment are absolutely necessary to keep the business operating by location and function during a pandemic. Operations critical to survival and recovery should be identified. Organizations should identify the suppliers, shippers, resources and other businesses they must interact with on a daily basis. Professional relationships with more than one supplier may be necessary should a primary contractor be unable to provide the required service. A disaster that shuts down a key supplier could be devastating to a business. In addition, organization-related domestic and international travel may be affected by a pandemic (e.g., quarantine, border closures). The analysis required for pandemic preparedness planning is not fundamentally different from that required for all-hazard COOP planning.

Protecting Personnel during a Pandemic

All organizations, whether government or private sector, large or small, are supported by three primary assets: people, communications, and physical infrastructure. Unlike other catastrophic events, an influenza pandemic will not directly affect the communications or physical infrastructure of an organization, but an influenza pandemic *will* directly affect an organization's people. Therefore, it is critical that organizations anticipate the potential impact of an influenza pandemic on personnel, and consequently, the organization's ability to continue essential functions. As part of that planning, organizations will need to ensure that reasonable measures are in place to protect the health of personnel during a pandemic.

Characteristics of Influenza Transmission

Understanding the characteristics of influenza transmission is important in order to assess the threat pandemic influenza poses to personnel in the workplace, as well as the efficacy and practicality of potential protective measures.

Human influenza virus is transmitted from person-to-person primarily via virus-laden large droplets (particles >5 μm in diameter) that are generated when infected persons cough, sneeze, or speak. These large droplets can then be directly deposited onto the mucosal surfaces of the upper respiratory tract of susceptible persons who are near (i.e., typically within 3 feet of) the droplet source. Transmission also may occur through direct and indirect contact with infectious respiratory secretions.

Patients with influenza typically become infectious after a latent period of about 1 to 1.5 days and prior to becoming symptomatic. At about 2 days, most infected persons will develop symptoms of illness although some remain asymptomatic throughout their infection. This is important because even seemingly healthy asymptomatic individuals in early stages of influenza could be infectious to others.

Vaccine and Antiviral Medications

The primary strategies for preventing pandemic influenza are the same as those for seasonal influenza: (1) vaccination; (2) early detection and treatment with antiviral medications; and (3) the use of infection control measures to prevent transmission. However, when a pandemic begins, only a limited stockpile of partially matched pandemic vaccine may be available. A virus-specific vaccine to protect personnel will not be available until 4 to 6 months after isolation of the pandemic virus. Finally, the supply of antiviral drugs will be limited throughout a pandemic. Until sufficient stockpiles of antiviral drugs have been established, these medications may be available for treatment of only some symptomatic individuals. Therefore, the appropriate and thorough application of infection control measures remains the key to limiting transmission, delaying the spread of a pandemic, and protecting personnel.

Infection Control Measures

A pandemic may come in waves, each lasting weeks or months. Not all susceptible individuals will be infected in the first wave of a pandemic. Therefore preventing transmission by limiting exposure during the first wave may offer several advantages. First, by limiting exposure, people who are not infected during the first wave may have an increased chance of receiving virus-specific vaccine as it becomes available. Second, limiting exposure and delaying transmission can change the shape of the epidemic curve and mitigate the social and economic impact of a pandemic by reducing the number of people who become ill at any given time.

Within the workplace, the systematic application of infection control and social distancing measures during a pandemic should reduce employee-to-employee disease transmission rates, increase employee safety and confidence, and possibly reduce absenteeism.

Given the characteristics of influenza transmission, a few simple infection control measures may be effective in reducing the transmission of infection. Persons who are potentially infectious should: stay home if they are ill; cover their nose and mouth when coughing or sneezing, and use facial tissues to contain respiratory secretions and dispose of them in a waste container (respiratory hygiene/cough etiquette); and wash their hands (with soap and water, an alcohol-based hand rub, or antiseptic handwash) after having contact with respiratory secretions and contaminated objects/materials (hand hygiene). Persons who are around individuals with influenza-like symptoms should: maintain spatial separation of at least 3 feet from that individual; turn their head away from direct coughs or sneezes; and wash their hands (with soap and water, alcohol-based hand rub, or antiseptic handwash) after having contact with respiratory secretions and contaminated objects/materials.

Hand washing should be facilitated by making hand hygiene facilities and products readily available in schools and workplaces. Antibacterial handwashing products do not appear to offer an advantage over soap and water in most settings for removing influenza virus from hands, however health care facilities should continue to follow hand hygiene guidelines that recommend use of antimicrobial soaps and alcohol-based hand cleaners to protect against transmission of other microorganisms. For the duration of a pandemic, the deployment of infection control measures requires the ready availability of soap and water, hand sanitizer, tissues and waste receptacles, and environmental cleaning supplies.

Minimizing workplace exposure to pandemic influenza can be facilitated by: developing policies and strategies for isolating and excusing employees who become ill at work; allowing unscheduled and non-punitive leave for employees with ill household contacts; restricting business-related travel to affected geographic areas; and establishing guidelines for when employees who have become ill can return to work.

Social Distancing Measures

Depending on the severity of a pandemic, and its anticipated effects on health care systems and the functioning of critical infrastructure, communities may recommend general measures to promote social distancing and the disaggregation of disease transmission networks. Within the workplace, social distancing measures could take the form of: guidelines modifying the frequency and type of face-to-face encounters that occur between employees (e.g., moratoriums on hand-shaking, substitution of teleconferences for face-to-face meetings, staggered breaks, posting of infection control guidelines in prominent locations); policies establishing flexible work hours or worksite, including telecommuting; and promotion of social distancing between employees and customers.

Some social distancing measures, such as the recommendation to maintain 3 feet of spatial separation between individuals or to otherwise limit face-to-face contact, may be adaptable to certain work environments and in appropriate settings should be sustainable indefinitely at comparatively minimal cost. Other community public health interventions (e.g., closure of schools and public transit systems, implementation of "snow day" restrictions) may increase rates of absenteeism and result in disruption of workflows and productivity. Low-cost or sustainable social distancing measures should be introduced within the workplace immediately after a community outbreak begins, and businesses should prepare for the possibility of measures that have the potential to disrupt their business continuity. Decisions as to how and when to implement community measures will be made on a case-by-case basis, with the Federal Government providing support and guidance to local officials.

Use of Face Masks

The benefit of wearing disposable surgical or procedure masks at school or in the workplace has not been established. Mask use by the public should be based on risk, including the frequency of exposure and closeness of contact with potentially infectious persons. Routine mask use in public should be permitted, but not required. The Federal Government will develop policies and guidance on the use and efficacy of masks. Other, more advanced respiratory protection may be indicated in certain instances, depending on the degree of exposure risk.

During a pandemic, persons who are diagnosed with influenza or who have a febrile respiratory illness should remain at home until the fever is resolved and the cough is resolving to avoid exposing others. If such symptomatic persons cannot stay home during the acute phase of their illness, consideration should be given to having them wear a surgical or procedure mask in public places when they may have close contact with other persons.

Although the use of surgical or procedure masks by asymptomatic individuals in community settings has not been demonstrated to be a public health measure to decrease infections during a community outbreak, persons may choose to wear a mask as part of individual protection strategies that include cough etiquette, hand hygiene, and avoiding public gatherings. If persons at risk for complications of influenza decide to wear masks during periods of increased respiratory illness activity in the community, it is likely they will need to wear them any time they are in a public place and when they are around other household members.

Any mask must be disposed of if it becomes moist. Individuals should wash their hands after touching or discarding a used mask. For more detailed information related to the use of face masks, the Department of Health and Human Services (HHS) has developed interim guidance on the use of masks to control influenza transmission, including the use of face masks and respirators in health care settings.

Cleaning of Facilities and Equipment

Given the concern regarding the spread of influenza through contaminated objects and surfaces, additional measures may be required to minimize the transmission of the virus through environmental surfaces such as sinks, handles, railings, and counters. Transmission from contaminated hard surfaces is unlikely, but influenza viruses may live up to 2 days on such surfaces. Surfaces that are frequently touched with hands should be cleaned at least daily during community outbreaks. At a minimum, organizations should develop procedures for cleaning facilities during an outbreak and develop procedures for employees to follow to keep work areas clean (e.g., disinfecting phones, keyboards, personal items). There is no evidence to support the efficacy of widespread disinfection of the environment or air.

HHS has developed recommendations regarding cleaning procedures as well as the handling of waste, eating utensils, and laundry for health care settings including home care. HHS will develop additional guidance regarding cleaning procedures and handling of potentially contaminated waste in non-health care settings such as the workplace.

International Travel

If an organization's employees or students travel outside the United States for business or educational reasons, plans should include consideration of the management of these personnel in the event of an influenza pandemic.[21] Once a pandemic emerges, international travel may be disrupted. It is also possible that containment measures may be instituted affecting airline passenger movement. Organizations should anticipate that such measures might further aggravate staffing shortages.

Risk Management in Occupational Settings

Organizations developing specific strategies to protect personnel should consider the factors that contribute to overall risk -- including the patterns of social contact entailed by specific positions, the health risk of employees for complications related to influenza, and other forms of social risk — and the feasibility of interventions designed to reduce social contacts or interrupt disease transmission. After completing such an assessment, organizations can tailor interventions to the particular needs of individuals, based on their personal health risk and the roles they play within the organization. To the extent possible, organizations should individualize the implementation of risk reduction strategies.

There are two basic categories of intervention: (1) *transmission interventions*, such as the use of facemasks and careful attention to cough etiquette and hand hygiene, which may reduce the likelihood that contacts with other people lead to disease transmission; and (2) *contact interventions*, such as substituting teleconferences for face-to-face meetings, telecommuting, the use of other social distancing techniques, and the implementation of liberal leave policies for persons with sick family members, which may eliminate or reduce the likelihood of contact with infected individuals. Interventions will have different costs and benefits, and be more or less appropriate or feasible, in different settings and for different individuals.

Social Contacts in the Workplace

The majority of Americans work in settings where social contacts occur. Some of these contacts, such as those between colleagues working on a joint project, may be regarded as voluntary or discretionary (i.e., face-to-face meetings are not absolutely necessary to maintain productivity), while others, such as those between sales clerks and customers, may be inherent to the nature of the position. Where feasible, voluntary or discretionary contacts may be reduced through contact interventions; where not, and in settings where social contacts are inherent to the nature of the position, risk reduction should be attempted through the implementation of transmission interventions. In theory, a contact intervention that reduces an individual's contacts by 30 percent is equivalent in terms of risk reduction to transmission interventions that reduce the probability of disease transmission by 30 percent.[22]

Some occupations can be classified as high risk because they will entail caring for persons with influenza (e.g., emergency medical services; police; fire and rescue; health care facility staff providers and support staff working in clinics, urgent care, and hospitals; and mortuary staff). The implementation of transmission interventions to protect personnel with such responsibilities is crucial, and organizations can additionally reduce risk by dedicating specific space and personnel for the care of patients with influenza and reducing or eliminating the connectivity of such areas and providers with the rest of the organization.

---

[21] All Federal Executive Branch employees abroad fall under Chief of Mission authority, regardless of their employment categories or location, except those under command of a U.S. area military commander or on the staff of an international organization. In coordination with the Department of State, each U.S. diplomatic mission abroad will prepare a mission-wide plan that will cover all mission personnel and their dependents. Individual agencies would not need to include their personnel serving abroad under Chief of Mission authority in their agency plans.

[22] In practice, the efficacy of contact interventions is easier to quantify than that of transmission interventions.

Individual Risk for Complications Related to Influenza

Risk group classifications will be modified as necessary in light of epidemiologic data collected during a pandemic. Individuals at high risk for severe and fatal infection cannot be predicted with certainty but are likely to include:

- Pregnant women;

- Persons with compromised immune systems due to cancer, AIDS, history of organ transplant, or other medical conditions;

- Persons less than age 65 with underlying chronic conditions;

- Persons age 65 or greater.

Organizations should consider providing additional protections for employees falling into categories identified as being at high risk for severe or fatal infection. Such protections could include reassignment from positions that entailed a high degree of unavoidable social contact or likely exposure to patients with influenza, and flexibility (where appropriate) in terms of worksite or work hours.

Social Risk

Some employees may be at increased personal risk during a pandemic because of limited access to health care services or other special needs not specified above. Risk reduction planning for such employees should be individualized.

Roles and Responsibilities

The responsibility for ensuring business continuity, COOP, and essential services, and providing for the health, safety, and security of employees, students, visitors, and customers is shared by the Federal, State, local, and tribal governments, private sector organizations, and academic institutions concerned. Federal, State, local, and tribal governments and the private sector have important and interdependent roles in preparing for, responding to, and recovering from a pandemic and ensuring that critical infrastructure is protected and sustained.

The Federal Government

The Federal Government will use all capabilities within its authority to support the private sector, State, local, and tribal entities, and schools and universities in preparedness and response activities. It will increase readiness to sustain critical infrastructure including essential Federal public health and medical functions during a pandemic and provide public health and medical support services under the *National Response Plan* (NRP). While HSPD-7 emphasizes protection of critical infrastructure from terrorism, it states that "all Federal departments and agencies shall work with the sectors relevant to their responsibilities to reduce the consequences of catastrophic failures not caused by terrorism." HSPD-7 assigns responsibilities for CIP as noted below. Each Sector-Specific Agency is responsible for developing, implementing, and maintaining a sector-specific plan for conducting CIP activities within the sector, which include collaborating with all relevant Federal departments and agencies, State, local, and tribal governments, and the private sector.

Department of Homeland Security: DHS's Office of National Security is the Government's Executive Lead for COOP. The Office of National Security will develop guidance, planning procedures, and exercises for an influenza pandemic and will monitor and report to the Executive Office of the President the readiness of departments and agencies to COOP during an influenza pandemic. DHS coordinates the overall national effort to enhance the protection of the critical infrastructure of the United States, and shall lead, integrate, and coordinate implementation of efforts among Federal departments and agencies, State, local, and tribal governments, and the private sector to protect critical infrastructure. DHS has overall coordination responsibilities for the 17 critical infrastructure sectors, and Sector-Specific Agencies, including DHS, have the lead for coordinating individual sectors. DHS coordinates protection activities for the following sectors: information technology; telecommunications; chemical; transportation systems (in collaboration with Department of Transportation), including mass transit, aviation, maritime, ground/surface, and rail and pipeline systems; emergency services; and postal and shipping. DHS coordinates with appropriate departments and agencies to ensure the protection of other key resources including dams, government facilities, and commercial facilities. DHS coordinates with the Nuclear Regulatory Commission (NRC) for the protection of nuclear power reactors, materials, and waste.

Department of Health and Human Services: HHS's primary responsibilities are those actions required to protect the health of all Americans and provide essential human services. Also, HHS in coordination with DHS will provide recommendations regarding measures Federal, State, local, and tribal agencies, private sector businesses, critical infrastructure entities, schools, and universities should employ to protect the health of personnel, customers, visitors, students, and teachers in order to aid in ensuring the continuity of essential services. HHS is the Sector-Specific Agency under HSPD-7 for public health, health care, and food (other than meat, poultry, and egg products).

Other Sector-Specific Agencies responsible under HSPD-7 for coordination with sector representatives are:

- Department of Agriculture for agriculture and food (meat, poultry, egg products);

- Environmental Protection Agency (EPA) for drinking water and water treatment systems;

- Department of Energy for energy, including the production refining, storage, and distribution of oil and gas, and electric power except for commercial nuclear power facilities (NRC);

- Department of the Treasury for banking and finance;

- Department of the Interior (DOI) for national monuments and icons; and

- Department of Defense (DOD) for the defense industrial base and defense critical infrastructure.

Other Important Federal Critical Infrastructure Responsibilities include:

- Department of State (DOS), in conjunction with DHS and other appropriate agencies, will work with foreign countries and international organizations to strengthen the protection of U.S. critical infrastructure.

- Department of Commerce (DOC), in coordination with DHS, will work with private sector, research, academic, and government organizations to promote critical infrastructure efforts, including using its authority under the Defense Production Act to ensure the timely availability of industrial products, materials, and services to meet homeland security requirements.

- Department of Education should coordinate with DHS and public and private education entities to collect and disseminate model pandemic influenza plans for adoption at the State, local, and tribal level, information on exercises and training, and monitor and share information on pandemic impacts.

- Department of Labor (DOL), in conjunction with HHS and other Sector-Specific Agencies, will work with the private sector to develop and disseminate information to promote the health and safety of personnel performing essential functions and roles.

State, Local, and Tribal Entities

State, local, and tribal entities should have credible pandemic preparedness plans that address key response issues and outline strategies to mitigate the human, social, and economic consequences of a pandemic. State and local governments have received Federal Emergency Management Agency (FEMA) guidance for COOP planning (*Introduction to State and Local EOP Planning*), and should incorporate pandemic influenza specific planning. State, local, and tribal entities should work to improve communication between public health departments and private sector partners as well among various private and public entities including schools and universities. Elements of State, local, and tribal entities should be prepared to support national efforts to ensure that critical infrastructure is sustained. State, local, and tribal entities may serve as owners or operators for specific critical infrastructure sectors. In addition, State, local, and tribal entities may play a critical role for those critical infrastructure entities located within their communities. A preparedness checklist for State and local governments is available at **www.pandemicflu.gov.**

The Private Sector

Because private industry owns and operates the vast majority of the critical infrastructure in the United States, its involvement is crucial for successful implementation of CIP and the National Infrastructure Protection Plan. The private sector will play an integral role in a community response to pandemic influenza by protecting employees' and customers' health and safety, and mitigating impact to the economy and the functioning of society. Many businesses already have continuity of business operations plans that: (1) identify and ensure continued performance of essential functions, and (2) provide for continued supply of products and services at as close to normal levels as possible. Businesses should review and update these plans as appropriate given the pandemic threat and integrate and coordinate their planning with those on whom they depend for essential services and products, and with those entities that depend on them for essential services and products. Such business continuity planning should ensure that essential functions and vital services can be performed in the setting of significant absenteeism. Businesses and corporations should be prepared for public health interventions and recommendations that may increase absenteeism. Elements of the private sector should be prepared to support Federal, State, local, and tribal efforts to ensure that critical infrastructure is sustained. A preparedness checklist for organizations and businesses is provided in Appendix A and is available at **www.pandemicflu.gov.**

Critical Infrastructure

Protecting critical infrastructure is a shared responsibility requiring cooperation among all levels of government — Federal, State, local, and tribal — and the involvement of the private sector. Over 85 percent of critical infrastructure is owned and operated by the private sector. Sector-Specific Agencies should work in coordination with critical infrastructure sectors to develop guidance for individual organization plans for maintaining continuity of essential services as part of pandemic influenza planning and preparedness. Movement of essential personnel, goods and services, and maintenance of critical infrastructure are necessary during an influenza pandemic that could span months in any given community. The critical infrastructure entities must respond in a manner that allows them to maintain the essential elements of their operations for a prolonged period of time, in order to prevent severe disruption of life in our communities. Given the interdependence among critical infrastructure entities, coordination and cooperation among critical infrastructure entities and sectors with respect to identifying essential functions and engaging in critical intra- and inter-sector and cross-border planning will be essential.

Schools and Universities

The roles and responsibilities of schools and universities in the area of continuity planning and protection of personnel are unique for several reasons. First, although there is no way to know the characteristics of a pandemic virus before it emerges, the planning assumptions suggest that in the absence of intervention influenza illness rates are likely to be highest among school-aged children (about 40 percent). Second, protecting and sustaining personnel in the workforce is of primary concern for effective continuity planning in public and private sector businesses and governmental entities. The focus in these sectors is on the workforce. In schools, the focus is primarily on protecting students. Third, universities must consider the potential impact of a pandemic on campus and dormitory closure, including the contingency plans for students who depend on student housing and campus food service. And fourth, schools and universities must also address continuity of instruction as part of continuity planning. Schools and universities (public and private) should review existing emergency response plans consistent with guidance provided by the Department of Education's Office of Safe and Drug-Free Schools, *Emergency Response and Crisis Management Guide*. Schools and universities should consider elements unique to pandemic influenza in their emergency response and crisis management plans to protect their faculty and students. Checklists for schools' and universities' actions for effective continuity planning are included in Appendix A and are available at **www.pandemicflu.gov.**

Faith-Based Organizations and Community-Based Organizations

Faith-based organizations (FBOs) and community-based organizations (CBOs) have a long tradition of helping Americans in need and together represent an integral part of our Nation's social service network. They help fill the needs of vulnerable populations and they help attend to the unmet needs that are not addressed by Federal disaster recovery programs. FBOs and CBOs have a long tradition of aiding victims of disasters. Communities should anticipate that in the event of multiple and widespread synchronous outbreaks during an influenza pandemic, the Federal Government may not possess sufficient resources or personnel to augment local capabilities. FBO/CBO and emergency management partnerships could be helpful in disaster mitigation, especially in a resource-constrained environment. FBOs and CBOs offer additional volunteer capacity; understanding of community needs and awareness of the most vulnerable populations; credibility with the community; access to social and population groups that may avoid interaction with government officials; and community influence. As locally based organizations with strong networks within communities, FBOs and CBOs are well situated to bring about grassroots involvement in mitigating the potential social and economic disruption associated with a pandemic. A preparedness checklist for FBOs and CBOs to ensure continuity of essential functions and protection of employees and volunteers is included in Appendix A and is available at **www.pandemicflu.gov.**

Individuals and Families

The critical role of individuals and families in controlling a pandemic cannot be overstated. The success or failure of infection control measures is ultimately dependent upon the acts of individuals -- practicing hand hygiene, cough etiquette, remaining home if ill or if a household member is ill, and complying with social distancing measures (see *Individual, Family, and Community Response to Pandemic Influenza* between Chapters 5 and 6). The collective response of all Americans will be crucial in mitigating the health, social, and economic impacts of a pandemic. A checklist of specific activities individuals and families can do now to prepare for a pandemic is included in Appendix A and is available at **www.pandemicflu.gov.**

Actions and Expectations

9.1. Pillar One: Preparedness and Communication

We must ensure preparedness, and the communication of roles and responsibilities for all levels of government and segments of societies including all Federal, State, local, and tribal governmental departments and agencies; private sector businesses and institutions; critical infrastructure entities; public and private schools and universities; and individuals and families.

a. Planning for a Pandemic

9.1.1. **Develop Federal implementation plans to include all components of the Federal Government and to address the full range of consequences of a pandemic, including human and animal health, security, transportation, economic, trade, and infrastructure considerations.**

9.1.1.1.   DHS, in coordination with HHS, DOD, and DOL, shall provide pandemic influenza COOP guidance to the Federal departments and agencies within 6 months. Measure of performance: COOP planning and personnel protection guidance provided to all departments for use, as necessary, in updating departmental pandemic influenza response plans.

9.1.1.2.   The Office of Personnel Management (OPM), in coordination with DHS, HHS, DOD, and DOL, shall provide guidance to the Federal departments and agencies on human capital management and COOP planning criteria related to pandemic influenza, within 3 months. Measure of performance: guidance provided to all departments for use, as necessary, in adjusting departmental COOP plans related to pandemic influenza.

9.1.1.3.   OPM, in coordination with DHS, HHS, DOD, and DOL, shall update the guides *Telework: A Management Priority, A Guide for Managers, Supervisors, and Telework Coordinators; Telework 101 for Managers: Making Telework Work for You; and, Telework 101 for Employees: Making Telework Work for You,* to provide guidance to Federal departments regarding workplace options during a pandemic, within 3 months. Measure of performance: updated telework guidance provided to all departments for use, as necessary, in updating departmental COOP plans related to pandemic influenza.

9.1.2. **Continue to work with States, localities, and tribal entities to integrate non-health sectors, including the private sector and critical infrastructure entities, in these planning efforts.**

9.1.2.1. DHS, in coordination with Sector-Specific Agencies, critical infrastructure owners and operators, and States, localities and tribal entities, shall develop sector-specific planning guidelines focused on sector-specific requirements and cross-sector dependencies, within 6 months. Measure of performance: planning guidelines developed for each sector.

9.1.2.2. DHS, in coordination with States, localities and tribal entities, shall support private sector preparedness with education, exercise, training, and information sharing outreach programs, within 6 months. Measure of performance: preparedness exercises established with private sector partners in all States and U.S. territories.

b. Communicating Expectations and Responsibilities

9.1.3. **Provide guidance to the private sector and critical infrastructure entities on their role in the pandemic response, and considerations necessary to maintain essential services and operations despite significant and sustained worker absenteeism.**

9.1.3.1. DHS, in coordination with all the Sector-Specific Agencies, shall conduct forums, conferences, and exercises with key critical infrastructure private sector entities and international partners to identify essential functions and critical planning, response and mitigation needs within and across sectors, and validate planning guidelines, within 6 months. Measure of performance: planning guidelines validated by collaborative exercises that test essential functions and critical planning, response, and mitigation needs.

9.1.3.2. DHS, in coordination with all the Sector-Specific Agencies, shall develop and coordinate guidance regarding business continuity planning and preparedness with the owners/operators of critical infrastructure and develop a Critical Infrastructure Influenza Pandemic Preparedness, Response, and Recovery Guide tailored to national goals and capabilities and to the specific needs identified by the private sector, within 6 months. Measure of performance: Critical Infrastructure Influenza Pandemic Preparedness, Response, and Recovery Guide developed and published on **www.pandemicflu.gov**.

9.1.4. **Provide guidance to individuals on infection control behaviors they should adopt pre-pandemic, and the specific actions they will need to take during a severe influenza season or pandemic, such as self-isolation and protection of others if they themselves contract influenza.**

9.1.4.1. 9.1.4.1. HHS, in coordination with DHS, DOL, OPM, Department of Education, VA, and DOD, shall develop sector-specific infection control guidance to protect personnel, governmental and public entities, private sector businesses, and CBOs and FBOs, within 6 months. Measure of performance: sector-specific guidance and checklists developed and disseminated on **www.pandemicflu.gov**.

9.1.4.2.   HHS, in coordination with DHS, DOL, EPA, Department of Education, VA, and DOD, shall develop interim guidance regarding environmental management and cleaning practices including the handling of potentially contaminated waste material, within 3 months, and revise as additional data becomes available. Measure of performance: development and publication of guidance and checklists on **www.pandemicflu.gov** and dissemination through other channels.

9.3. Pillar Three: Response and Containment

We recognize that a virus with pandemic potential anywhere represents a risk to populations everywhere. Once health authorities signal that sustained and efficient human-to-human spread of the virus has occurred, a cascade of response mechanisms will be initiated, from the site of the documented transmission to locations around the globe. This response must ensure that critical infrastructure, essential services, and the economy are sustained.

a. Sustaining Infrastructure, Essential Services, and the Economy

9.3.1.   Encourage the development of coordination mechanisms across American industries to support the above activities during a pandemic.

9.3.1.1.   DHS shall map and model critical infrastructure interdependencies across and within sectors to share critical information with sectors and identify national challenges during a pandemic, within 6 months. Measure of performance: critical infrastructure modeling capability established and mapping of critical infrastructure interdependencies completed.

9.3.1.2.   DHS shall develop and operate a national-level monitoring and information-sharing system for core essential services to provide status updates to critical infrastructure dependent on these essential services, and aid in sharing real-time impact information, monitoring actions, and prioritizing national support efforts for preparedness, response, and recovery of critical infrastructure sectors within 12 months. Measure of performance: national-level critical infrastructure monitoring and information-sharing system established and operational.

9.3.2.   Provide guidance to activate contingency plans to ensure that personnel are protected, that the delivery of essential goods and services is maintained, and that sectors remain functional despite significant and sustained worker absenteeism.

9.3.2.1.   DHS shall coordinate Federal, State, local, and tribal actions/options/capability requirements (legislative and regulatory additions/changes and waivers, personnel and material resources, and financial) to develop and implement tailored support packages to address critical infrastructure systems and essential operational requirements at each phase of the pandemic: planning, preparedness, response, mitigation, and recovery. Measure of performance: support packages ensure essential functions of all critical infrastructure sectors sustained during a pandemic.

APPENDIX A

Guidance for Federal Department Planning

Federal departments and agencies are expected to develop their own pandemic plans. This guidance is intended to facilitate department and agency planning.

Relationship between the *Strategy*, the Implementation Plan, and Department Plans

The *National Strategy for Pandemic Influenza (Strategy)*: The *Strategy* articulates the high-level principles and approach of the Federal Government to the threat of an influenza pandemic.

Implementation Plan for the National Strategy (Plan): This Plan proposes actions across the Federal Government in support of the Strategy, and describes expectations of non-Federal entities, including State, local, and tribal governments, the private sector, international partners, and individuals. While the Strategy is built upon pillars (preparedness, surveillance, response), this Plan segregates action on a functional basis (international efforts, transportation and borders, human health, animal health). It also addresses crosscutting issues such as economic issues and the relevant legal authorities in each of these functional areas. Finally, it provides a "playbook" and algorithm that the Federal Government will follow in its response to a pandemic.

Department Plans: Department plans should be operational documents. They should first articulate the manner in which the Department will discharge its responsibilities as defined in this Plan. In addition to describing the manner in which the Department will support the Federal Government efforts, plans should address the operational approach to employee safety, continuity of operations, and the manner in which the Department will communicate to its stakeholders as described below.

Guidance for Department Planning

Unlike other catastrophic events, a pandemic will not be geographically or temporally bounded, and will not directly affect the physical infrastructure of an organization. These facts lead to unique planning considerations. Institutional planning efforts should build upon existing continuity of operations planning by the organization, but be expanded to address the following questions:

1. How will the Department protect the health and safety of its employees?

2. What are the Department's essential functions and services, and how will these be maintained in the event of significant and sustained absenteeism?

3. How will the Department support the Federal response to a pandemic, and States, localities, and tribal entities?

4. How and what will the Department communicate to its stakeholders during a pandemic?

Protecting the Health of Employees

This portion of the plan should build upon existing employee health and safety efforts. HHS, in coordination with the Department of Labor, and other departments and agencies, will provide recommendations on the protection of employee health to inform this planning.

Maintaining Essential Functions and Services

Maintaining essential functions and services relates to continuity of operations. While some of the guidance in Federal Preparedness Circular - 65, Federal Executive Branch Continuity of Operations (FPC-65) may not seem to be directly relevant to pandemic planning, most of the principles are relevant to the continuity considerations raised by a pandemic.

Supporting the Federal Response and States, Localities and Tribal Entities

This Plan provides high-level direction to departments and agencies for the actions that they are to take in support of the Strategy. Department plans should articulate the manner in which these actions will be executed by the Department, including the roles and responsibilities of operating divisions and more detailed descriptions of the ways the Department will support the Federal, State, local, and tribal response.

Communicating to Stakeholders

Every department and agency has connections to a unique group of stakeholders, whether private sector entities, non-governmental organizations (NGOs), or individuals. As the "face of the Federal Government" for these stakeholders, departments should identify the messages that it will communicate during a pandemic.

Guidance for Organizations and Businesses

Federal departments and agencies; State, local, and tribal governments and organizations; and public and private businesses must ensure preparedness and the communication of roles and responsibilities related to continuity planning and protection of personnel. In the event of pandemic influenza, organizations and businesses will play a key role in protecting employees' health and safety as well as limiting the negative impact to the economy and society. Planning for pandemic influenza is critical. The Department of Health and Human Services (HHS) has developed the following checklist for large organizations and businesses. It identifies important, specific activities organizations and businesses can do now to prepare. Further information can be found at **www.pandemicflu.gov.** This checklist is applicable to all organizations and businesses, public or private.

1. **Plan for the impact of a pandemic on your business or organization**

    1.1. Identify a pandemic coordinator and/or team with defined roles and responsibilities for preparedness and response planning. The planning process should include input from labor representatives.

    1.2. Identify essential employees and other critical inputs (e.g., raw materials, suppliers, subcontractor services/products, logistics) required to maintain business operations by location and function during a pandemic.

    1.3. Train and prepare ancillary workforce (e.g., contractors, employees in other job titles/descriptions, retirees).

1.4. Develop and plan for scenarios likely to result in an increase or decrease in demand for your products and/or services during a pandemic (e.g., effect of restrictions on mass gatherings, need for hygiene supplies).

1.5. Determine potential impact of a pandemic on organization or business financials using multiple possible scenarios that affect different product lines and/or production sites.

1.6. Determine potential impact of a pandemic on organization-related domestic and international travel (e.g., quarantine, border closures).

1.7. Find up-to-date reliable pandemic information from community public health, emergency management, and other sources and make sustainable links.

1.8. Establish an emergency communications plan and revise periodically. This plan includes identification of key contacts (with back-ups), chain of communications (including suppliers and customers), and processes for tracking and communicating business and employee status.

1.9. Implement an exercise/drill to test your plan and revise periodically.

2. **Plan for the impact of a pandemic on your employees and customers**

2.1. Forecast and allow for employee absence during a pandemic due to factors such as personal illness, family member illness, community containment measures and quarantines, school and/or business closures, and public transportation closures.

2.2. Implement guidelines to modify frequency and type of face-to-face contact (e.g., handshaking, seating in meetings, office layout, shared workstation) among employees and between employees and customers.

2.3. Encourage and track annual influenza vaccination for employees during regular influenza seasons.

2.4. Evaluate employee access and availability to health care services during a pandemic, and improve services as needed.

2.5. Evaluate and improve access to and availability to mental health and social services during a pandemic, including corporate, community, and faith-based resources, and improve services as needed.

2.6. Identify employees and key customers with special needs, and incorporate the requirements of such person into your preparedness plan.

3. **Establish policies to be implemented during a pandemic**

3.1. Establish policies for employee compensation and sick leave absences unique to a pandemic (e.g., non-punitive, liberal leave), including policies on when a previously ill person is no longer infectious and can return to work after illness.

3.2. Establish policies for flexible worksite (e.g., telecommuting) and flexible work hours (e.g., staggering shifts).

3.3. Establish policies for preventing influenza spread at the worksite (e.g., promoting respiratory hygiene/cough etiquette, increasing social distancing among employees and between employees and customers, and prompt exclusion of people with influenza symptoms).

3.4. Establish policies for personnel who have been exposed to pandemic influenza, are suspected to be ill, or become ill at the worksite (e.g., infection control response, immediate mandatory sick leave).

3.5. Establish policies for restricting travel to affected geographic areas (consider both domestic and international sites) and for evacuating employees working in or near an affected area when an outbreak begins, and establish guidance for employees returning from affected areas.

3.6. Set up authorities, triggers, and procedures for activating and terminating the organization's response plan, altering business operations (e.g., shutting down operations in affected areas), and transferring business knowledge to key employees.

4. Allocate resources to protect your employees and customers during a pandemic

4.1. Provide sufficient and available infection control supplies. The deployment of infection control measures requires the ready availability of soap and water, hand sanitizer, tissues and waste receptacles, environmental cleaning supplies, for the duration of a pandemic.

4.2. Enhance communications and information technology infrastructure as needed to support employee telecommuting and remote customer access.

4.3. Ensure availability of medical consultation and advice for emergency response.

5. Communicate to and educate your employees

5.1. Develop and disseminate programs and materials covering pandemic fundamentals (e.g., signs and symptoms of influenza, modes of transmission), personal and family protection, and response strategies (e.g., hand hygiene, cough/sneeze etiquette, contingency plans).

5.2. Anticipate employee fear and anxiety, rumors, and misinformation and plan communications accordingly.

5.3. Ensure communications are culturally and linguistically appropriate.

5.4. Disseminate information to employees about the organizational pandemic preparedness plan.

5.5. Provide information for the at-home care of ill employees and family members.

5.6. Develop platforms (e.g., hotlines, dedicated websites) for communicating pandemic status and actions to employees, vendors, suppliers, and customers inside and outside the worksite in a consistent and timely way, including redundancies in the emergency contact system.

5.7. Identify community sources for timely and accurate pandemic information (domestic and international) and resources for obtaining countermeasures (e.g., vaccines and antiviral medications).

6.   Coordinate with external organizations and help your community

    6.1.   Collaborate with insurers, health plans, and major health care facilities to share your pandemic plans and understand their capabilities and plans.

    6.2.   Collaborate with Federal, State, and local public health agencies and/or emergency responders to participate in their planning processes, share your pandemic plans, and understand their capabilities and plans.

    6.3.   Communicate with local and/or State public health agencies and/or emergency responders about the assets and/or services your business could contribute to the community.

    6.4.   Share best practices with other businesses in your community, chambers of commerce, and associations to improve community response efforts.

Guidance for Schools (K-12)

Schools (K-12) must ensure preparedness, and the communication of roles and responsibilities related to ensuring continuity of instruction and protection of students and personnel. Local educational agencies (LEAs) play an integral role in protecting the health and safety of their district's staff, students, and their families. HHS, in coordination with the Department of Education, has developed the following checklist to assist LEAs in developing and/or improving plans to prepare for and respond to an influenza pandemic.

Building a strong relationship with the local health department is critical for developing a meaningful plan. The key planning activities in this checklist build upon existing contingency plans recommended for school districts by the Department of Education *(Practical Information on Crisis Planning: A Guide For Schools and Communities)*. Further information can be found at **www.pandemicflu.gov.**

1.   Planning and Coordination

    1.1.   Identify the authority responsible for declaring a public health emergency at the State and local levels and for officially activating the district's pandemic influenza response plan.

    1.2.   Identify for all stakeholders the legal authorities responsible for executing the community operational plan, especially those authorities responsible for case identification, isolation, quarantine, movement restriction, health care services, emergency care, and mutual aid.

    1.3.   As part of the district's crisis management plan, address pandemic influenza preparedness, involving all relevant stakeholders in the district (e.g., lead emergency response agency, district administrators, local public health representatives, school health and mental health professionals, teachers, food services directors, and parent representatives). This committee is accountable for articulating strategic priorities and overseeing the development and execution of the district's operational pandemic plan.

    1.4.   Work with local and/or State health departments and other community partners to establish organizational structures such as the Incident Command System (ICS), to manage the execution of the district's pandemic influenza plan. An ICS is a standardized organization structure that establishes a line of authority and common terminology and procedures to be followed in response to an incident. Ensure compatibility between the district's established ICS and the local/State health department's and State education department's ICS.

1.5. Delineate accountability and responsibility as well as resources for key stakeholders engaged in planning and executing specific components of the operational plan. Ensure that the plan includes timelines, deliverables, and performance measures.

1.6. Work with your local and/or State health department and State education agencies to coordinate with their pandemic plans. Ensure that pandemic planning is coordinated with the community's pandemic plan as well as the State department of education's plan.

1.7. Test the linkages between the district's ICS and the local/State health department's and State education department's ICS.

1.8. Contribute to the local health department's operational plan for surge capacity of health care and other services to meet the needs of the community (e.g., schools designated as contingency hospitals, schools feeding vulnerable populations, community utilizing LEA's health care and mental health staff). In an affected community, at least two pandemic disease waves (about 6-8 weeks each) are likely over several months.

1.9. Incorporate into the pandemic influenza plan the requirements of students with special needs (e.g., low income students who rely on the school food service for daily meals), those in special facilities (e.g., juvenile justice facilities), as well as those who do not speak English as their first language.

1.10. Participate in exercises of the community's pandemic plan.

1.11. Work with the local health department to address provision of psychosocial support services for the staff, students, and their families during and after a pandemic.

1.12. Consider developing in concert with the public health department a surveillance system that would alert the public health department to a substantial increase in absenteeism among students.

1.13. Implement an exercise/drill to test your pandemic plan and revise it periodically.

1.14. Share what you have learned from developing your preparedness and response plan with other LEAs as well as private schools within the community to improve community response efforts.

2. **Continuity of Student Learning and Core Operations**

2.1. Develop scenarios describing the potential impact of a pandemic on student learning (e.g., student and staff absences), school closings, and extracurricular activities based on having various levels of illness among students and staff.

2.2. Develop alternative procedures to ensure continuity of instruction (e.g., web-based distance instruction, telephone trees, mailed lessons and assignments, instruction via local radio or television stations) in the event of district school closures.

2.3. Develop a continuity of operations plan for essential central office functions (including payroll, ongoing communication with students and parents).

3.   Infection Control Policies and Procedures

3.1. Work with local health department to implement effective infection prevention policies and procedures that help limit the spread of influenza at schools in the district (e.g., promotion of hand hygiene, cough/sneeze etiquette). Make good hygiene a habit now in order to help protect children from many infectious diseases such as influenza.

3.2. Provide sufficient and accessible infection prevention supplies (e.g., soap, alcohol-based/waterless hand hygiene products, tissues and receptacles for their disposal).

3.3. Establish policies and procedures for students and staff sick leave absences unique to a pandemic influenza (e.g., non-punitive, liberal leave).

3.4. Establish sick leave policies for staff and students suspected to be ill or who become ill at school. Staff and students with known or suspected pandemic influenza should not remain at school and should return only after their symptoms resolve and they are physically ready to return to school.

3.5. Establish policies for transporting ill students.

3.6. Ensure that the LEA pandemic plan for school-based health facilities conform to those recommended for health care settings.

4.   Communications Planning

4.1. Assess readiness to meet communications needs in preparation for an influenza pandemic, including regular review, testing, and updating of communications plans.

4.2. Develop a dissemination plan for communication with staff, students, and families, including lead spokespersons and links to other communication networks.

4.3. Ensure language, culture, and reading level appropriateness in communications by including community leaders representing different language and/or ethnic groups on the planning committee, asking for their participation in both document planning and the dissemination of public health messages within their communities.

4.4. Develop and test platforms (e.g., hotlines, telephone trees, dedicated websites, local radio or TV stations) for communicating pandemic status and actions to school district staff, students, and families.

4.5. Develop and maintain up-to-date communications contacts of key public health and education stakeholders and use the network to provide regular updates as the influenza pandemic unfolds.

4.6. Ensure the provision of redundant communication systems/channels that allow for the expedited transmission and receipt of information.

4.7. Advise district staff, students, and families where to find up-to-date and reliable pandemic information from Federal, State, and local public health sources.

4.8. Disseminate information about the LEA's pandemic influenza preparedness and response plan (e.g., continuity of instruction, community containment measures).

4.9. Disseminate information from public health sources covering routine infection control (e.g., hand hygiene, cough/sneeze etiquette), pandemic influenza fundamentals (e.g., signs and symptoms of influenza, modes of transmission), as well as personal and family protection and response strategies (e.g., guidance for the at-home care of ill students and family members).

4.10. Anticipate the potential fear and anxiety of staff, students, and families as a result of rumors and misinformation and plan communications accordingly.

Guidance for Colleges and Universities

Colleges and universities must ensure preparedness, and the communication of roles and responsibilities related to ensuring continuity of instruction and protection of students and personnel. In the event of an influenza pandemic, colleges and universities will play an integral role in protecting the health and safety of students, employees and their families. HHS, in coordination with the Department of Education, has developed the following checklist as a framework to assist colleges and universities to develop and/or improve plans to prepare for and respond to an influenza pandemic. Further information can be found at www.pandemicflu.gov.

1.   Planning and Coordination

1.1. Identify a pandemic coordinator and response team (including campus health services and mental health staff, student housing personnel, security, communications staff, physical plant staff, food services director, academic staff, and student representatives) with defined roles and responsibilities for preparedness, response, and recovery planning.

1.2. Delineate accountability and responsibility as well as resources for key stakeholders engaged in planning and executing specific components of the operational plan. Ensure that the plan includes timelines, deliverables, and performance measures.

1.3. Incorporate into the pandemic plan scenarios that address college/university functioning based upon having various levels of illness in students and employees and different types of community containment interventions. Plan for different outbreak scenarios including variations in severity of illness, mode of transmission, and rates of infection in the community. Issues to consider include:

- cancellation of classes, sporting events, and/or public events;

- closure of campus, student housing, and/or public transportation;

- assessment of the suitability of student housing for quarantine of exposed and/or ill students;

- contingency plans for students who depend on student housing and food services (e.g., international students or students who live too far away to travel home);

- contingency plans for maintaining research laboratories, particularly those using animals; and

- stockpiling non-perishable food and equipment that may be needed in the case of an influenza pandemic.

1.4. Work with local public health authorities to identify legal authority, decision makers, trigger points, and thresholds to institute community containment measures such as closing (and re-opening) the college/university. Identify and review the college/university's legal responsibilities and authorities for executing infection control measures, including case identification, reporting information about ill students and employees, isolation, movement restriction, and provision of health care on campus.

1.5. Ensure that pandemic influenza planning is consistent with any existing college/university emergency operations plan, and is coordinated with the pandemic plan of the community and of the State higher education agency.

1.6. Work with the local health department to discuss an operational plan for surge capacity for health care and other mental health and social services to meet the needs of the college/university and community during and after a pandemic.

1.7. Establish an emergency communication plan and revise regularly. This plan should identify key contacts with local and State public health officials as well as the State's higher education officials (including back-ups) and the chain of communications, including alternate mechanisms.

1.8. Test the linkages between the college/university's ICS and the ICS of the local and/or State health department and the State's higher education agency.

1.9. Implement an exercise/drill to test your plan, and revise it regularly.

1.10. Participate in exercises of the community's pandemic plan.

1.11. Share what you have learned from developing your preparedness and response plan with other colleges/universities to improve community response efforts.

2. **Continuity of Student Learning and Operations**

2.1. Develop and disseminate alternative procedures to ensure continuity of instruction (e.g., web-based distance instruction, telephone trees, mailed lessons and assignments, instruction via local radio or television stations) in the event of college/university closures.

2.2. Develop a continuity of operations plan for maintaining the essential operations of the college/university including payroll; ongoing communication with employees, students and families; security; maintenance; as well as housekeeping and food service for student housing.

3. **Infection Control Policies and Procedures**

3.1. Implement infection control policies and procedures that help limit the spread of influenza on campus (e.g., promotion of hand hygiene, cough/sneeze etiquette). Make good hygiene a habit now in order to help protect employees and students from many infectious diseases such as influenza. Encourage students and staff to get annual influenza vaccine.

3.2. Procure, store, and provide sufficient and accessible infection prevention supplies (e.g., soap, alcohol-based hand hygiene products, tissues and receptacles for their disposal).

3.3. Establish policies for employee and student sick-leave absences unique to pandemic influenza (e.g., non-punitive, liberal leave).

3.4. Establish sick leave policies for employees and students suspected to be ill or who become ill on campus. Employees and students with known or suspected pandemic influenza should not remain on campus and should return only after their symptoms resolve and they are physically ready to return to campus.

3.5. Establish a pandemic plan for campus-based health care facilities that addresses issues unique to health care settings. Ensure health services and clinics have identified critical supplies needed to support a surge in demand and take steps to have those supplies on hand.

3.6. Adopt CDC travel recommendations during an influenza pandemic, and be able to support voluntary and mandatory movement restrictions. Recommendations may include restricting travel to and from affected domestic and international areas, recalling non-essential employees working in or near an affected area when an outbreak begins, and distributing health information to persons who are returning from affected areas.

4.   Communications Planning

4.1. Assess readiness to meet communications needs in preparation for an influenza pandemic, including regular review, testing, and updating of communications plans that link with public health authorities and other key stakeholders.

4.2. Develop a dissemination plan or communication with employees, students, and families, including lead spokespersons and links to other communication networks. Ensure language, culture, and reading level appropriateness in communications.

4.3. Develop and test platforms (e.g., hotlines, telephone trees, dedicated websites, local radio or television) for communicating college/university response and actions to employees, students, and families.

4.4. Ensure the provision of redundant communication systems/channels that allow for the expedited transmission and receipt of information.

4.5. Advise employees and students where to find up-to-date and reliable pandemic information from Federal, State, and local public health sources.

4.6. Disseminate information about the college/university's pandemic preparedness and response plan. This should include the potential impact of a pandemic on student housing closure, and the contingency plans for students who depend on student housing and campus food service, including how student safety will be maintained for those who remain in student housing.

4.7. Disseminate information from public health sources covering routine infection control (e.g., hand hygiene, cough/sneeze etiquette), pandemic influenza fundamentals (e.g., signs and symptoms of influenza, modes of transmission), personal and family protection and response strategies, and the at-home care of ill students or employees and their family members.

4.8. Anticipate and plan communications to address the potential fear and anxiety of employees, students, and families that may result from rumors or misinformation.

Guidance for Faith-Based and Community-Based Organizations

The collaboration of faith-based organizations (FBOs) and community-based organizations (CBOs) with public health agencies will be essential in providing the public's health and safety if and when an influenza pandemic occurs. HHS has developed the following checklist for FBOs and CBOs. This checklist identifies important, specific activities FBOs and CBOs can do now to prepare. Further information can be found at **www.pandemicflu.gov.**

1. **Plan for the impact of a pandemic on your organization and its mission**

    1.1. Assign key staff with the authority to develop, maintain, and act upon an influenza pandemic preparedness and response plan.

    1.2. Determine the potential impact of a pandemic on your organization's usual activities and services. Plan for situations likely to require increasing, decreasing, or altering the services your organization delivers.

    1.3. Determine the potential impact of a pandemic on outside resources that your organization depends on to deliver its services (e.g., supplies, travel).

    1.4. Outline what the organizational structure will be during an emergency and revise periodically. The outline should identify key contacts with multiple back-ups, roles and responsibilities, and who is supposed to report to whom.

    1.5. Identify and train essential staff (including full-time, part-time, and unpaid or volunteer staff) needed to carry on your organization's work during a pandemic. Include back up plans, cross-train staff in other jobs so that if staff are sick, others are ready to come in to carry on the work.

    1.6. Test your response and preparedness plan using an exercise or drill, and review and revise your plan as needed.

2. **Communicate with and educate your staff, members, and persons in the community that you serve**

    2.1. Find up-to-date, reliable pandemic information and other public health advisories from State and local health departments, emergency management agencies, and HHS. Make this information available to your organization and others.

    2.2. Distribute materials with basic information about pandemic influenza: signs and symptoms, how it is spread, ways to protect yourself and your family (e.g., respiratory hygiene and cough etiquette), family preparedness plans, and how to care for ill persons at home.

2.3. When appropriate, include basic information about pandemic influenza in public meetings (e.g., sermons, classes, trainings, small group meetings, announcements).

2.4. Share information about your pandemic preparedness and response plan with staff, members, and persons in the communities that you serve.

2.5. Develop tools to communicate to staff, members, and persons in the communities that you serve information about pandemic status and your organization's actions. This might include websites, flyers, local newspaper announcements, pre-recorded widely distributed phone messages, etc.

2.6. Consider your organization's unique contribution to addressing rumors, misinformation, fear, and anxiety.

2.7. Advise staff, members, and persons in the communities you serve to follow information provided by public health authorities -- State and local health departments, emergency management agencies, and HHS.

2.8. Ensure that what you communicate is appropriate for the cultures, languages, and reading levels of your staff, members, and persons in the communities that you serve.

3. Plan for the impact of a pandemic on your staff, members, and the communities that you serve

3.1. Plan for staff absences during a pandemic due to personal and/or family illnesses, quarantines, and school, business, and public transportation closures. Staff may include full-time, part-time, and volunteer personnel.

3.2. Work with local health authorities to encourage yearly influenza vaccination for staff, members, and persons in the communities that you serve.

3.3. Evaluate access to mental health and social services during a pandemic for your staff, members, and persons in the communities that you serve; improve access to these services as needed.

3.4. Identify persons with special needs (e.g., elderly, disabled, limited English speakers) and be sure to include their needs in your response and preparedness plan. Establish relationships with them in advance so they will expect and trust your presence during a crisis.

4. Set up policies to follow during a pandemic

4.1. Set up policies for non-penalized leave for personal illness or care for sick family members during a pandemic.

4.2. Set up mandatory sick-leave policies for staff suspected to be ill, or who become ill at the worksite. Employees should remain at home until their symptoms resolve and they are physically ready to return to duty.

4.3. Set up policies for flexible work hours and working from home.

4.4. Evaluate your organization's usual activities and services (including rites and religious practices if applicable) to identify those that may facilitate virus spread from person to person. Set up policies to modify these activities to prevent the spread of pandemic influenza (e.g., guidance for respiratory hygiene and cough etiquette, and instructions for persons with influenza symptoms to stay home and phone the organization rather than visit in person).

4.5. Follow HHS travel recommendations during an influenza pandemic. Recommendations may include restricting travel to affected domestic and international sites, recalling non-essential staff working in or near an affected site when an outbreak begins, and distributing health information to persons who are returning from affected areas.

4.6. Set procedures for activating your organization's response plan when an influenza pandemic is declared by public health authorities and altering your organization's operations accordingly.

5. **Allocate resources to protect your staff, members, and persons in the communities that you serve during a pandemic**

5.1. Determine the amount of supplies needed to promote respiratory hygiene and cough etiquette and how they will be obtained.

5.2. Consider focusing your organization's efforts during a pandemic to providing services that are most needed during the emergency (e.g., mental/spiritual health or social services).

6. **Coordinate with external organizations and help your community**

6.1. Understand the roles of Federal, State, and local public health agencies and emergency responders and what to expect and what not to expect from each in the event of a pandemic.

6.2. Work with local and/or State public health agencies, emergency responders, local health care facilities, and insurers to understand their plans and what they can provide, share about your preparedness and response plan and what your organization is able to contribute, and take part in their planning. Assign a point of contact to maximize communication between your organization and your State and local public health systems.

6.3. Coordinate with emergency responders and local health care facilities to improve availability of medical advice and timely/urgent health care services for your staff, members, and persons in the communities that you serve.

6.4. Share what you've learned from developing your preparedness and response plan with other FBOs and CBOs to improve community response efforts.

6.5. Work together with other FBOs and CBOs in your local area and through networks (e.g., denominations, associations) to help your communities prepare for pandemic influenza.

Planning Guidance for Individuals and Families

Individuals and families can prepare for an influenza pandemic now. This guidance is designed to help you understand the threat of a pandemic influenza outbreak in our country and your community.

It describes common sense actions that you can take in preparing for a pandemic. Each individual and family should know both the magnitude of what can happen during a pandemic outbreak and what actions you can take to help lessen the impact of an influenza pandemic on you and your community. Further information including a planning checklist can be found at **www.pandemicflu.gov.**

Pandemic Influenza: What Individuals Need to Know

An influenza (flu) pandemic is a widespread outbreak of disease that occurs when a new influenza virus appears that people have not been exposed to before. Pandemics are different from seasonal outbreaks of influenza. Seasonal influenza outbreaks are caused by viruses that people have already been exposed to; influenza shots are available to help prevent widespread illness, and impacts on society are less severe. Pandemic influenza spreads easily from person to person and can cause serious illness because people do not have immunity to the new virus.

Some Differences between Seasonal Flu and Pandemic Flu

Seasonal Flu	**Pandemic Flu**
Caused by influenza viruses that are similar to those already affecting people.	Caused by a new influenza virus that people have not been exposed to before. Likely to be more severe, affect more people, and cause more deaths than seasonal influenza because people will not have immunity to the new virus.
Symptoms include fever, cough, runny nose, and muscle pain. Deaths can be caused by complications such as pneumonia.	Symptoms similar to the common flu may be more severe and complications more serious.
Healthy adults usually not at risk for serious complications (the very young, the elderly, and those with certain underlying health conditions at increased risk for serious complications).	Healthy adults may be at increased risk for serious complications.
Generally causes modest impact on society (e.g., some school closings, encouragement of people who are sick to stay home).	A severe pandemic could change the patterns of daily life for some time. People may choose to stay home to keep away from others who are sick. Also, people may need to stay home to care for ill family and loved ones. Travel and public gatherings could be limited. Basic services and access to supplies could be disrupted.

A pandemic may come and go in waves, each of which can last for months at a time. Everyday life could be disrupted due to people in communities across the country becoming ill at the same time. These disruptions could include everything from school and business closings to interruption of basic services such as public transportation and health care. An especially severe influenza pandemic could lead to high levels of illness, death, social disruption, and economic loss.

Importance and Benefits of Being Prepared

It is difficult to predict when the next influenza pandemic will occur or how severe it will be. The effects of a pandemic can be lessened if preparations are made ahead of time. When a pandemic starts, everyone around the world could be at risk. The United States has been working closely with other countries and the World Health Organization (WHO) to strengthen systems to detect outbreaks of influenza that might cause a pandemic.

A pandemic would touch every aspect of society, and so every aspect of society must begin to prepare. State, tribal, and local governments are developing, improving, and testing their plans for an influenza pandemic. Businesses, schools, universities, and other community organizations are preparing plans as well.

As you begin your individual or family planning, you may want to review your State's planning efforts and those of your local public health and emergency preparedness officials. Many of the State plans and other planning information can be found at **www.pandemicflu.gov.**

The Department of Health and Human Services (HHS) and other Federal agencies are providing funding, advice, and other support to your State. The Federal Government will provide up-to-date information and guidance to the public if an influenza pandemic unfolds. For reliable, accurate, and timely information, visit the Federal Government's official website at **www.pandemicflu.gov.**

The benefits of preparation will be many. States and communities will be better prepared for any disaster. Preparation will bring peace of mind and the confidence that we are ready to fight an influenza pandemic.

Pandemic Influenza - Challenges and Preparation

As you plan, it is important to think about the challenges that you might face, particularly if a pandemic is severe. It may take time to find the answers to these challenges. The following are some situations that could be caused by a severe pandemic and possible ways to address them. A series of checklists have been prepared to help guide those efforts, to organize our national thinking, and bring consistency to our efforts. You will find two checklists (Pandemic Flu Planning Checklist for Individuals and Families; Family Emergency Health Information Sheet) to help you plan at **www.pandemicflu.gov.**

Social Disruption May Be Widespread

- Plan for the possibility that usual services may be disrupted. These could include services provided by hospitals and other health care facilities, banks, stores, restaurants, government offices, and post offices.

- Prepare backup plans in case public gatherings, such as volunteer meetings and worship services, are canceled.

- Consider how to care for people with special needs in case the services they rely on are not available.

Being Able to Work May Be Difficult or Impossible

- Find out if you can work from home.

- Ask your employer about how business will continue during a pandemic. (A Business Pandemic Influenza Planning Checklist is available at **www.pandemicflu.gov.**)

- Plan for the possible reduction or loss of income if you are unable to work or your place of employment is closed.

- Check with your employer or union about leave policies.

Schools May Be Closed for an Extended Period of Time

- Help schools plan for pandemic influenza. Talk to the school nurse or the health center. Talk to your teachers, administrators, and parent-teacher organizations.

- Plan home learning activities and exercises. Have materials, such as books, on hand. Also plan recreational activities that your children can do at home.

- Consider childcare needs.

Transportation Services May Be Disrupted

- Think about how you can rely less on public transportation during a pandemic. For example, store food and other essential supplies so you can make fewer trips to the store.

- Prepare backup plans for taking care of loved ones who are far away.

- Consider other ways to get to work, or, if you can, work at home.

People Will Need Advice and Help at Work and Home

- Think about what information the people in your workplace will need if you are a manager. This may include information about insurance, leave policies, working from home, possible loss of income, and when not to come to work if sick. (A Business Pandemic Influenza Planning Checklist is available at **www.pandemicflu.gov.**)

- Meet with your colleagues and make lists of things that you will need to know and what actions can be taken.

- Find volunteers who want to help people in need, such as elderly neighbors, single parents of small children, or people without the resources to get the medical help they will need.

- Identify other information resources in your community, such as mental health hotlines, public health hotlines, or electronic bulletin boards.

- Find support systems-people who are thinking about the same issues you are thinking about. Share ideas.

Be Prepared

Stock a supply of water and food. During a pandemic you may not be able to get to a store. Even if you can get to a store, it may be out of supplies. Public waterworks services may also be interrupted. Stocking supplies can be useful in other types of emergencies, such as power outages and disasters. Store foods that:

- are nonperishable (will keep for a long time) and don't require refrigeration.

- are easy to prepare in case you are unable to cook.

- require little or no water, so you can conserve water for drinking.

Stay Healthy

Take common-sense steps to limit the spread of germs. Make good hygiene a habit.

- Wash hands frequently with soap and water.

- Cover your mouth and nose with a tissue when you cough or sneeze.

- Put used tissues in a waste basket.

- Cough or sneeze into your upper sleeve if you don't have a tissue.

- Clean your hands after coughing or sneezing. Use soap and water or an alcohol-based hand cleaner.

- Stay at home if you are sick.

It is always a good idea to practice good health habits.

- Eat a balanced diet. Be sure to eat a variety of foods, including plenty of vegetables, fruits, and whole grain products. Also include low-fat dairy products, lean meats, poultry, fish, and beans. Drink lots of water and go easy on salt, sugar, alcohol, and saturated fat.

- Exercise on a regular basis and get plenty of rest.

Will the seasonal flu shot protect me against pandemic influenza?

- No, it won't protect you against pandemic influenza. But flu shots can help you to stay healthy.

- Get a flu shot to help protect yourself from seasonal influenza.

- Get a pneumonia shot to prevent secondary infection if you are over the age of 65 or have a chronic illness such as diabetes or asthma.

- Make sure that your family's immunizations are up-to-date.

Get Informed

- Knowing the facts is the best preparation. Identify sources you can count on for reliable information. If a pandemic occurs, having accurate and reliable information will be critical.

- Reliable, accurate, and timely information is available at **www.pandemicflu.gov.**

- Another source for information on pandemic influenza is the Centers for Disease Control and Prevention (CDC) Hotline at: 1-800-CDC-INFO (1-800-232-4636). This line is available in English and Spanish, 24 hours a day, 7 days a week.

- Look for information on your local and State government websites. Links are available to each State department of public health at **www.pandemicflu.gov.**

- Listen to local and national radio, watch news reports on television, and read your newspaper and other sources of printed and web-based information.

- Talk to your local health care providers and public health officials.

Pandemic Influenza - Prevention and Treatment

You have an essential role in preparing and making sure you are informed of prevention activities in your local area. Each community must have plans, each State and each agency of the Federal Government must work together. The Federal Government is working to boost our international and domestic disease monitoring, rebuild our vaccine industry, build stockpiles of medicines, and support research into new treatments and medicines. Your State will be taking steps to monitor and build supplies too.

Vaccine

Influenza vaccines are designed to protect against specific influenza viruses. While there is currently no pandemic influenza in the world, the Federal Government is making vaccines for several existing bird influenza viruses that may provide some protection should one of these viruses change and cause an influenza pandemic. A specific pandemic influenza vaccine cannot be produced until a pandemic influenza virus strain emerges and is identified. Once a pandemic influenza virus has been identified, it will likely take 4-6 months to develop, test, and begin producing a vaccine.

Efforts are being made to increase vaccine-manufacturing capacity in the United States so that supplies of vaccines would be more readily available. In addition, research is underway to develop new ways to produce vaccines more quickly.

Treatment

A number of antiviral drugs are approved by the U.S. Food and Drug Administration to treat and sometimes prevent seasonal influenza. Some of these antiviral medications may be effective in treating pandemic influenza. These drugs may help prevent infection in people at risk and shorten the duration of symptoms in those infected with influenza. However, it is unlikely that antiviral medications alone would effectively contain the spread of pandemic influenza. The Federal Government is stockpiling antiviral medications that would most likely be used in the early stages of an influenza pandemic. There are efforts to find new drugs and to increase the supply of antiviral medications. Antiviral medications are available by prescription only and not over the counter.

Questions and Answers

Will bird flu cause the next influenza pandemic?

Avian influenza (bird flu) is a disease of wild and farm birds caused by influenza viruses. Bird flu viruses do not usually infect humans, but since 1997 there have been a number of confirmed cases of human infection from bird flu viruses. Most of these resulted from direct or close contact with infected birds (e.g., domesticated chickens, ducks, turkeys).

The spread of bird flu viruses from an infected person to another person has been reported very rarely and has not been reported to continue beyond one person. A worldwide pandemic could occur if a bird flu virus were to change so that it could easily be passed from person to person. Experts around the world are watching for changes in bird flu viruses that could lead to an influenza pandemic.

Is it safe to eat poultry?

Yes, it is safe to eat properly cooked poultry. Cooking destroys germs, including the bird flu virus. The United States bans imports of poultry and poultry products from countries where bird flu has been found.

Guidelines for the safe preparation of poultry include the following:

- Wash hands before and after handling food.

- Keep raw poultry and its juices away from other foods.

- Keep hands, utensils, and surfaces, such as cutting boards, clean.

- Use a food thermometer to ensure poultry has been fully cooked. More information on how to properly cook poultry can be found at www.usda.gov/birdflu.

What types of birds can carry bird flu viruses?

Wild birds can carry bird flu viruses but usually do not get sick from them. Domesticated birds (e.g., farm-raised chickens, ducks, and turkeys) can become sick with bird flu if they come into contact with an infected wild bird. Domesticated birds usually die from the disease.

What is the U.S. Government doing to prepare for pandemic influenza?

The U.S. Government has been preparing for pandemic influenza for several years. In November 2005, the President announced the *National Strategy for Pandemic Influenza*. Ongoing preparations include the following:

- Working with WHO and with other nations to help detect human cases of bird flu and contain an influenza pandemic, if one begins.

- Supporting the manufacturing and testing of influenza vaccines, including finding more reliable and quicker ways to make large quantities of vaccines.

- Developing a national stockpile of antiviral drugs to help treat and control the spread of disease.

- Supporting the efforts of Federal, State, tribal, and local health agencies to prepare for and respond to pandemic influenza.

- Working with Federal agencies to prepare and to encourage communities, businesses, and organizations to plan for pandemic influenza.

APPENDIX B

Glossary of Terms

For the purposes of the National Pandemic Influenza Implementation Plan (Plan):

Acronyms

AHPA	Animal Health Protection Act
AIDS	Acquired immunodeficiency syndrome
APEC	Asia Pacific Economic Cooperation Forum
APHIS	Animal and Plant Health Inspection Service
ASEAN	Association of Southeast Asian Nations
ATF	Bureau of Alcohol, Tobacco, Firearms, and Explosives
ATSA	Aviation and Transportation Security Act
CBO	Community-based organization
CBP	Customs and Border Protection
CDC	Centers for Disease Control and Prevention
CFR	Code of Federal Regulations
CIP	Critical infrastructure protection
CITES	Convention on International Trade in Endangered Species of Wild Fauna and Flora
CONUS	Continental United States
COOP	Continuity of operations
DEA	Drug Enforcement Administration
DHS	Department of Homeland Security
DOC	Department of Commerce
DOD	Department of Defense
DOE	Department of Energy
DOI	Department of the Interior
DOJ	Department of Justice
DOL	Department of Labor
DOS	Department of State
DOT	Department of Transportation
DPA	Defense Production Act
EIP	Emerging Infections Program
EIS	Epidemic Intelligence Service
EMAC	Emergency Management Assistance Compact

EMS	Emergency Medical Services
EMTALA	Emergency Medical Treatment and Active Labor Act
EPA	Environmental Protection Agency
ESA	Endangered Species Act
ESAR-VHP	Emergency System for the Advanced Registration of Volunteer Health Professionals
ESF	Emergency Support Function
ESF #1	Emergency Support Function #1 - Transportation
ESF #8	Emergency Support Function #8 - Public Health and Medical Services
ESF #11	Emergency Support Function #11 - Agriculture and Natural Resources
ESF #13	Emergency Support Function #13 - Public Safety and Security
ESSENCE	Electronic Surveillance System for Early Notification of Community-based Epidemics
FAA	Federal Aviation Administration
FAMS	Federal Air Marshal Service
FAO	United Nations Food and Agriculture Organization
FBI	Federal Bureau of Investigation
FBO	Faith-based organization
FDA	Food and Drug Administration
FEMA	Federal Emergency Management Agency
FHWA	Federal Highway Administration
FMCSA	Federal Motor Carrier Safety Administration
FMS	Federal medical station
FOAA	Federal Operations, Export Financing, and Related Programs Appropriations Act
FPC	Federal Preparedness Circular
FRA	Federal Railroad Administration
FWA	Fish and Wildlife Act
G-8	Group of Eight (major industrialized nations) including the United States, France, Italy, Germany, Japan, United Kingdom, Canada, Russia
GEIS	Global Emerging Infections Surveillance and Response System
GHSAG	Global Health Security Action Group
GOARN	Global Outbreak Alert and Response Network
HAvBED	National Hospital Available Beds for Emergencies and Disasters
HCA	Humanitarian and Civic Assistance
HHS	Department of Health and Human Services
HIPAA	Health Insurance Portability and Accountability Act
HPAI	Highly pathogenic avian influenza
HSC	Homeland Security Council

HSPD-5	Homeland Security Presidential Directive 5
HSPD-7	Homeland Security Presidential Directive 7
HSPD-8	Homeland Security Presidential Directive 8
ICAO	International Civil Aviation Organization
ICLN	Integrated Consortium of Laboratory Networks
ICU	Intensive care unit
IFI	International financial institution
IHR	International Health Regulations
IMO	International Maritime Organization
IPAPI	International Partnership on Avian and Pandemic Influenza
LBMS	Live bird marketing system
LEA	Local education agencies
LRN	Laboratory Response Network
MARAD	Maritime Administration
MBTA	Migratory Bird Treaty Act
MDB	Multilateral development banks
MTF	Medical treatment facility
NAHLN	National Animal Health Laboratory Network
NAMRU	Naval Medical Research Unit
NBIS	National Biosurveillance Integration System
NDMS	National Disaster Medical System
NEC	National Economic Council
NGO	Non-governmental organization
NHTSA	National Highway Traffic Safety Administration
NIMS	National Incident Management System
NPIP	National Poultry Improvement Program
NRC	Nuclear Regulatory Commission
NRP	National Response Plan
NSC	National Security Council
NVS	National Veterinary Stockpile
NVSL	National Veterinary Services Laboratories
NVSN	New Vaccine Surveillance Network
NWHC	National Wildlife Health Center
OCONUS	Outside the continental United States
OHDCA	Overseas Humanitarian, Disaster, and Civic Aid

OIE	World Organization for Animal Health (formerly named the "Office International des Epizooties")
OPM	Office of Personnel Management
Partnership	International Partnership on Avian and Pandemic Influenza
PHEO	Public Health Emergency Officer
PHS	U.S. Public Health Service
PHSA	Public Health Service Act
PHSBPR	Public Health Security and Bioterrorism Preparedness and Response Act
PPE	Personal protective equipment
PPIA	Poultry Products Inspection Act
PSAP	Public safety answering point
REDI	Regional Emerging Disease Intervention Center in Singapore
RT-PCR	Reverse transcriptase - polymerase chain reaction
SAFETEA-LU	Safe, Accountable, Flexible, Efficient Transportation Equity Act: A Legacy for Users
SARS	Severe acute respiratory syndrome
SCHIP	State Children's Health Insurance Program
SLEP	Shelf Life Extension Program
SNS	Strategic National Stockpile
SPN	Sentinel Provider Network
SPP	Security and Prosperity Partnership
STB	Surface Transportation Board
TIGR	The Institute for Genomic Research
Treasury	Department of the Treasury
TSA	Transportation Security Administration
UN	United Nations
USACE	U.S. Army Corps of Engineers
USAID	U.S. Agency for International Development
USCG	U.S. Coast Guard
USDA	Department of Agriculture
USTR	U.S. Trade Representative
VA	Department of Veterans Affairs
VHA	Veterans Health Administration
WHO	World Health Organization

Definition of Terms

Adjuvants. Substances that can be added to a vaccine to increase the effectiveness of the vaccine.

Affected country. An at-risk country experiencing endemic (widespread and recurring) or epidemic (isolated) cases in humans or domestic animals of influenza with human pandemic potential.

Antiviral medications. Medications presumed to be effective against potential pandemic influenza virus strains. These antiviral medications include the neuraminidase inhibitors oseltamivir (Tamiflu®) and zanamivir (Relenza®).

Arrival screening. Medical screening upon arrival to detect individuals who have signs of illness or who are at high risk of developing illness.

Asymptomatic. Asymptomatic means without symptoms of influenza.

At-risk country. An unaffected country with insufficient medical, public health, or veterinary capacity to prevent, detect, or contain influenza with pandemic potential.

Colleges. Educational institutions post 12th grade (post high school).

Community-based organization. A private nonprofit organization, Indian tribe or tribally sanctioned organization, or other type of group that works within a community for the improvement of some aspect of that community. Community-based organizations include non-profit organizations (501 c(3)), faith-based organizations, tribes, and their subsidiaries.

Containment. Contain an outbreak to the affected region(s) and limit of spread of the pandemic through aggressive attempts to contain.

Continuity of operations. Refers to the capability to ensure the performance of essential functions during any emergency or situation that may disrupt normal operations.

Cough etiquette. Covering ones mouth and nose while coughing or sneezing; using tissues and disposing in no-touch receptacles; and washing your hands to avoid spreading an infection to others.

Countermeasures. Refers to pre-pandemic and pandemic influenza vaccine and antiviral medications.

Critical infrastructure. Systems and assets, whether physical or virtual, so vital to the United States that the incapacity or destruction of such systems and assets would have a debilitating impact on security, national economic security, national public health or safety, or any combination of those matters. Specifically, it refers to the critical infrastructure sectors and key resources identified in Homeland Security Presidential Directive 7 (HSPD-7). As defined by HSPD-7, critical infrastructure includes the following sectors and key resources: agriculture and food; public health and health care; drinking water and water treatment systems; energy (including the production, refining, storage, and distribution of oil and gas, and electric power except for nuclear facilities); banking and finance; national monuments and icons; defense industrial base; information technology; telecommunications; chemical; transportation systems (including mass transit, aviation, maritime, ground/surface, and rail and pipeline systems); emergency services; postal and shipping; dams; government facilities; commercial facilities; and nuclear reactors, material, and waste. Critical infrastructure in this Plan is used to refer to the 17 critical infrastructure and key resources included in the National Infrastructure Protection Plan.

Delegation of authority. Identification, by position, the authorities for making policy determinations and decisions at headquarters, field levels, and other organizational locations, as appropriate. Generally, pre-determined delegations of authority will take effect when normal channels of direction are disrupted and terminate when these channels have resumed.

Departure screening. Medical screening prior to departure from a high-risk area to identify individuals who have signs of illness (influenza) or who are at high risk of developing illness.

Devolution. The capability to transfer and sustain authority and responsibility for essential functions from an organization's primary operating staff and facilities, to other employees and facilities.

Disaggregation of disease transmission networks. The disruption of activities and social interactions that facilitate transmission of influenza (e.g., closure of schools, canceling public meetings or large social gatherings, keeping schoolchildren home, and restriction of travel).

Domestic animals. Livestock, including poultry, and other farmed birds or mammals; does not include companion animals such as dogs, cats, or pet birds.

Dose sparing strategies. Strategies to increase influenza vaccine immunogenicity and minimize the dose of vaccine necessary to confer immunity.

En route screening. Surveillance (typically by non-medical personnel) to detect individuals who develop signs of illness (influenza) while en route.

Epidemic. A pronounced clustering of cases of disease within a short period of time; more generally, a disease whose frequency of occurrence is in excess of the expected frequency in a population during a given time interval.

ESAR-VHP. Emergency System for Advance Registration of Volunteer Health Professionals.

Essential functions. Functions that are absolutely necessary to keep a business operating during an influenza pandemic, and critical to survival and recovery.

Face mask. Disposable surgical or procedure face mask (see definitions of both below).

Faith-based organization. Any organization that has a faith-inspired interest.

Geographic quarantine (cordon sanitaire). The isolation, by force if necessary, of localities with documented disease transmission from localities still free of infection.

Hand hygiene. Hand washing with either plain soap or antimicrobial soap and water and use of alcohol-based products (gels, rinses, foams) containing an emollient that do not require the use of water.

High-throughput rapid diagnostic kit. Medical technology to accurately and rapidly detect influenza strains. The technology is currently being used to rapidly detect avian influenza employing nucleic acid diagnostic primers (short strands of DNA/RNA).

High-risk country. An at-risk country that is located in proximity to an affected country, or in which a wildlife case of influenza with pandemic potential has been detected.

Highly pathogenic avian influenza (HPAI). An infection of poultry caused by any influenza A virus that meets the World Organization for Animal Health (OIE) definition for high pathogenicity based on the mortality rate of chickens exposed to the virus intravenously or on the amino acid sequence of the cleavage site of the virus' hemagglutinin molecule.

Installations. Refers to military posts, installation, bases, stations, and activities.

International financial institution. Usually refers to intergovernmental organizations dealing with financial issues, most often the International Monetary Fund and/or the World Bank.

International Partnership for Avian and Pandemic Influenza (the Partnership; IPAPI). Partnership announced by President Bush at the UN General Assembly on September 14, 2005. Over 80 countries and 8 international organizations are working in the Partnership to fight pandemic influenza nationally and globally.

Isolation. Separation of infected individuals from those who are not infected.

Key assets. Subset of key resources that are "individual targets whose destruction could cause large scale injury, death, or destruction of property, and/or profoundly damage our national prestige or confidence."

Key resources. Publicly or privately controlled resources essential to the minimal operations of the economy and government. This refers to the four key resources identified in HSPD-7 and the National Infrastructure Protection Plan. These four key resources include: dams; government facilities; commercial facilities; and nuclear reactors, material, and waste.

Laboratory Response Network. National network of local, State, and Federal public health, food testing, veterinary diagnostic, and environmental testing laboratories supported by CDC that provide the laboratory infrastructure and capacity to respond to biological and chemical terrorism, and other public health emergencies.

Layered protective measures. Rather than focusing on a single measure for mitigation, a layered approach uses an array of measures deployed in tandem, to reduce overall risk. A layered, system-wide, integrated approach to risk reduction includes redundant measures and is designed to avoid a single point of failure. Examples include, implementing pre-departure, en route, and arrival screening measures for international travel.

Live bird marketing system (LBMS). Live poultry markets in the United States and the poultry distributors and poultry production premises that supply those markets.

Local education agencies (LEAs). Local (State, county, city, district) school boards.

Localities. Refers to local (county, city, municipal) governments and agencies.

Multilateral development banks. Multilateral development banks are institutions that provide financial support and professional advice for economic and social development activities in developing countries.

National Animal Health Laboratory Network (NAHLN). Refers to a cooperative effort among the American Association of Veterinary Laboratory Diagnosticians, the USDA Animal and Plant Health Inspection Service, and the USDA Cooperative State Research, Education and Extension Service to coordinate the capabilities of Federal, State, and university veterinary diagnostic laboratories to enhance the response to animal health events.

National Poultry Improvement Plan (NPIP). Cooperative industry-State-Federal program that establishes standards for the evaluation of poultry with respect to freedom from certain diseases.

National veterinary services. The national veterinary administration, all the veterinary authorities, and all persons authorized, registered, or licensed by the veterinary statutory body of a country to prevent and/or control animal diseases.

National Veterinary Stockpile (NVS). Refers to the supply of materiel, including vaccine, that is appropriate for a response to a damaging animal disease and capable of deployment within 24 hours of an outbreak; the stockpile is maintained by USDA's Animal and Plant Health Inspection Service.

Orders of succession. Refers to the sequential order or ranking of individuals who would assume authority and responsibility if the leadership is incapacitated or unavailable.

Outbreak. An epidemic limited to localized increase in the incidence of disease, e.g., in a village, town, or closed institution; a cluster of cases of an infectious disease.

Outbreak containment. Disruption of epidemic amplification through the use of medical countermeasures and infection control techniques; "containment" also refers more generally to delaying the geospatial spread of an epidemic.

Pandemic. A worldwide epidemic when a new or novel strain of influenza virus emerges in which humans have little or no immunity, and develops the ability to infect and be passed between humans.

Pandemic vaccine. Vaccine for specific influenza virus strain that has evolved the capacity for sustained and efficient human-to-human transmission. This vaccine can only be developed once the pandemic strain emerges.

Pathogenicity. Refers to the condition or quality of being pathogenic, or the ability to cause disease.

Plan. Refers to the Implementation Plan for the National Strategy for Pandemic Influenza.

Post-exposure prophylaxis. The use of antiviral medications in individuals exposed to others with influenza to prevent disease transmission.

Pre-pandemic vaccine. Vaccine against strains of influenza virus in animals that have caused isolated infections in humans of pandemic potential. This vaccine is prepared prior to the emergence of a pandemic strain and may be a good or poor match (and hence of greater or lesser protection) for the pandemic strain that ultimately emerges.

Priority country. A priority country is a high-risk or affected country that merits special attention because of the severity of the outbreak, its strategic importance, its regional role, or foreign policy priorities.

Procedure mask. Disposable face mask that is either flat or pleated and is affixed to the head with ear loops.

Prophylaxis. Prevention of disease or of a process that can lead to disease. With respect to pandemic influenza this specifically refers to the administration of antiviral medications to healthy individuals for the prevention of influenza.

Quarantine. Separation of individuals who have been exposed to an infection but are not yet ill from others who have not been exposed to the transmissible infection.

Rapid diagnostic test. Medical test for rapidly confirming the presence of infection with a specific influenza strain.

Reconstitution. Refers to the process by which an organization resumes normal operations.

Respirator. Refers to a particulate respirator, commonly known as N-95 respirator, often used in hospitals to protect against infectious agents. Particulate respirators are "air-purifying respirators" because they clean particles out of the air as one breathes.

R_0. Represents the basic reproductive rate of a pathogen, i.e., the average number of secondary infections caused by an infected individual within a given social context. An $R_0 = 2$ means that infected individuals, on average, transmit infection to two other people, so that every generation of disease transmission doubles the number of people infected. R_0 will change during an epidemic as public health interventions are applied, the behavior of individuals changes, and as the pool of persons susceptible to the disease is depleted.

Schools (K-12). Refers to schools, both public and private, spanning the grades kindergarten through 12th grade (elementary through high school).

Sector. Part or division of the national economy.

Sector-Specific Agency. Federal departments and agencies identified under HSPD-7 as responsible for infrastructure protection activities in a designated critical infrastructure sector or key resources category.

Situational awareness. Situational awareness is the ability to identify, process, and comprehend the critical elements of information about what is happening during an evolving influenza pandemic.

Snow days. Refers to days which the authorities recommend that individuals and families limit social contacts by remaining within their households to reduce community disease transmission of infection.

Social distancing. Infection control strategies that reduce the duration and/or intimacy of social contacts and thereby limit the transmission of influenza. There are two basic categories of intervention: transmission interventions, such as the use of facemasks, may reduce the likelihood of casual social contacts resulting in disease transmission; contact interventions, such as closing schools or canceling large gatherings, eliminate or reduce the likelihood of contact with infected individuals.

Standard of care. The level of care that is reasonably expected under the extant circumstances.

States. Refers to State governments and State agencies.

Strategy. Refers to the *National Strategy for Pandemic Influenza*.

Surge capacity. Refers to the ability to expand provision of services beyond normal capacity to meet transient increases in demand. Surge capacity within a medical context denotes the ability of health care or laboratory facilities to provide care or services above their usual capacity, or to expand manufacturing capacity of essential medical materiel (e.g., vaccine) to meet increased demand.

Surgical mask. Refers to disposable face masks that comes in two basic types: one type is affixed to the head with two ties, conforms to the face with the aid of a flexible adjustment to the nose bridge, and may be flat/pleated or duck-billed in shape; the second type of surgical mask is pre-molded, adheres to the head with a single elastic and has a flexible adjustment for the nose bridge.

Symptomatic. Symptomatic means with symptoms of influenza.

Targeted passenger travel restrictions. Travel restrictions to the United States targeting travelers from a high-risk area or from areas unable to meet U.S. criteria for departure and en route screening.

Telecommuting. Working from home or an alternate site and avoiding coming to the workplace through telecommunication (computer access).

Telework. Refers to the activity of working away (home) from the workplace through telecommunication (computer access).

T_g. Generation time of a pathogen, or how long it takes for infected individuals to infect others. Epidemics caused by a pathogen with an $R_0 = 2$ and a $T_g = 2$ days will double in size about every 2 days, epidemics caused by a pathogen with an $R_0 = 3$ and a $T_g = 9$ days will triple in size about every 9 days, etc.

Treatment course (antiviral medications). The course of antiviral medication prescribed as treatment (not prophylaxis) for a person infected with an agent susceptible to the antiviral medication. For oseltamivir, a treatment course for seasonal influenza is 10 capsules, administered twice daily for 5 days (a prophylaxis course is much greater, typically 42 capsules taken once daily for 42 days).

Treatment course (vaccine). The course of vaccine (typically two injections) required to induce protective immunity against the target of the vaccine.

TRICARE. Department of Defense's worldwide health care program for active duty and retired uniformed services members and their families.

Universities. Refers to educational institutions post 12th grade (post high school).

U.S. travelers from affected areas. U.S. citizens traveling to the United States from countries or region where an outbreak (influenza pandemic) has occurred.

Virulence. Virulence refers to the disease-evoking severity of influenza.

Wave. The period during which an outbreak or epidemic occurs either within a community or aggregated across a larger geographical area. The disease wave includes the time during which disease occurrence increases rapidly, peaks, and declines back toward baseline.

APPENDIX C

Authorities and References

Various Federal statutes, regulations, orders, directives, and plans authorize or otherwise enable Federal departments and agencies to engage in actions to support the three pillars of the *National Strategy for Pandemic Influenza (Strategy)*: Preparedness and Communication; Surveillance and Detection; and Response and Containment. The major statutes, regulations, directives, and plans discussed in this Implementation Plan (Plan) are those summarized below.[23]

Chapter 2 - U.S. Government Planning for a Pandemic

Executive Order 12656, Assignment of Emergency Preparedness Responsibilities (November 18, 1988). This Executive Order assigns responsibilities to each Federal agency for national security and emergency preparedness.

Homeland Security Presidential Directive 5 (HSPD-5) Management of Domestic Incidents (February 28, 2003). This Presidential Directive is intended to enhance the ability of the United States to manage domestic incidents by establishing a single, comprehensive national incident management system. In HSPD-5 the President designates the Secretary of Homeland Security as the Principal Federal Official for Domestic Incident Management and empowers the Secretary to coordinate Federal resources used in response to or recovery from terrorist attacks, major disasters, or other emergencies in specific cases. The directive assigns specific responsibilities to the Attorney General, Secretary of Defense, Secretary of State, and the Assistants to the President for Homeland Security and National Security Affairs, and directs the heads of all Federal departments and agencies to provide their "full and prompt cooperation, resources, and support," as appropriate and consistent with their own responsibilities for protecting national security, to the Secretary of Homeland Security, Attorney General, Secretary of Defense, and Secretary of State in the exercise of leadership responsibilities and missions assigned under HSPD-5. The directive also notes that it does not alter, or impede the abilities of Federal departments and agencies to carry out their responsibilities under law.

National Response Plan (NRP). In HSPD-5, the President directed the development of a new NRP to align Federal coordination structures, capabilities, and resources into a unified, all-discipline, and all-hazards approach to domestic incident management. The NRP, released in December 2004 and fully implemented in April 2005, is such a plan. It provides the structure and mechanisms for the coordination of Federal support to State, local, and tribal incident managers and for exercising direct Federal authorities and responsibilities. The NRP assists in the important homeland security mission of preventing terrorist attacks within the United States; reducing the vulnerability to all natural and manmade hazards; and minimizing the damage and assisting in the recovery from any type of incident that occurs.

Chapter 3 - Federal Government Response to a Pandemic

The Economy Act, 31 U.S.C. §§ 1535-1536 (2002). The Economy Act authorizes Federal agencies to provide goods or services on a reimbursable basis to other Federal agencies when more specific statutory authority to do so does not exist.

---

[23] Some of the authorities and references described in this appendix are applicable to actions discussed in more than one chapter but may only be set forth in the section they are primarily applicable to.

Robert T. Stafford Disaster Relief and Emergency Assistance Act of 1974, codified as amended at 42 U.S.C. §§ 5121-5206, and scattered sections of 12 U.S.C., 16 U.S.C., 20 U.S.C., 26 U.S.C., 38 U.S.C. (2002). The Stafford Act establishes programs and processes for the Federal Government to provide disaster and emergency assistance to States, local governments, tribal nations, individuals, and qualified private nonprofit organizations. The provisions of the Stafford Act are broad and may cover many situations, including natural disasters and terrorist events. In a major disaster or emergency as defined in the Stafford Act, the President "may direct any Federal agency, with or without reimbursement, to utilize its authorities and the resources granted to it under Federal law (including personnel, equipment, supplies, facilities, and managerial, technical, and advisory services) in support of State and local assistance efforts."

Under the Act, the Federal Emergency Management Agency (FEMA) of the Department of Homeland Security (DHS), is authorized to coordinate the activities of Federal agencies in response to a Presidential declaration of a major disaster or emergency, if warranted, with the Department of Health and Human Services (HHS) having the lead for health and medical services. The President could declare either an emergency or a major disaster with respect to an influenza pandemic.

The National Emergencies Act, 50 U.S.C. §§ 1601-1651 (2003), establishes procedures for Presidential declaration and termination of national emergencies. The act requires the President to identify the specific provision of law under which he or she will act in dealing with a declared national emergency and contains a sunset provision requiring the President to renew a declaration of national emergency to prevent its automatic expiration. The Presidential declaration of a national emergency under the act is a prerequisite to exercising any special or extraordinary powers authorized by statute for use in the event of national emergency.

The Defense Production Act (DPA) of 1950, codified as amended by the Defense Production Act Reauthorization of 2003 at 50 U.S.C. app.§§ 2061-2171 (2002), is the primary authority to ensure the timely availability of resources for national defense and civil emergency preparedness and response. Among other things, the DPA authorizes the President to demand that companies accept and give priority to government contracts that the President "deems necessary or appropriate to promote the national defense." The DPA defines "national defense" to include critical infrastructure protection and restoration, as well as activities authorized by the emergency preparedness sections of the Stafford Act. Consequently, DPA authorities are available for activities and measures undertaken in preparation for, during, or following a natural disaster or accidental or man-caused event. The President's authority has been delegated to various agencies, depending on the product, with the Department of Commerce (DOC) providing overall coordination of the Defense Priorities and Allocations System. The DOC has redelegated DPA authority under Executive Order 12919, National Defense Industrial Resource Preparedness (June 7, 1994), as amended, to the Secretary of Homeland Security to place and, upon application, to authorize State and local governments to place priority-rated contracts in support of Federal, State, and local emergency preparedness activities.

The Public Health Security and Bioterrorism Preparedness and Response Act of 2002 (PHSBPR), Pub. L. No. 107-188, 116 Stat. 294 (2002) (codified in scattered sections of 7 U.S.C., 18 U.S.C., 21 U.S.C., 29 U.S.C., 38 U.S.C., 42 U.S.C., and 47 U.S.C. (2002)), is designed to improve the ability of the United States to prevent, prepare for, and respond to bioterrorism and other public health emergencies. Key provisions of the PHSBPR, 42 U.S.C. §§ 247d and 300hh among others, address the development of a national preparedness plan by HHS designed to provide effective assistance to State and local governments in the event of bioterrorism or other public health emergencies; operation of the National Disaster Medical

System (NDMS) to mobilize and address public health emergencies; grant programs for the education and training of public health professionals and improving State, local, and hospital preparedness for and response to bioterrorism and other public health emergencies; streamlining and clarifying communicable disease quarantine provisions; enhancing controls on dangerous biological agents and toxins; and protecting the safety and security of food and drug supplies.

Flood Control and Coastal Emergencies Act, 33 U.S.C § 701n (2002), authorizes the U.S. Army Corps of Engineers (USACE) to use an emergency fund for preparation for emergency response to natural disasters, flood fighting and rescue operations, rehabilitation of flood control and hurricane protection structures, temporary restoration of essential public facilities and services, advance protective measures, and provision of emergency supplies of water. The USACE receives funding for such activities under this authority from the Energy and Water Development Appropriation.

Volunteer Services. There are statutory exceptions to the general statutory prohibition against accepting voluntary services under 31 U.S.C. § 1342 (2002) that can be used to accept the assistance of volunteer workers. Such services may be accepted in "emergencies involving the safety of human life or the protection of property." Additionally, provisions of the Stafford Act, 42 U.S.C. §§ 5152(a), 5170a(2) (2002), authorize the President to, with their consent, use the personnel of private disaster relief organizations and to coordinate their activities. Under the Congressional Charter of 1905, 36 U.S.C. §§ 300101-300111 (2002), the American Red Cross and its chapters are a single national corporation. The Charter mandates that the American Red Cross maintain a system of domestic and international disaster relief. The American Red Cross qualifies as a nonprofit organization under section 501(c)(3) of the Internal Revenue Code.

Chapter 4 - International Efforts

Clearance of Proposed International Agreements. The Department of State (DOS) must ensure that all proposed international agreements of the United States are fully consistent with U.S. foreign policy objectives. The requirements for this coordination with and clearance from DOS are codified, in part, at sections 181.1-8 of Title 22 of the Code of Federal Regulations (CFR). The C-175 clearance requirements are specifically referenced in 22 C.F.R. § 181.4 (and Volume 11 of the Foreign Affairs Manual, Chapter 700).

Foreign Assistance. Relevant foreign assistance authorities for health and disasters authorize the provision of assistance "notwithstanding any other provision of law." These authorities would permit the provision of aid, such as medical goods and services, and even security details to ensure delivery of these items. Annual foreign operations appropriations acts reenact this special health authority annually, as follows:

Section 522 of the FY06 Foreign Operations, Export Financing, and Related Programs Appropriations Act (FOAA), Pub. L. No. 109-102, funds child survival and health activities and includes robust authority that would enable us to overcome any country-specific and other assistance limitations (e.g., North Korea, Iran, Burma, China). In cases of emergency to health and human welfare, there is an exceptional authority reenacted annually from the usual 15-day Congressional notification period (required for reprogramming notifications). Any assistance appropriated as economic assistance (i.e., not just funds appropriated for health) may be used pursuant to this authority to provide assistance for health.

The Foreign Assistance Act of 1961, as amended, provides relevant authorities for disaster assistance, with a full "notwithstanding" authority, and for health, with a more limited "notwithstanding" authority, as follows:

- FAA § 491 authorizes provision of assistance for natural and man-made disasters, "notwithstanding any other provision of law."

- FAA §104(c) (22 U.S.C. § 2151b-4) authorizes "[a]ssistance for [h]ealth and [d]isease [p]revention." Such assistance "may be made available notwithstanding any other provision of law that restricts assistance to foreign countries." There are some limitations on the "notwithstanding" authority (e.g., the notwithstanding clause does not trump limitations on assistance to organizations that support or participate in a program of coercive abortion or involuntary sterilization), but we do not foresee such exceptions constraining our ability to respond to a pandemic influenza.

- Title IV of the Emergency Supplemental Appropriations Act for Defense, the Global War on Terror, and Tsunami Relief, Pub. L. No. 109-13, 119 Stat. 231 (2005), appropriates $656 million for emergency relief, rehabilitation, and reconstruction aid to countries affected by the Asian tsunami and earthquakes of December 2004 and March 2005, and the avian influenza virus, to remain available until September 30, 2006. Additional funding is being sought as part of the President's $7.1 billion pandemic influenza legislative request.

Foreign Assistance to Address Civil Unrest Abroad. If foreign assistance were required for police to address civil unrest abroad associated with an outbreak, such assistance could be provided for police forces under various authorities, most notably, under FAA § 481(a)(4). Assistance for military forces for such purposes could also be provided under certain authorities, e.g., section 551 of the FAA for peace-keeping and other programs in the national security interest of the United States and section 23 of the Arms Export Control Act codified in 22 U.S.C. § 2751 et seq. (2000) for military assistance.

Title 11, Emergency Supplemental Appropriation to address Pandemic Influenza of the Department of Defense Appropriations Act of 2006, Pub. L. No. 109-148 (2006). This Act provides $10 million and additional authority for the Department of Defense (DOD) to assist military partner nations in pandemic influenza response preparedness.

The Public Health Service Act (PHSA), 42 U.S.C. § 201 note (2005). The PHSA authorizes HHS to engage in international biomedical research, health care technology, and specified health services research and statistical activities "to advance the status of the health sciences in the United States" and thereby the health of the American people (42 U.S.C. 242). HHS has interpreted this authority to support numerous international surveillance and research activities as well.

Military assistance. The major authorities that DOD may rely on to provide assistance outside the United States, include:

- 10 U.S.C. § 401 (Humanitarian and Civic Assistance (HCA). This section of the Code provides for HCA projects, approved in coordination with the Combatant Commanders and DOS that improve operational readiness skills of participating U.S. forces and are conducted in conjunction with military operations.

- 10 U.S.C. § 402 (Transportation). Subject to certain exceptions, DOD may transport supplies provided by non-governmental, U.S. sources without charge on a space-available basis.

- 10 U.S.C. §404 (Foreign Disaster Assistance). Under certain circumstances and subject to certain congressional notice requirements, the President may direct the Secretary of Defense to provide disaster assistance outside the United States in order to respond to manmade or natural disasters when necessary to prevent the loss of life.

- 10 U.S.C. § 2557 (Excess Nonlethal Supplies: Humanitarian Relief). This provision authorizes excess supplies to be made available to DOS for humanitarian relief. DOS will be responsible for distribution.

- 10 U.S.C. § 2561(Transportation and Other Humanitarian Support). DOD also may provide fully funded transportation (on an other-than space-available basis), if it pays such transportation costs with its operation and maintenance funds earmarked for Overseas Humanitarian, Disaster, and Civic Aid (OHDCA) purposes.

Chapter 5 - Transportation and Borders

Transportation Authorities

General Transportation Security Authorities. DHS has broad authority to protect transportation security, including authorities that could keep quarantinable diseases from reaching the United States. The Transportation Security Administration (TSA) is "responsible for security in all modes of transportation" (49 U.S.C. § 114). If the TSA Assistant Secretary "determines that a regulation or security directive must be issued immediately in order to protect transportation security the [Assistant Secretary] shall issue the regulation or security directive without providing notice or an opportunity for comment and without prior approval of the Secretary [of Homeland Security]" (49 U.S.C. § 114(l)(2)(A)). TSA interprets these provisions on transportation security to provide authority for TSA to keep a flight destined for the United States from landing in the United States if it is determined that a flight may be transporting persons with a quarantinable disease. These TSA authorities are also sufficiently broad to allow TSA to direct an air carrier to temporarily avoid deplaning its passengers until HHS or other medical authorities can screen the passengers. Finally, pursuant to 49 U.S.C. § 114(q), the Federal Air Marshal Service (FAMS) of TSA has the authority to exercise law enforcement powers in the transportation domain.

Emergency Transportation Security Authorities. In the case of a national emergency, the Aviation and Transportation Security Act (ATSA) provides DHS with additional authorities. ATSA confers four specific national emergency responsibilities upon DHS: "(A) To coordinate domestic transportation, including aviation, rail, and other surface transportation, and maritime transportation (including port security); (B) To coordinate and oversee the transportation-related responsibilities of other departments and agencies of the Federal Government other than the DOD and the military departments; (C) To coordinate and provide notice to other departments and agencies of the Federal Government, and appropriate agencies of State and local governments, including departments and agencies for transportation, law enforcement, and border control, about threats to transportation; (D) To carry out such other duties, and exercise such other powers, related to transportation during a national emergency as the Secretary shall prescribe" (49 U.S.C. § 114(g) (1) (A)-(D)). ATSA qualifies this authority by adding: "(2) AUTHORITY OF OTHER DEPARTMENTS AND AGENCIES. The authority of the [Secretary of Homeland Security] under this subsection shall not supersede the authority of any other department or agency of the Federal Government under law with respect to transportation or transportation-related matters, whether or not during a national emergency (49 U.S.C. § 114(g) (2)). ATSA also adds: "(3) CIRCUMSTANCES. The Secretary [of Homeland Security] shall prescribe the circumstances constituting a national emergency for purposes of this subsection" (49 U.S.C. § 114(g) (3)).

During a national emergency declared by the President, the Department of Transportation (DOT), through the Maritime Administration (MARAD), can enhance U.S. sealift capacity by taking control of vessels, containers, and chassis through requisitioning (46 App. U.S.C. § 1242; 50 U.S.C. §§ 196-198).

Aviation. The Federal Aviation Administration (FAA) is the lead agency for aviation safety regulation and oversight and is responsible for the operation and maintenance (to include personnel, physical, and cyber) of the Air Traffic Control System (Title 49 U.S.C., subtitle VII, Aviation Programs). Any movement in the navigable airspace of the United States can be stopped, redirected, or excluded by the FAA, regardless of the commodity involved (49 U.S.C. § 44701). Additionally, the FAA can order U.S.-flag air carriers not to enter designated airspace of a foreign country (e.g., to keep airspace clear for rescue operations). If the FAA determines that an emergency exists related to safety in air commerce that requires immediate action, the FAA may prescribe regulations and issue orders immediately to meet that emergency (49 U.S.C. § 46105(c)). FAA interprets these provisions on aviation security or safety to provide authority for FAA to close airspace to, or redirect, a flight if it is determined that a flight may be transporting persons with a quarantinable disease.

Subject to the direction and control of the Secretary of Homeland Security, the TSA has the authority to cancel a flight or series of flights if a decision is made that a particular security threat cannot be addressed in a way adequate to ensure, to the extent feasible, the safety of passengers and crew (49 U.S.C. § 44905(b)). TSA is required to work in conjunction with the FAA with respect to any actions or activities that may affect aviation safety or air carrier operations (49 U.S.C. § 114(f)(13); 6 U.S.C. § 233(a)). TSA interprets these provisions to authorize TSA to cancel flights in the case of a pandemic influenza.

Chicago Convention. The Chicago Convention, a multilateral treaty establishing the framework for the operation of international civil aviation, provides authority to deny entry to flights that do not comply with U.S. laws and regulations, including those relating to entry, clearance, customs, and quarantine. The Chicago Convention articles that may be relevant include 11, 13, 14, 16, 29, and 89.

Rail. Any movement in the United States by rail carrier (including commuter rail but excluding urban rapid transit not connected to the general system of rail transportation) may be stopped, redirected, or limited by the authority of the Surface Transportation Board (STB) or the Federal Railroad Administration (FRA), or both, irrespective of commodity involved. The FRA may issue an emergency order imposing any restrictions or prohibitions necessary to abate what the FRA determines is an emergency situation involving a hazard of death or personal injury caused by unsafe conditions or practices (49 U.S.C. § 20104). For a period of 270 days, the STB may direct the movement and prioritization of freight traffic necessary to alleviate an emergency situation involving the failure of traffic movement having substantial adverse impacts on shippers or on rail service in any region of the United States (49 U.S.C. § 11123), and may also order that preference be given to certain traffic, when the President so directs in time of war or threatened war (49 U.S.C. § 11124).

Mass Transit. In general, DOT is forbidden from regulating the operation, routes, schedules, rates, fares, tolls, rentals, or other charges of public transportation system grantees of the Federal Transit Administration. However, the Safe, Accountable, Flexible, Efficient, Transportation Equity Act: A Legacy for Users, Pub. L. No. 109-59, 119 Stat. 1144 (2005) (SAFETEA_LU), amended section 5334 of title 49 of the United States Code to create an express exception to the above prohibition when needed for national defense or in the event of a national or regional emergency.

Highways. The Federal Highway Administration (FHWA) possesses no authority to operate the Nation's highway system during times of emergency. States, local governments, and other Federal agencies own, control, and operate the Nation's roads and bridges. The Federal Motor Carrier Safety Administration (FMCSA) can order a vehicle to cease operation and relocate to a safe place if there is reason to believe it would constitute a security threat because it carries a hazardous material (49 U.S.C. § 521(b)(5); 49 U.S.C. § 5103(b), Section 1711, Homeland Security Act of 2002, Pub. L. 107-296).

Pipelines. The operation of any pipeline facility used to transport gas or hazardous liquid can be stopped by the Pipeline and Hazardous Materials Safety Administration if continued operation of the facility is or would become hazardous (49 U.S.C. § 60112).

Hazardous Materials. Any aspect of hazardous materials transportation that presents an "imminent hazard" may be halted by court order (49 U.S.C. § 5122(b)). An "imminent hazard" is a condition that presents a substantial likelihood that death, serious illness, severe personal injury, or a substantial endangerment to health, property, or the environment may occur before the reasonable foreseeable completion date of a formal proceeding begun to lessen the risk of that death, illness, injury, or endangerment (49 U.S.C. § 5102). DOT is also authorized to issue or impose emergency restrictions, prohibitions, recalls, or out-of-service orders, without notice or an opportunity for a hearing, but only to the extent necessary to abate an imminent hazard (49 U.S.C. §5121(d)).

Transportation Authorities Relating Specifically to Vessels. In the case of vessels, if there is evidence that a vessel is carrying a person or persons with a quarantinable disease that would present a public health threat to the port if the ship or the person were allowed to enter, the U.S. Coast Guard (USCG) has authority to prevent the vessel from entering a U.S. port or place until the infected person(s) can be dealt with by HHS/CDC personnel so as to prevent the spread of the disease in the United States (50 U.S.C. §§ 191–195; 33 U.S.C. §§ 1221–1232; 33 C.F.R. part 6; 33 C.F.R. § 160.111).

The Saint Lawrence Seaway Development Corporation may halt traffic through those portions of the Saint Lawrence Seaway subject to the jurisdiction of the United States, if required for safety or security of the seaway or for national security (e.g., deepwater vessels could be barred from entering or leaving the Seaway) (33 U.S.C. §§ 984, 1226).

Defense Production Act of 1950, 50 U.S.C. App. §§ 2061-2171 (2002). The DPA is the primary authority to ensure the timely availability of resources for national defense and civil emergency preparedness and response. Under the DPA, the Secretary of Transportation has been delegated the authority to marshal civil transportation in a defined area if national defense or domestic emergency conditions require civil transportation materials, services, or facilities that are not being provided by the marketplace. However, formal findings must be made by DOD, Department of Energy (DOE), or DHS, before DOT can exercise its DPA authority.

Border Authorities

General Border Authorities. DHS has broad authority to protect U.S. borders, including specific statutory provisions designating USCG and the United States Customs and Border Protection (CBP) to assist in the enforcement of State health laws and Federal quarantine regulations (42 U.S.C. §§ 97, 268). CBP has general authority pursuant to the customs and immigration laws (e.g., 19 U.S.C. §§ 482, 1461, 1496, 1589a, 1499, 1581, 1582, 1595a, and 8 U.S.C. §§ 1157, 1357) to examine merchandise, cargo, conveyances and persons upon their entry to, and exit from, the United States to ensure compliance with U.S. law, and to seize and forfeit conveyances, animals, or other things imported contrary to law or used in the unlawful importation, exportation, or subsequent transportation of articles imported contrary to U.S. law (18 U.S.C. § 545, 19 U.S.C. § 1595a). Section 421 of the Homeland Security Act transferred to the

Secretary of Homeland Security certain agricultural import and entry inspection functions originally assigned to the Secretary of Agriculture under the Animal Health Protection Act. This transfer included the authority to enforce prohibitions or restrictions on the entry of livestock diseases into the United States. Finally, the Secretary of Homeland Security and the Commissioner of CBP may temporarily close ports of entry "when necessary to respond to a national emergency or to [respond to] a specific threat to human life or national interests" (19 U.S.C. § 1318(b)). Such closings would effectively stop the legal entry of persons and conveyances and the legal importation and exportation of articles at those places.

Border Authorities Relating to Travelers. DHS has authority to find inadmissible any alien "who is determined (in accordance with the regulations prescribed by the Secretary of Health and Human Services) to have a communicable disease of public health significance" (8 U.S.C. § 1182(a)(1)). Under 8 U.S.C. § 1222(a), DHS could detain aliens for the purpose of determining whether they have a communicable disease listed in section 1182(a). The list of communicable diseases of public health significance as defined in HHS regulations is, however, limited, and does not generally include quarantinable diseases, including pandemic influenza, listed in Executive Order 13295.

Aliens with pandemic influenza could be excluded pursuant to 8 U.S.C. § 1182(f), which provides that "[w]henever the President finds that the entry of any aliens or of any class of aliens into the United States would be detrimental to the interests of the United States, he may by proclamation, and for such period as he shall deem necessary, suspend the entry of all aliens or any class of aliens as immigrants or nonimmigrants, or impose on the entry of aliens any restrictions he may deem to be appropriate." The President may not delegate the authority to issue such a proclamation. Accordingly, if the President determined that the entry of any aliens or class of aliens was detrimental to the interests of the United States, for reasons that may include the threatened spread of a pandemic into the United States, he may issue a proclamation suspending such entry and directing enforcement by all Federal agencies.

Control of Communicable Diseases. The Public Health Service Act (PHSA), 42 U.S.C. § 264, authorizes the Secretary of Health and Human Services to make and enforce regulations necessary to prevent the introduction, transmission, or spread of communicable diseases from foreign countries into the United States, or from one State or possession into any other State or possession. Under section 362 of the PHSA, 42 U.S.C. § 265, the Secretary of Health and Human Services may prohibit, in whole or in part, the introduction of persons and property from such countries or places as he/she shall designate for the purpose of averting a serious danger of the introduction of a communicable disease into the United States if he determines that such a prohibition is in the interest of the public health.

Vessels en route to the United States. Section 366 of the PHSA (42 U.S.C. § 269) requires vessels at foreign ports clearing or departing for the United States to obtain a bill of health from a U.S. consular officer, U.S. Public Health Service officer, or other U.S. medical officer, unless otherwise prescribed in regulations. Historically, a bill of health was a document required from ships in international traffic that set forth the sanitary history and condition of the vessel and, in some cases, the condition of the port during the time of departure. Foreign quarantine regulations in part 71 currently state that a bill of health is not required. Under the CDC's proposed rule, the CDC Director, to the extent permitted by law and in consultation with such other Federal agencies as the Director may deem necessary, would be authorized to require a foreign carrier clearing or departing for a U.S. port to obtain a bill of health from a U.S. consular officer or a medical officer designated for such purpose.

Animals, Poultry, and Wildlife

The Animal Health Protection Act (AHPA) of 2002, 7 U.S.C. 8301 et seq. The AHPA, described in detail in Authorities Chapter 7, gives the Secretary of Agriculture a broad range of authorities to use in the event of an outbreak of avian influenza in the United States and to prevent the introduction of such a disease into the United States.

The Poultry Products Inspection Act, 21 U.S.C. 451 et seq. This Act requires the inspection of poultry products and provides for criminal penalties for adulteration and misbranding of poultry products.

Importation of wild bird species parts and products. The importation of these items must comply with conservation laws and treaties enforced by the Department of the Interior (DOI), including the Wild Bird Conservation Act, the Migratory Bird Treaty Act of 1918, 16 U.S.C. 703-712, the Endangered Species Act of 1973 (ESA), 16 U.S.C. 1531-1544, which implements the Convention on International Trade in Endangered Species of Wild Fauna and Flora (CITES), T.I.A.S. 8249; the Lacey Act Amendments of 1981, 16 U.S.C. 3371-3378; and the Bald Eagle Protection Act of 1940, 16 U.S.C.668-668d. The DOI has the authority to take measures to restrict trade in wild birds based on threats to wildlife populations. In the event of an outbreak of highly pathogenic avian influenza (HPAI) in domestic or wild exotic birds in the United States, DOI has the authority (under 50 C.F.R. Part 13) to suspend the issuance of export and re-export permits under CITES and the ESA if such action is deemed necessary after coordination with USDA.

Chapter 6 - Protecting Human Health

The Public Health Service Act (PHSA), 42 U.S.C. §§ 201 et seq. (1994). The Secretary of Health and Human Services is authorized to develop and take such action as may be necessary to implement a plan under which the personnel, equipment, medical supplies, and other resources of the Department may be effectively used to control epidemics of any disease or condition and to meet other health emergencies and problems, (see 42 U.S.C. § 243). During an emergency proclaimed by the President, the President has broad authority to direct the services of the Public Health Service, (42 U.S.C. § 217). Under that section, the President is authorized to "utilize the [Public Health] Service to such extent and in such manner as shall in his judgment promote the public interest."

- **Research.** Section 301 of the PHSA, 42 U.S.C. § 241, authorizes the Secretary to conduct and encourage, cooperate with, and render assistance to other appropriate public authorities, scientific institutions, and scientists in the conduct of, and promote the coordination of, research, investigations, experiments, demonstrations and studies relating to the causes, diagnosis, treatment, control, and prevention of physical and mental impairments of man. The Secretary is also authorized to collect and make available through publications and other appropriate means, information as to, and the practical application of, such research and other activities.

- **Public Health Emergency.** Section 319(a) of the PHSA, 42 U.S.C. 247d, authorizes the Secretary of Health and Human Services to declare a public health emergency and "take such action as may be appropriate to respond" to that emergency consistent with his authorities. Appropriate action may include making grants, entering into contracts, and conducting and supporting investigation into the cause, treatment, or prevention of the disease or disorder that presents the emergency. The Secretary's declaration also can be the first step in authorizing emergency use of unapproved products or approved products for unapproved uses under section 564 of the Food, Drug, and Cosmetic Act (21 U.S.C. 360bbb-3), or waiving certain regulatory requirements of the Department, such as select agents requirements, or -- when the President also declares an emergency -- waiving certain Medicare, Medicaid, and State Children's Health Insurance Program (SCHIP) provisions.

- **Vaccines and therapeutics.** The PHSA provides additional authorities for core activities of HHS that will be needed to plan and implement an emergency response. For example, sections 301, 319F-1, 402, and 405 of the PHSA authorize the Secretary of Health and Human Services to conduct and support research and development of vaccines and therapeutics. Section 351 of the PHSA and provisions of the Federal Food, Drug, and Cosmetics Act authorize the Secretary and the Food and Drug Administration (FDA) to regulate vaccine development and production. Infrastructure support for preventive health services such as immunization activities, including vaccine purchase assistance, is provided under section 317 of the PHSA.

- **Liability protection.** Section 319F-3 of the PHSA provides immunity to manufacturers, distributors, program planners, "qualified persons," and their employees for claims for loss caused by, arising out of, relating to, or resulting from the administration or use of any "covered countermeasure" that is the subject of a declaration made by the Secretary. A covered countermeasure is a drug, device, or biological that is (1) subject to an emergency use authorization under section 564 of the Federal Food Drug and Cosmetic Act, (2) used against an epidemic or pandemic and either approved or subject to an IND, or (3) a security countermeasure as defined under the Project BioShield Act. Section 319F-4 allows the Secretary to, by declaration, establish an emergency fund in the Treasury which will be used to provide compensation for injuries directly caused by administration of a covered countermeasure.

- **Strategic National Stockpile.** Section 319F-2 of the PHSA authorizes the Secretary, in coordination with the Secretary of Homeland Security, to maintain the Strategic National Stockpile to provide for the emergency health security of the United States.

- **Quarantine.** Section 361 of the PHSA (42 U.S.C. § 264), authorizes the Secretary of Health and Human Services to make and enforce regulations necessary to prevent the introduction, transmission, or spread of communicable diseases from foreign countries into the United States, or from one State or possession into any other State or possession. Implementing regulations are found at 42 C.F.R. Parts 70 and 71. The HHS Centers for Disease Control and Prevention (CDC) administers these regulations as they relate to quarantine of humans. Diseases for which individuals may be quarantined are specified by Executive Order; the most recent change to the list of quarantinable diseases was Executive Order 13375 of April 1, 2005, which amended Executive Order 13295 by adding "influenza caused by novel or re-emergent influenza viruses that are causing, or have the potential to cause, a pandemic" to the list. CDC issued a new proposed rule updating these regulations on November 30, 2005. 70 Fed. Reg. 71892 (www.cdc.gov/ncidod/dq/nprm/index.htm). Other provisions in Title III of the PHSA permit HHS to establish quarantine stations, provide care and treatment for persons under quarantine, and provide for quarantine enforcement by specified components of DHS and cooperating State and local entities.

- **Vaccine Development.** Further, HHS has broad authority to coordinate vaccine development, distribution, and use activities under section 2102 of the PHSA, describing the functions of the National Vaccine Program. The Secretary has authority for health information and promotion activities under title XVII and other sections of the PHSA. HHS can provide support to States and localities for emergency health planning under title III of the PHSA.

- **National Goals.** Under section 1701 of the PHSA, 42 U.S.C. § 300u, the Secretary is authorized to formulate national goals for health information, promotion, health services, and education and to undertake activities, including training, support, planning, and technical assistance, to carry out those goals.

- **Mobilizing the Commissioned Corps.** Section 203 of the PHSA, 42 U.S.C. § 204, authorizes the Federal Government to mobilize officers of the United States Public Health Service Regular Commissioned Corps and the Reserve Commissioned Corps, including commissioned corps officers who are veterinarians, in times of emergencies.

Department of Veterans Affairs (VA) Authorities. The primary function of the Veterans Health Administration (VHA) is to provide a complete medical and hospital service for the medical care and treatment of veterans. Section 8111A of title 38 of the U.S. Code authorizes the Secretary to provide care to members of the Armed Forces during a time of war or national emergency. Section 1784 of title 38 authorizes the Secretary to furnish hospital care or medical services as a humanitarian service to non-VA beneficiaries in emergency cases. Section 1785 of title 38 authorizes the Secretary to provide hospital care and medical services to non-VA beneficiaries responding to, involved in, or otherwise affected by a disaster or emergency. This provision codifies VA's existing obligations under the Federal Response Plan (now National Response Plan). These include VA's obligations under the Robert T. Stafford Disaster Relief and Emergency Assistance Act, 42 U.S.C. § 5121, et seq., and during activation of the National Disaster Medical System (NDMS), 42 U.S.C. § 300hh-11.

- The explicit language in section 8111A and the legislative history of section 1785 indicate that during declared major disasters and emergencies and activation of NDMS, the highest priority for receiving VA care and services goes to service-connected veterans, followed by members of the Armed Forces receiving care under section 8111A and then by individuals affected by a disaster or emergency described in section 1785 (i.e., individuals requiring care during a declared disaster or emergency, or during activation of the NDMS). As a practical matter, when faced with individuals who require emergency medical treatment (e.g., during a disaster or emergency situation), VHA practitioners must prioritize based on medical need. This may require deferring routine or elective care for veterans in order to treat medical emergencies. Life-threatening conditions are treated prior to less severe or routine conditions, regardless of priority. Such prioritization is not dictated by statute or regulation. Rather, it is derived from the general authority granted to the Secretary (and through delegation to the Under Secretary for Health and to health care providers) to provide "needed care" to veterans. Thus, during a disaster or an emergency, VA has flexibility and discretion in providing needed care.

Exemption of Certain International Persons from Quarantine or other Restrictions. There are certain legal bases pursuant to which Federal authorities could insist that certain people on an aircraft be released from quarantine (e.g., diplomats and their families are "inviolable" under the Vienna Convention on Diplomatic Relations; United Nations (UN) diplomats are "inviolable" under the UN General Convention on Privileges and Immunities and the HQ Agreement; diplomats attending UN conferences are "inviolable" under the General Convention; consular officers (not families) are potentially "inviolable" under Articles 40 and 41 of the Vienna Convention on Consular Relations; and heads of States are generally subject to immunity).

ENHANCE 911 Act of 2004. Pub. L. No. 108-494. This Act requires officials of the Department of Transportation and the Department of Commerce to establish a joint program to facilitate coordination and communication between Federal, State, and local communications systems, emergency personnel, public safety organizations, telecommunications carriers, and telecommunications equipment manufacturers and vendors. The Act also requires those agencies to create an E-911 Implementation Coordination Office to implement that program. The Office will be housed at the Department of Transportation, National Highway Traffic Safety Administration (NHTSA) and is required to: develop, collect, and disseminate information concerning practices, procedures, and technology used in the implementation of E-911 services.

Other Authorities

The Defense Production Act, 50 U.S.C. p. §§ 2601-2171 (2002). Under the DPA, agencies can: (1) issue rated orders to manufacturers to give Government orders priority over all other orders, (2) issue rated orders to non-influenza countermeasure manufacturing facilities to manufacture influenza vaccine or antiviral medications, or (3) pursuant to DHS/FEMA regulations, and in consultation with Department of Justice (DOJ) and the Federal Trade Commission, convene industry and execute voluntary agreements as to how industry might meet the Government's vaccine and antiviral requirements.

Chapter 7 - Protecting Animal Health

The Animal Health Protection Act (AHPA) of 2002, 7 U.S.C. 8301 et seq. The AHPA enables the Secretary of Agriculture to prevent, detect, control, and eradicate diseases and pests of animals, such as avian influenza, in order to protect animal health, the health and welfare of people, economic interests of livestock and related industries, the environment, and interstate and foreign commerce in animals and other articles. The AHPA provides a broad range of authorities to use in the event of an outbreak of avian influenza in the United States and to prevent the introduction of such a disease into the United States. The Secretary is specifically authorized to carry out operations and measures to detect, control, or eradicate any pest or disease of livestock, which includes poultry, 7 U.S.C. 8308, and to promulgate regulations and issue orders to carry out the AHPA (see 7 U.S.C. 8315). The Secretary may also prohibit or restrict the importation, entry, or interstate movement of any animal, article, or means of conveyance to prevent the introduction into or dissemination within the United States of any pest or disease of livestock (7 U.S.C. 8303 8305). Section 421 of the Homeland Security Act, 6 U.S.C. 231, transferred to the Secretary of Homeland Security certain agricultural import and entry inspection functions under the AHPA, including the authority to enforce the prohibitions or restrictions imposed by USDA. Under certain specified circumstances, the Secretary of Agriculture may declare an extraordinary emergency to regulate intrastate activities or commerce (7 U.S.C. 8306). The Secretary also has authority to cooperate with other Federal agencies, States, or political subdivisions of States, national or local governments of foreign countries, domestic or international organizations or associations, Indian tribes, and other persons to prevent, detect, control, or eradicate avian influenza (7 U.S.C. 8310).

The Poultry Products Inspection Act (PPIA) of 1957, 21 U.S.C. 452. The PPIA provides for the inspection of poultry and poultry products and otherwise regulates the processing and distribution of such articles to prevent the movement or sale in interstate or foreign commerce of, or the burdening of such commerce by, poultry products which are adulterated or misbranded. It is essential in the public interest that the health and welfare of consumers be protected by assuring that poultry products distributed to them are wholesome, not adulterated, and properly marked, labeled, and packaged. Unwholesome, adulterated, or misbranded poultry products impair the effective regulation of poultry products in interstate or foreign commerce, are injurious to the public welfare, destroy markets for wholesome, not adulterated, and properly labeled and packaged poultry products, and result in sundry losses to poultry producers and processors of poultry and poultry products, as well as injury to consumers. All articles and poultry which are regulated under the PPIA are either in interstate or foreign commerce or substantially affect such commerce, and that regulation by the Secretary of Agriculture and cooperation by the States and other jurisdictions are appropriate to prevent and eliminate burdens upon such commerce, to effectively regulate such commerce, and to protect the health and welfare of consumers. USDA statutory authorities to inspect and condemn animal carcasses and parts that may become adulterated or otherwise unfit may be relied upon for government action in appropriate situations.

The Virus-Serum-Toxin Act, 21 U.S.C. 151 et seq. The Secretary of Agriculture is authorized under this act to regulate veterinary biological products. These products generally act through a specific immune process and are intended for use in the treatment, including prevention, diagnosis, or cure, of diseases in animals. They include, but are not limited to, vaccines, bacterins, sera, antisera, antitoxins, toxoids, allergens, diagnostic antigens prepared from, derived from, or prepared with microorganisms, animal tissues, animal fluids, or other substances of natural or synthetic origin.

Public Health Security and Bioterrorism Preparedness and Response Act of 2002, Pub. L. 107-188, 116 Stat. 594 (2002). Title II of this act, "Enhancing Controls on Dangerous Biological Agents and Toxins" (sections 201-231), provides for the regulation of certain biological agents and toxins by HHS (subtitle A, sections 201-204) and USDA (subtitle B, sections 211-213, also known as the Agricultural Bioterrorism Protection Act of 2002). The Act also provides for interagency coordination between the two departments regarding certain agents and toxins that present a threat to both human and animal health. The regulations governing HHS's select agent program are found at part 73 of title 42 of the CFR; the regulations governing USDA's select agent program are found at part 331 of title 7 of the CFR (plants) and part 121 of title 9 of the CFR (animals). For HHS, the CDC is designated as the agency with primary responsibility for the select agent program. The Animal and Plant Health Inspection Service (APHIS) is the USDA agency fulfilling that role for the provisions applicable to animals and plants. These statutes and their implementing regulations require entities, such as private, State, and Federal research laboratories, universities, and vaccine companies, that possess, use, or transfer biological agents or toxins which are determined to pose a severe threat to public health and safety, to animal or plant health, or to animal or plant products register these agents with APHIS or CDC. USDA's select agent regulations may be applicable in the event of an outbreak of avian influenza, as HPAI is listed as select agent under USDA regulations. For example, the USDA regulations will govern the possession, use, or movement of an HPAI virus in connection with any research attendant to a response to the outbreak. At the same time, it should be noted that the Agricultural Bioterrorism Protection Act provides that the Secretary may grant exemptions from the applicability of provisions of the regulations, in the case of listed agents or toxins, if the Secretary determines that such exemptions are consistent with protecting animal and plant health, and animal and plant products.

Animal Damage Control Act of 1931, 46 Stat. 1468, codified as amended at 7 U.S.C. §§ 426-426b (2000), and the **Rural Development, Agriculture, and Related Agencies Appropriations Act of 1988,** Pub. L. No. 100-202, 101 Stat. 1329-133 (codified at 7 U.S.C. § 426c (2000). Under these acts, USDA has authority to cooperate with other Federal agencies, States, local jurisdictions, individuals, public and private agencies, organizations, and institutions while conducting a program involving animal species that are injurious and/or a nuisance to, among other things, agriculture, horticulture, forestry, animal husbandry, wildlife, and human health and safety, as well as conducting a program involving mammal and bird species that are reservoirs for zoonotic diseases.

The Fish and Wildlife Act (FWA) of 1956, 16 U.S.C. § 742a et seq. The FWA establishes a comprehensive national fish and wildlife policy and authorizes the Secretary of the Interior to take steps required for the development, management, conservation, and protection of fish and wildlife resources through research, land acquisition, facilities development, and other means. The FWA authorizes the Secretary to direct a program of continuing research, extension, and information services on fish and wildlife matters, both domestically and internationally.

The Migratory Bird Treaty Act (MBTA) of 1918, 16 U.S.C. §§ 703-712. The MBTA places with the Secretary of the Interior Federal responsibility for protection and management of migratory birds and implements four international treaties that affect migratory birds common to the United States, Canada, Mexico, Japan, and the former Soviet Union. The MBTA makes it unlawful to hunt, kill, capture, possess, or otherwise take migratory birds, including their feathers, other parts, nests, or eggs, except as allowed by the Secretary through permit or regulation.

The Fish and Wildlife Coordination Act of 1934, 16 U.S.C. 661-667e. This act authorizes the Secretary of the Interior to provide assistance to, and cooperate with, Federal, State, and public or private agencies and organizations in the conservation of wildlife and in controlling losses of wildlife from disease and other causes. It also authorizes the Secretary to make surveys and investigations of wildlife of the public domain, including lands and waters or interests therein acquired or controlled by any agency of the United States.

Commissioned Corps. Section 203 of the PHSA, 42 U.S.C. § 204, authorizes the Federal Government to mobilize officers of the United States Public Health Service Regular Commissioned Corps and the Reserve Commissioned Corps, including commissioned corps officers who are veterinarians, in times of emergencies. Under section 361 of the PHSA, 42 U.S.C. § 264, HHS may make and enforce regulations to prevent the introduction, transmission, or spread of communicable diseases from foreign countries into States or possessions or from one State or possession into any other State or possession. For purposes of carrying out and enforcing such regulations, the Secretary may provide for such inspection, fumigation, disinfection, sanitation, pest extermination, destruction of animals or articles found to be so infected or contaminated as to be sources of dangerous infection to human beings, and other measures as in his judgment may be necessary.

Chapter 8 - Law Enforcement, Public Safety, and Security

Protecting Federal Facilities and Property. DHS is charged with protecting the buildings, grounds, and property that are owned, occupied, or secured by the Federal Government (including any agency, instrumentality, or wholly-owned or mixed-ownership corporation thereof) and the persons on the property (40 U.S.C. 1315). DHS may designate employees of the Department of Homeland Security, including employees transferred to the Department from the Office of the Federal Protective Service of the General Services Administration pursuant to the Homeland Security Act of 2002, as officers and agents for duty in connection with the protection of property owned or occupied by the Federal Government and persons on the property, including duty in areas outside the property to the extent necessary to protect the property and persons on the property. While engaged in the performance of official duties, an officer or agent designated under this section may enforce Federal laws and regulations for the protection of persons and property, and carry out such other activities for the promotion of homeland security as the Secretary may prescribe.

Strategic National Stockpile. In accordance with Public Law 108-276 (Project BioShield Act of 2004) and Emergency Support Function #8 - Public Health and Medical Services (ESF #8), DHS will coordinate with HHS and DOJ in ensuring the adequate physical security of the stockpile. ESF #8 instructs DOJ to provide stockpile security and quarantine enforcement upon request of HHS.

Assistance to States in Maintaining Order

Emergency Federal Law Enforcement Assistance Act. Upon written request by a Governor, the Attorney General can coordinate and deploy emergency Federal law enforcement assistance to State and local law enforcement authorities (42 U.S.C. § 10501). Federal law enforcement agencies that are authorized to provide assistance to State and local government officials by enforcing State and local law should be duly deputized to do so under State and local statutes.

Robert T. Stafford Disaster Relief and Emergency Assistance Act. In disaster and emergency situations, this Act authorizes Federal agencies to assist in the provision of State and local public health measures, including by providing logistical or materials support to State and local law enforcement (42 U.S.C. §§ 5170, 5192-5193, 5195a). The Act also authorizes DHS/FEMA to *"procure by condemnation or otherwise, construct, lease, transport, store, maintain, renovate, or distribute* materials and facilities for emergency preparedness," (emphasis added). The term "materials" includes "raw materials, supplies, medicines, equipment, component parts, and technical information and processes necessary for emergency preparedness," (*id.* § 5195a(5)); the term "facilities" includes "buildings, shelters, utilities, and land," (*id.* § 5195(a)(6)). The term "emergency preparedness" includes measures to be undertaken in preparation for anticipated hazards, during a hazard, or following a hazard. An influenza pandemic would fit within the broad definition of "hazard" (see, *id.* § 5195a(a)(1), 5195a(a)(3)).

The Insurrection Act, 10 U.S.C. §§ 331-335. The President may, upon request of a State legislature, or the Governor when the legislature cannot be convened, send the Armed Forces as necessary to suppress an insurrection against State authority (*id.* at § 331). Ordinarily requests under this provision specify that the violence cannot be brought under control by State and local law enforcement agencies and the State National Guard troops. In addition, the President may use the Armed Forces or the federalized National Guard as he considers it necessary to suppress any insurrection, domestic violence, unlawful combination, or conspiracy if it (1) so hinders the execution of State and Federal law that people are deprived of their rights secured by the Constitution and laws, or (2) opposes or obstructs the execution of Federal law (*id.* at § 333). The President may also use the Armed Forces of the federalized National Guard to enforce Federal law (*id.* at 332). This statutory authority is an exception to the Posse Comitatus Act, 18 U.S.C. § 1385 (2002), authorizing the military to make arrests, conduct searches, and perform other traditional law enforcement functions.

Under the Insurrection Act, the President may use the National Guard (when called into Federal service), reserves (when called to active duty), and members of the Armed Forces to enforce Federal laws or to suppress the insurrection. DOD has an established protocol, the Commander, U.S. Joint Forces Command Civil Disturbance Plan ("Garden Plot"). Under this plan, the Attorney General is responsible for receiving and coordinating requests for military assistance. The military on-scene commander acts in coordination with the Senior Civilian Representative of the Attorney General, most likely the U.S. Attorney in the given area.

Military Support for Civilian Law Enforcement Agencies. The Secretary of Defense may, in accordance with other applicable law, make available any equipment (including associated supplies or spare parts), base facility, or research facility of the DOD to any Federal, State, or local civilian law enforcement official for law enforcement purposes (10 U.S.C. § 372(a)). Training and personnel to maintain and operate equipment may also be provided (10 U.S.C. §§ 373-4).

Enforcement of Quarantines

State and local Quarantines. State and local officials draw their authority to enforce State and local quarantines from State and local law. Under section 311 of the PHSA, 42 U.S.C. § 243(a), the Secretary of Health and Human Services is authorized to accept State and local authorities' assistance in the enforcement of Federal quarantine rules and regulations, and is required to assist State and local authorities in the enforcement of their quarantines and other health regulations.

The U.S. Coast Guard, and "military officers commanding in any fort or station upon the seacoast," as well as Customs officers, which may include Customs and Border Protection officers and Immigration and Customs Enforcement special agents, must, at the direction of the Secretary of Health and Human Services, aid in the execution of such State quarantines and other health laws "according to their respective powers and within their respective precincts" (42 U.S.C. § 97).

The President also could use the Insurrection Act (see above) and use the Armed Forces or federalized National Guard to help suppress violence arising out of a State quarantine, as for any other law enforcement activity permitted under the Insurrection Act, 10 U.S.C. §§ 331-335, provided the requirements for using the Act described above are met (e.g., if the President is asked by a State to assist and if the defiance to the State quarantine orders amounts to an insurrection against State authority that the State cannot handle (see 10 U.S.C. § 331), or there is widespread unlawful activity that has the effect of depriving people of rights secured by the Constitution and laws) (see 10 U.S.C. § 333).

Federal Quarantines. Customs officers, which may include Customs and Border Protection officers and Immigration and Customs Enforcement special agents, and the U.S. Coast Guard have specific authority and responsibility to assist with the enforcement of quarantines at ports of entry (42 U.S.C. § 268). With regard to other Federal law enforcement officers, the United States Marshals Service has the broadest of Federal law enforcement missions, 28 U.S.C. § 565; and, along with other Department of Justice agencies (FBI, DEA, ATF) can be directed by the Attorney General to enforce quarantines. The U.S. Marshals Service can also deputize other Federal law enforcement officers throughout the executive branch to give them law enforcement powers in circumstances that extend beyond those for which they are otherwise statutorily authorized to exercise them, as was done during Hurricane Katrina.

Under the Insurrection Act the President may direct the military to enforce quarantines, or conduct security functions such as guarding stockpiles and pharmaceuticals, when he finds it necessary to enforce Federal law (see 10 U.S.C. §§ 332-334), or other prerequisites for use of the Act described above are met.

Criminal Sanctions. The violation of Federal quarantine regulations is a crime punishable by a fine of not more $1,000 or by imprisonment for not more than 1 year, or both (42 U.S.C. § 271). Additionally, individuals may be fined up to $250,000 if a violation of the regulation results in death, or up to $100,000 if a violation of the regulation does not result in death (18 U.S.C. §§ 3559, 3571(c)).

Chapter 9 - Institutions: Protecting Personnel and Ensuring Continuity of Operations

The Occupational Safety and Health Act of 1970 authorizes the Secretary of Labor to promote the safety and health of America's workers by setting and enforcing standards; providing training, outreach, and education; and establishing partnerships. The Occupational Safety and Health Administration has promulgated several standards to protect workers that would be particularly important in the event of a pandemic influenza outbreak. These standards include, but are not limited to: 29 CFR 1910.120 (Hazardous Waste Operations and Emergency Response), 29 CFR 1910.132 (Personal Protective Equipment), 29 CFR 1910.134 (Respiratory Protection), and 29 CFR 1910.1030 (Bloodborne Pathogens).